# Lippincott's

# *Fast Facts* for
# *NCLEX-PN*®

Wolters Kluwer | Lippincott Williams & Wilkins
Health

Philadelphia · Baltimore · New York · London
Buenos Aires · Hong Kong · Sydney · Tokyo

## Staff

Clinical Director
Joan M. Robinson, RN, MSN

Clinical Editors
Joanne Bartelmo, RN, MSN
Anita Lockhart, RN, MSN
Leigh Ann Trujillo, RN, BSN

Acquisitions Editor
Bill Lamsback

Product Director
David Moreau

Product Manager
Rosanne Hallowell

Copy Editor
Christine Dahlin

Editorial Assistants
Karen J. Kirk, Jeri O'Shea, Linda K. Ruhf

Art Director
Elaine Kasmer

Vendor Manager
Cynthia Rudy

Manufacturing Manager
Beth J. Welsh

Production and Indexing Services
SPi Global

The clinical treatments described and recommended in this publication are based on research and consultation with nursing, medical, and legal authorities. To the best of our knowledge, these procedures reflect currently accepted practice. Nevertheless, they can't be considered absolute and universal recommendations. For individual applications, all recommendations must be considered in light of the patient's clinical condition and, before administration of new or infrequently used drugs, in light of the latest package-insert information. The authors and publisher disclaim any responsibility for any adverse effects resulting from the suggested procedures, from any undetected errors, or from the reader's misunderstanding of the text.

Printed in China

LFFNCLEXPN010612

---

**Library of Congress Cataloging-in-Publication Data**
Lippincott's fast facts for NCLEX-PN.
    p. ; cm.
  Fast facts for NCLEX-PN
  Includes bibliographical references.
  ISBN 978-1-4511-7629-2
  I. Lippincott Williams & Wilkins. II. Title: Fast facts for NCLEX-PN.
  [DNLM: 1. Nursing, Practical—Examination Questions. 2. Nursing, Practical—Handbooks. 3. Nursing Care—Examination Questions. 4. Nursing Care—Handbooks. WY 18.2]
  610.73076—dc23
                                    2012000007

RRS1203

# Contents

# Advisory board

# Contributors
# and consultants

Kathy Cochran, RN, MSN
Assistant Dean of Nursing and Allied
  Health
PN Program Director/Instructor
Georgia Northwestern Technical
  College
Rome, Georgia

Dolores Cotton, RN, MSN
Practical Nursing Coordinator
Meridian Technology Center
Stillwater, Oklahoma

Lauren Mixon, RN, BSN
PN Instructor
Nunez Community College
Chalmette, Louisiana

Ann C. Nobles, RN, BBA, MSN, CHE
Practical Nursing Instructor
Reid State Technical College
Evergreen, Alabama

Beverly Skloss, RN, MSN
Director—School of Vocational
  Nursing and Nursing Education
Valley Baptist Medical Center
Harlingen, Texas

Brigitte Thiele, RN, BSN
Nursing Instructor
Three Rivers Community College
Poplar Bluff, Missouri

Peggy Thweatt, RN, MSN
Nursing Faculty
Medical Careers Institute
LPN Program
Newport News, Virginia

# How to use this book

*Lippincott's Fast Facts for NCLEX-PN®* is designed as a quick and easy review to use when studying for the NCLEX-PN. With over 4,500 bulleted facts, this book covers all aspects of nursing care, organized around the major subject areas tested on the exam: adult health, maternal-neonatal nursing, pediatric nursing, psychiatric nursing, pharmacology, coordinated care, and patient safety.

Within each chapter, you'll find hundreds of facts grouped according to key clinical topics that are specific to the subject area. For example, in Chapter 1, Adult Care, bullets are grouped by body system (such as cardiovascular system, respiratory system, musculoskeletal system, and integumentary system). In Chapter 2, Maternal-Neonatal Care, they're arranged according to stages of pregnancy and delivery (antepartum, intrapartum, postpartum, neonatal). In Chapter 6, Coordinated Care, facts are organized according to client-focused concepts and nursing responsibilities, including advance directives, client rights, and information technology.

Each fact is accurate and up to date and has been thoroughly reviewed by nursing experts well versed in the NCLEX-PN test plan to ensure that the most likely content areas have been addressed. And each fact has been concisely worded to provide a kernel of valuable information that you'll be able to easily understand and readily recall while taking the exam. A small open box precedes each stand-alone fact, serving to keep each point separate and distinct. You may use the box to check off the fact as "studied" when you feel you've sufficiently learned or mastered the information, or leave it blank to return to later when you need a refresher or further review.

Two appendices have been included to help prepare you for the types and style of questions found on the NCLEX and to teach you key strategies for how to answer questions correctly. Samples are also provided to graphically simulate how questions, including new alternate-format type questions (graphic option, chart/exhibit, drag-and-drop, hot spot, fill-in-the-blank, audio, and multiple-response/multiple choice), might appear on the actual exam.

You're busy, and finding the right time and place to study can sometimes be difficult. Because of its convenient size and portability, *Lippincott's Fast Facts for NCLEX-PN®* is the perfect tool to have on hand when studying alone or in group settings. Tuck it in your purse or backpack and carry it with you wherever you go to review facts—a few at a time, section by section, or whenever you have a few minutes—between classes, during lunch breaks, or even while waiting for a bus or train. You'll be sure to make the most of your study time and increase your chance of success with this excellent review.

# Adult care

## Cardiovascular system

❑ A client's electrocardiogram showing ST elevation in leads $V_2$, $V_3$, and $V_4$ suggests an anterior-wall myocardial infarction.

❑ The left anterior descending artery is the primary source of blood for the anterior wall of the heart.

❑ The circumflex artery supplies the lateral wall of the heart.

❑ The internal mammary artery supplies the breast.

❑ The coronary arteries may receive a minute portion of blood during systole.

❑ Most of the blood flow to the coronary arteries is supplied during diastole.

❑ Breathing patterns are irrelevant to blood flow.

❑ Coronary artery disease accounts for 30% of all deaths in the United States.

❑ Atherosclerosis, or plaque formation, is the leading cause of coronary artery disease.

❑ A myocardial infarction is commonly a result of coronary artery disease.

❑ In atherosclerosis, hardened blood vessels can't dilate properly; therefore, they constrict blood flow and block oxygen transport. As a result, oxygen can't reach the heart muscle, resulting in angina.

❑ Diabetes mellitus is a risk factor for coronary artery disease that can be controlled with diet, exercise, and medication.

❑ Cholesterol levels above 240 mg/dL are considered excessive and are a risk factor for developing coronary artery disease.

❑ Total cholesterol levels below 240 mg/dL are considered below the nationally accepted levels and carry a lesser risk of coronary artery disease.

❑ A lipid panel tests the amount of total cholesterol, low-density lipoprotein cholesterol, high-density lipoprotein cholesterol, and triglycerides.

❑ Sublingual nitroglycerin is administered to treat acute angina.

❑ Coronary artery bypass surgery and percutaneous transluminal coronary angioplasty are invasive, surgical treatments for coronary artery disease.

❑ An electrocardiogram showing ST elevation in leads II, III, and aVF suggests occlusion of the right coronary artery.

❑ The right coronary artery supplies the right ventricle, or the inferior portion of the heart.

❑ Occlusion of the right coronary artery could produce an infarction in that area.

❑ The most common symptom of a myocardial infarction is chest pain, resulting from deprivation of oxygen to the heart.

❑ The correct landmark for obtaining an apical pulse is the left fifth intercostal space in the midclavicular line.

❑ The apex of the heart is the point of maximal impulse where heart sounds are heard loudest.

❑ Rescuers of adult victims should begin compressions rather than opening the airway and delivering breaths.

❑ The sequence for cardiopulmonary resuscitation is CAB (compressions, airway, breathing) rather than ABC (airway, breathing, compressions).

❑ Chest compression depth on an adult should be at least 2 inches (5 cm).

❑ All rescuers, trained or not, should deliver high-quality chest compressions by pushing hard to a depth of at least 2 inches (5 cm), at a rate of at least 100 compressions per minute, allowing full chest recoil after each compression, and minimizing interruptions in chest compressions.

❑ Trained rescuers should also provide cardiopulmonary resuscitation with a compression to ventilation ratio of 30:2.

❑ The outermost layer of the heart is called the epicardium.

❑ The epicardium is made up of squamous epithelial cells overlying connective tissue.

❑ The myocardium is the middle layer of the heart and forms most of the heart wall.

❑ The myocardium has striated muscle fibers that cause the heart to contract.

❑ The heart's inner layer is called the endocardium.

❑ The endocardium consists of endothelial tissue with blood vessels and bundles of smooth muscle.

❑ The serous pericardium has two layers: the parietal and the visceral layer.

❑ The pericardium surrounds the heart and the roots of the great vessels.

❑ The pericardium has two layers: the fibrous and serous pericardium.

❑ Pulmonic sounds can be auscultated at the left second intercostal space in the midclavicular line.

❑ Abnormalities of the pulmonic valve are auscultated at the left second intercostal space along the left sternal border.

❑ Aortic valve abnormalities are heard at the second intercostal space to the right of the sternum.

❑ Mitral valve abnormalities are heard at the fifth intercostal space in the midclavicular line.

- ❑ Tricuspid valve abnormalities are heard at the third and fourth intercostal spaces along the sternal border.
- ❑ Troponin I levels rise rapidly and are detectable within 1 hour of myocardial injury.
- ❑ Lactate dehydrogenase isoenzymes may be useful in diagnosing cardiac injury.
- ☑ Because creatine kinase levels may rise with skeletal muscle injury, increased creatine kinase levels may help detect cardiac injury.
- ☑ Measuring for an increase in troponin I levels is the best indicator for determining myocardial injury.
- ❑ An aneurysm is an outpouching of a vessel.
- ❑ Systemic hypertension or increased atrial contraction can result in a fourth heart sound.
- ❑ Aortic valve malfunction is heard as a murmur.
- ❑ The left ventricle is responsible for most of the cardiac output.
- ❑ An anterior-wall myocardial infarction may result in a decrease in left ventricular function.
- ❑ When the left ventricle doesn't function properly, resulting in left-sided heart failure, fluid accumulates in the interstitial and alveolar spaces in the lungs and causes crackles.
- ❑ Pulmonic and tricuspid valve malfunction cause right-sided heart failure.
- ❑ Because the myocardium is deprived of oxygen during a myocardial infarction, additional oxygen is administered to assist in oxygenation and prevent further damage.
- ❑ Arrhythmias caused by oxygen deprivation to the myocardium are the most common complication of a myocardial infarction.
- ❑ Because the pumping function of the heart is compromised by a myocardial infarction (MI), heart failure is the second most common complication of MI.
- ❑ Pericarditis most commonly results from a bacterial or viral infection, but may also occur after a myocardial infarction.
- ❑ Jugular vein distention isn't a symptom of abdominal aortic aneurysm or pneumothorax.
- ❑ A myocardial infarction, if severe enough, can progress to heart failure.
- ❑ Jugular venous pressure is measured with the head of the bed inclined between 15 and 30 degrees. A centimeter ruler is used to obtain the vertical distance between the sternal angle and the point of highest pulsation.
- ❑ The apical pulse is the most accurate pulse point in the body.

- ❏ The radial pulse rate can be affected by cardiac and vascular disease; therefore, it won't always accurately depict the heart rate.

- ❏ The heart contains four valves: two atrioventricular valves (mitral and tricuspid) and two semilunar valves (pulmonic and aortic).

- ❏ The aortic valve prevents backflow from the aorta into the left ventricle.

- ❏ The pulmonic valve prevents backflow from the pulmonary artery into the right ventricle.

- ❏ The tricuspid valve prevents backflow from the right ventricle into the right atrium.

- ❏ The mitral valve prevents backflow from the left ventricle into the left atrium.

- ❏ The mitral valve is also known as the bicuspid or left atrioventricular valve.

- ❏ Because the atria only have to pump blood into the ventricles, their walls are relatively thin.

- ❏ The walls of the left ventricle are the thickest of any of the chambers of the heart because the left ventricle pumps blood against the resistance of the systemic circulation.

- ❏ The walls of the right ventricle are thicker than those of the atria because the right ventricle pumps blood against the resistance of the pulmonary circulation.

- ❏ Crackles in the lungs are a classic sign of left-sided heart failure.

- ❏ The most accurate area on the body to assess dependent edema in a bedridden client is the sacral area.

- ❏ Sacral, or dependent, edema is secondary to right-sided heart failure.

- ❏ Inadequate deactivation of aldosterone by the liver after right-sided heart failure leads to fluid retention, which causes oliguria.

- ❏ Adequate urine output, polyuria, and polydipsia aren't associated with right-sided heart failure.

- ❏ The interatrial septum divides the atrial chambers, helping them to contract and force blood into the ventricles below.

- ❏ The right and left atria serve as volume reservoirs for blood being sent into the ventricles.

- ❏ Weight gain, nausea, and a decrease in urine output are secondary effects of right-sided heart failure.

- ❏ Cardiomyopathy is usually identified as a symptom of left-sided heart failure.

- ❏ Left-sided heart failure causes primarily pulmonary symptoms rather than systemic ones.

- ❏ Angina pectoris doesn't cause weight gain, nausea, or a decrease in urine output.

❑ An increased PR interval is indicative of a first-degree atrioventricular block.

❑ Normal sinus rhythm and sinus arrhythmia produce normal PR intervals.

❑ The PR interval (if present) is less than 0.12 second in accelerated junctional rhythm.

❑ The portion of the aorta distal to the renal arteries is more prone to an aneurysm because the vessel isn't surrounded by stable structures, unlike the proximal portion of the aorta.

❑ Abdominal pain is the most common symptom in a client with an abdominal aortic aneurysm as a result of disruption of normal circulation in the abdominal region.

❑ An aortogram clearly delineates the vessels and any abnormalities.

❑ An abdominal aortic aneurysm will only be visible on an X-ray if it is calcified.

❑ Computed tomography scan and ultrasound don't give a direct view of the vessels and don't yield as accurate a diagnosis as the aortogram.

❑ Rupture of an abdominal aortic aneurysm is a life-threatening emergency.

❑ Hypertension should be avoided or controlled in a client with an abdominal aortic aneurysm because it can cause the weakened vessel to rupture.

❑ Cardiac arrhythmias aren't directly linked to an abdominal aortic aneurysm.

❑ The aorta lies directly left of the umbilicus.

❑ When assessing a client for an abdominal aortic aneurysm, the area of the abdomen that is most commonly palpated is the middle lower abdomen to the left of the midline.

❑ Continuous pressure on the vessel walls from hypertension causes the walls to weaken and an aneurysm to occur.

❑ Atherosclerotic changes can occur with peripheral vascular diseases and are linked to aneurysms, but the link isn't as strong as it is with hypertension.

❑ Hypertension is linked to more than 50% of clients with abdominal aortic aneurysms.

❑ A bruit is a vascular sound that reflects partial arterial occlusion.

❑ Severe lower back pain indicates an aneurysm rupture, secondary to pressure being applied within the abdominal cavity.

❑ Blood pressure decreases due to the loss of blood when an aneurysm ruptures.

❑ After an abdominal aortic aneurysm ruptures, the vasculature is interrupted and blood volume is lost, so blood pressure doesn't increase.

❑ The red blood cell count is decreased after the abdominal aortic aneurysm ruptures because the vasculature is interrupted and blood volume is lost.

- The white blood cell count increases after the abdominal aortic aneurysm ruptures as cells migrate to the site of injury.

- Symptoms of severe lower back pain, decreased blood pressure, decreased red blood cell count, and increased white blood cell count indicate a ruptured abdominal aortic aneurysm.

- Rupture of a repaired abdominal aortic aneurysm is most commonly caused by leakage at the repair site.

- Marfan syndrome results in degeneration of the elastic fibers of the aortic media.

- In most cases of cardiomyopathy, the etiology is a viral or bacterial infection or cardiotoxic effects of drugs or alcohol.

- Although the cause isn't entirely known, cardiac dilation and heart failure may develop in the mother during the last month of pregnancy or the first few months after birth.

- In hypertrophic obstructive cardiomyopathy, hypertrophy of the ventricular septum is apparent.

- Heart failure most commonly occurs in clients with cardiomyopathy because the structure and function of the heart muscle are affected.

- Myocardial infarction results from prolonged myocardial ischemia due to reduced blood flow through one of the coronary arteries.

- Pericardial effusion is most predominant in clients with pericarditis.

- Atrial fibrillation is defined as chaotic, asynchronous, electrical activity in the atrial tissue.

- Ventricular fibrillation is a chaotic rhythm with no QRS complexes.

- In atrial flutter there are flutter waves that are "sawtooth" in appearance.

- P waves are present in sinus tachycardia.

- Dyspnea, cough, weight gain, weakness, and edema are classic symptoms of heart failure.

- Pericarditis is exhibited by a feeling of fullness in the chest and auscultation of a pericardial friction rub.

- Hypertension is usually exhibited by headaches, visual disturbances, and a flushed face.

- An $S_4$ heart sound occurs as a result of increased resistance to ventricular filling after atrial contraction.

- Increased resistance to ventricular filling is related to decreased compliance of the ventricle.

- A dilated aorta causes a murmur.

- An $S_4$ heart sound isn't heard in a normally functioning heart.

❏ The primary goals in the treatment of cardiomyopathy are to improve myocardial filling and cardiac output.

❏ The only definitive treatment for cardiomyopathy that can't be controlled medically is a heart transplant because the damage to the heart muscle is irreversible.

❏ Coronary artery bypass grafting is a surgical intervention used for atherosclerotic vessels.

❏ Ischemic changes are represented on an electrocardiogram by T-wave inversion.

❏ An increased QRS complex duration suggests a bundle-branch block.

❏ A shortened PR interval indicates a junctional rhythm.

❏ Pathologic Q waves are present with myocardial infarction.

❏ Inadequate oxygen supply to the myocardium is responsible for the pain accompanying angina.

❏ Decreased afterload causes increased cardiac output.

❏ It is most important for the nurse to determine if the client has allergies to iodine or shellfish before cardiac catheterization because catheterization involves the injection of a radiopaque dye.

❏ Percutaneous transluminal coronary angioplasty can alleviate the blockage in the coronary arteries and restore blood flow and oxygenation.

❏ Cardiogenic shock is related to reduced cardiac output and ineffective pumping of the heart.

❏ Distributive shock results from changes in the intravascular volume distribution and is usually associated with increased cardiac output.

❏ Of all clients with an acute myocardial infarction, 15% suffer cardiogenic shock secondary to the myocardial damage and decreased function.

❏ At least 40% of the heart muscle must be involved for cardiogenic shock to develop.

❏ The cardiac index is a figure derived by dividing the cardiac output by the client's body surface area.

❏ The cardiac index is used for identifying whether the cardiac output is meeting a client's needs.

❏ Heart rate, blood pressure, and decreased cerebral blood flow are less useful in detecting the risk of cardiogenic shock.

❏ The most useful factor in detecting a client's risk of developing cardiogenic shock is the cardiac index.

❏ Initially, the decrease in cardiac output results in a decrease in cerebral blood flow.

❑ A decrease in cerebral blood flow causes restlessness, agitation, or confusion.

❑ Arterial blood gas analysis is the diagnostic study that can determine when cellular metabolism becomes anaerobic and when pH decreases.

❑ The first treatment goal for cardiogenic shock is to increase myocardial oxygen supply.

❑ In a shock state, the myocardium requires more oxygen; if it doesn't receive more oxygen, the shock worsens.

❑ Increasing the oxygen supply to the myocardium will play a large role in correcting metabolic acidosis and hypoxia.

❑ A systolic blood pressure of 140 to 159 mm Hg or a diastolic pressure of 90 to 99 mm Hg represents stage 1 hypertension.

❑ Systolic blood pressure greater than or equal to 160 mm Hg or diastolic pressure greater than or equal to 100 mm Hg represents stage 2 hypertension.

❑ A systolic blood pressure of 120 to 139 mm Hg or a diastolic pressure of 80 to 89 mm Hg represents prehypertension.

❑ A systolic blood pressure less than 120 mm Hg and a diastolic pressure less than 80 mm Hg are considered normal.

❑ Peripheral chemoreceptors in the aorta and carotid arteries are primarily stimulated by oxygen.

❑ Decreases in pulsatile pressure cause a reflex increase in heart rate.

❑ Primary hypertension describes persistently elevated blood pressure with an unknown cause; it accounts for approximately 90% of hypertension cases.

❑ Primary hypertension is characterized by a progressive, usually asymptomatic blood pressure increase over several years.

❑ Malignant hypertension is rapidly progressive, uncontrollable, and causes a rapid onset of complications.

❑ Secondary hypertension occurs secondary to a known, correctable cause.

❑ An occipital headache is typical of hypertension secondary to continued increased pressure on the cerebral vasculature.

❑ The most common symptom of hypertension is headache.

❑ The brachial artery is most commonly used to measure blood pressure due to its easy accessibility and location.

❑ The radial and ulnar arteries can be used in extraordinary circumstances to obtain a blood pressure reading, but the measurement may not be as accurate.

❑ Primary varicose veins have a gradual onset and progressively worsen.

❑ Fatigue and pressure are classic signs of varicose veins, secondary to increased blood volume and edema.

❑ Passive filling of the ventricles begins with diastole.

❑ The right atrium receives deoxygenated blood returning from the body through the inferior and superior venae cavae and from the heart through the coronary sinus.

❑ The left atrium receives oxygenated blood from the lungs through the four pulmonary veins.

❑ The right atrium receives deoxygenated blood returning from the body through the inferior and superior venae cavae and from the heart through the coronary sinus.

❑ The atria pump their blood through the two atrioventricular valves (mitral and tricuspid) directly into their respective ventricles.

❑ The right ventricle pumps blood through the pulmonic valve into the pulmonary arteries and then into the lungs.

❑ Oxygenated blood returns to the left atrium.

❑ The left ventricle pumps blood through the aortic valve into the aorta and then throughout the body.

❑ Deoxygenated blood returns to the right atrium.

❑ The firing of the sinoatrial node sets off a chain reaction in cardiac conduction.

❑ When an impulse leaves the sinoatrial node, it travels through the atria along Bachmann's bundle and the internodal pathways on its way to the atrioventricular node.

❑ After the impulse passes through the atrioventricular node, it travels to the ventricles, first down the bundle of His, then along the bundle branches and, finally, down the Purkinje fibers.

❑ The sinoatrial node has a firing rate of 60 to 100 beats/minute.

❑ The atrioventricular node has a firing rate of 40 to 60 beats/minute.

❑ Purkinje fibers have a firing rate of 20 to 40 beats/minute.

❑ Automaticity is the ability to spontaneously initiate an impulse (pacemaker cells have this ability).

❑ Excitability is a cell's response to an electrical stimulus (results from ion shifts across the cell membrane).

❑ Conduction is the ability of a cell to transmit an electrical impulse to another cardiac cell.

❑ Contractility is the ability of a cell to contract after receiving a stimulus.

☒ Preload is the stretching of muscle fibers in the ventricles as the ventricles fill with blood.

❑ Contractility is influenced by preload.

☒ Afterload refers to the pressure that the ventricular muscles must generate to overcome the higher pressure in the aorta to get the blood out of the heart.

❑ Electrical stimulation causes troponin to expose actin-binding sites, which allows muscle contraction to occur in the heart.

❑ Valves in the veins prevent blood backflow, and most are located in smaller, more distal veins.

❑ The largest vein, the vena cava, has no valves.

❑ Arteries have thick, muscular walls to accommodate the high speed and pressure of blood flow.

❑ Arterioles have thinner walls than arteries and control blood flow to capillaries.

❑ Capillaries have microscopic walls composed of a single layer of endothelial cells.

❑ Conductive arteries typically have few branches and follow relatively straight lines.

❑ Distributive arteries typically have multiple branches and arise from the conductive arteries.

❑ The heart relies on the coronary arteries and their branches for its supply of oxygenated blood; it also depends on the cardiac veins to remove oxygen-depleted blood.

❑ During diastole, blood flows out of the heart and into the coronary arteries.

❑ The right coronary artery supplies blood to the right atrium, part of the left atrium, most of the right ventricle, and the inferior part of the left ventricle.

❑ The left coronary artery, which splits into the left anterior descending and circumflex arteries, supplies blood to the left atrium, most of the left ventricle, and most of the interventricular septum.

❑ Syncope is a brief loss of consciousness caused by a lack of blood to the brain; it usually occurs abruptly and can last for seconds to minutes.

❑ In the aortic area, sounds reflect blood moving from the left ventricle during systole, crossing the aortic valve, and flowing through the aortic arch.

❑ In the pulmonic area, sounds reflect blood being ejected from the right ventricle during systole, crossing the pulmonic valve and flowing through the main pulmonary artery.

❑ In the tricuspid area, sounds reflect movement of blood from the right atrium across the tricuspid valve and right ventricular filling during diastole.

❑ In the mitral area, also called the apical area, sounds reflect blood flow across the mitral valve and left ventricular filling during diastole.

❑ Listen for heart murmurs over the same precordial areas used in auscultation for heart sounds.

- ☒ An $S_3$ heart sound, also known as ventricular gallop, is commonly heard in children and may be normal in women during the last trimester of pregnancy; however, it may be a cardinal sign of heart failure in other adults.

- ❏ Also called an atrial gallop, an $S_4$ heart sound is an adventitious heart sound that you'll hear best over the tricuspid or mitral area when the client lies on his left side.

- ❏ A pericardial friction rub has a scratchy, rubbing quality.

- ❏ A weak pulse has decreased amplitude with a slower upstroke and downstroke. It may be a result of increased peripheral vascular resistance, as occurs in cold weather or with severe heart failure, or decreased stroke volume, as occurs with hypovolemia or aortic stenosis.

- ❏ A bounding pulse has a sharp upstroke and downstroke with a pointed peak and elevated amplitude and may result from increased stroke volume, as with aortic insufficiency, or arterial wall stiffness, which can occur with aging.

- ❏ Pulsus alternans is a regular, alternating pattern of weak and strong pulses and is associated with left-sided heart failure.

- ❏ Pulsus bigeminus is similar to pulsus alternans but occurs at irregular intervals and is caused by premature atrial or ventricular beats.

- ❏ Pulsus paradoxus has increases and decreases in amplitude associated with the respiratory cycle; marked decreases occur when the client inhales.

- ❏ Pulsus paradoxus is associated with pericardial tamponade, advanced heart failure, and constrictive pericarditis.

- ❏ Pulsus biferiens shows an initial upstroke, a subsequent downstroke, and then another upstroke during systole.

- ❏ Pulsus biferiens is caused by aortic stenosis and aortic insufficiency.

- ❏ Activated partial thromboplastin time, prothrombin time, bleeding time, and activated clotting time are tests that measure clotting time.

- ❏ Increased International Normalized Ratio (INR) values may indicate disseminated intravascular coagulation, cirrhosis, hepatitis, vitamin K deficiency, salicylate intoxication, or uncontrolled oral anticoagulation.

- ❏ Electrophysiology studies are used to help determine the cause of an arrhythmia and the best treatment for it.

- ❏ In transesophageal echocardiography, ultrasonography is combined with endoscopy to provide a better view of the heart's structures.

- ❏ Transesophageal echocardiography is used to evaluate valvular disease or repairs, but it's also used to diagnose thoracic and aortic disorders, endocarditis, congenital heart disease, intracardiac thrombi, and tumors.

❑ Cardiac blood pool imaging (also called multiple-gated acquisition, or MUGA, scanning) is used to evaluate regional and global ventricular performance.

❑ In arterial pressure–based cardiac output monitoring, a client's existing arterial catheter is used to continuously calculate and display cardiac output.

❑ Arterial pressure-based cardiac output helps to determine a client's fluid status and potential response to a fluid challenge before significant changes in blood pressure occur.

❑ Endocarditis is an inflammation of the endocardium, the heart valves, or a cardiac prosthesis; it typically results from bacterial invasion and therefore may also be referred to as infective endocarditis.

❑ Sharp pain and cool feet are symptoms of alteration in arterial blood flow.

❑ Varicose veins occur most commonly in the saphenous veins of the lower extremities.

❑ Edema and pigmentation are signs and symptoms of secondary varicose veins.

❑ Ligation and stripping of the vein can rid the vein of varicosity, but it won't prevent other varicose veins from forming.

❑ Sitting and bed rest are contraindicated in the postoperative management of a client who has undergone ligation and stripping because both promote decreased blood return to the heart and venous stasis.

❑ Although ice packs would help reduce edema for a client who has undergone ligation and stripping, they would also cause vasoconstriction and impede blood flow.

❑ Pulmonary embolism is manifested by dyspnea, chest pain, and diminished breath sounds.

❑ A pulmonary embolism is a blood clot that forms in a vein, travels to the lungs, and lodges in the pulmonary vasculature.

❑ A hemothorax refers to blood in the pleural space.

❑ A pneumothorax is caused by an opening in the pleura.

❑ Pulmonary hypertension is an increase in pulmonary artery pressure, which increases the workload of the right ventricle.

❑ Hypercoagulability, along with venous stasis and venous wall injury, accounts for the formation of deep vein thrombosis.

❑ An embolus is a blood clot or fatty globule that forms in one area of the body and is carried through the bloodstream to another area.

❑ Deep vein thrombosis is associated with deep leg pain of sudden onset.

❑ Production of pink, frothy sputum is a classic sign of acute pulmonary edema.

❑ Hypocapnia is a blood gas abnormality that is initially most suggestive of pulmonary edema.

❑ In an attempt to compensate for increased work of breathing due to hyperventilation, carbon dioxide decreases, causing hypocapnia.

❑ The left ventricle is responsible for the majority of force for cardiac output.

❑ If the left ventricle is damaged, the output decreases and fluid accumulates in the interstitial and alveolar spaces, causing pulmonary edema.

❑ Damage to the left atrium would contribute to heart failure but wouldn't affect cardiac output or the onset of pulmonary edema.

❑ If the right atrium and right ventricle were damaged, right-sided heart failure would result.

❑ Pulmonary edema is a life-threatening complication of heart failure.

❑ Pulmonary edema can develop in minutes, secondary to a sudden fluid shift from the pulmonary vasculature into the interstitium and alveoli of the lung.

❑ The volume of blood in the ventricle at the end of diastole determines preload.

❑ Cardiac index is the individualized measurement of cardiac output, based on the client's body surface area.

❑ Cardiac output is the amount of blood the heart expels per minute.

❑ Tachycardia, finger clubbing, and a loud $S_2$ suggest transposition of the great arteries (a cyanotic congenital heart defect).

❑ Dyspnea, cough, and palpitations occur with mitral insufficiency.

❑ Dyspnea, fatigue, and syncope indicate aortic insufficiency.

❑ In a client with atrial fibrillation, warfarin reaches therapeutic levels when the International Normalized Ratio (INR) is 2 to 3.

❑ With atrial tachycardia, the rhythm is regular, the P wave is hidden in the preceding T wave, and the rate ranges from 140 to 250 beats/minute.

❑ A ventricular rate that varies with the degree of atrioventricular block, along with sawtooth P waves, characterizes atrial flutter.

❑ Irregular ventricular response and absent P waves characterize atrial fibrillation.

❑ Regular and equal atrial and ventricular rhythms and a rate of 100 to 160 beats/minute characterize sinus tachycardia.

❑ Cardiac tamponade is associated with decreased cardiac output, which in turn reduces blood pressure.

❑ Shortness of breath, tachypnea, low blood pressure, tachycardia, diffuse crackles, and a cough producing pink, frothy sputum are late signs of pulmonary edema.

- ❏ The murmur of aortic stenosis is low-pitched, rough, and rasping.
- ❏ The murmur of aortic stenosis is heard loudest in the second intercostal space to the right of the sternum.
- ❏ Atrial fibrillation occurs with irregular and rapid discharge from multiple ectopic atrial foci that cause quivering of the atria without atrial systole.

## Hematologic and immune systems

- ❏ For an adult client to be diagnosed with AIDS, he must test positive for human immunodeficiency virus (HIV), have a CD4+ T-cell count below 200 cells/μl, and have one or more specific opportunistic infections or cancers along with the HIV infection.
- ❏ Human immunodeficiency virus is most easily transmitted in blood, semen, and vaginal secretions and has also been found in urine, feces, saliva, tears, and breast milk.
- ❏ A gastrectomy can cause pernicious anemia due to the client's inability to absorb vitamin $B_{12}$.
- ❏ A client who has had a gastrectomy is at high risk for developing anemia.
- ❏ Antinuclear antibody titer is commonly used as a screening tool for rheumatoid arthritis (RA) but is not a diagnostic tool for RA.
- ❏ Complete blood count, erythrocyte sedimentation rate, and rheumatoid factor are all used as diagnostic tools for rheumatoid arthritis (RA) and are also used to monitor progress of RA or response to therapy.
- ❏ In adults, thrombocytopenia is indicated when the platelet count is less than 100,000/μl.
- ❏ Normal platelet count ranges from 140,000 to 400,000/μl.
- ❏ Thrombocytopathy is platelet dysfunction.
- ❏ Thrombocytosis is an excess number of platelets.
- ❏ The classic symptoms for thrombocytopenia are petechiae and bruising.
- ❏ Pancytopenia is a reduction in all blood cells.
- ❏ Idiopathic thrombocytopenic purpura and disseminated intravascular coagulation cause platelet aggregation and bleeding.
- ❏ Heparin-associated thrombosis and thrombocytopenia may be suspected when a decrease in platelet count from 230,000 μl to 5,000 μl is noted in a client who has had coronary artery bypass graft surgery.
- ❏ A xenogeneic transplant is a transplant between two different species.
- ❏ An allogeneic transplant is between two humans.
- ❏ A syngeneic transplant is between identical twins.
- ❏ An autologous transplant is a transplant from the same individual.

❑ Systemic lupus erythematosus affects women eight times more often than men; usually strikes during childbearing age; is three times more common in black women than in white women; and is a chronic, inflammatory, autoimmune disorder that primarily affects connective tissue.

❑ Systemic lupus erythematosus affects the skin and kidneys, and may also affect the respiratory, cardiac, neurologic, and renal systems.

❑ In stage I of Hodgkin's disease, symptoms include a single enlarged lymph node (usually), unexplained fever, night sweats, malaise, and generalized pruritus.

❑ Kidney failure is the most common cause of death for clients with systemic lupus erythematosus.

❑ The classic sign of systemic lupus erythematosus (SLE) is the butterfly rash (superficial lesions over the cheeks and nose).

❑ Other common signs of SLE include vomiting, weight loss, and difficulty urinating.

❑ Pancytopenia and elevated antinuclear antibody titer support the diagnosis of systemic lupus erythematosus.

❑ Chronic lymphocytic leukemia shows a proliferation of small abnormal mature B cells and decreased antibody response.

❑ Thrombocytopenia is often present in chronic lymphocytic leukemia.

❑ Uncontrolled proliferation of granulocytes occurs in myelogenous leukemia.

❑ The initial phase of chemotherapy for acute lymphocytic leukemia, called the induction phase, is designed to put the client into remission by giving high doses of drugs and administering doses closer together than once each month.

❑ The hematologic system functions as an important part of the body's defenses.

❑ Blood components play a vital role in transporting electrolytes and regulating acid-base balance.

❑ Lymphatic vessels prevent edema by moving fluid and proteins from interstitial spaces to venous circulation; they also reabsorb fats from the small intestine.

❑ Lymph nodes are tissues that filter out bacteria and other foreign cells and are grouped by region.

❑ Lymph nodes are grouped by region: cervicofacial, supraclavicular, axillary, epitrochlear, inguinal, and femoral.

❑ The spleen destroys bacteria, filters blood, serves as a blood reservoir, forms lymphocytes and monocytes, and traps formed particles.

❑ Hematopoiesis occurs in the spleen and is the process by which red blood cells, white blood cells, and platelets are produced.

❑ Bone marrow may be described as either red or yellow; red bone marrow is a source of lymphocytes and macrophages. Hematopoiesis is carried out by red bone marrow.

❑ Yellow bone marrow is red bone marrow that has changed to fat.

❑ Bone marrow contains stem cells, which may develop into several different cell types during hematopoiesis.

❑ Some stem cells evolve into lymphocytes; lymphocytes may become B cells or T cells; other stem cells evolve into phagocytes.

❑ Erythrocytes (also called red blood cells, or RBCs) are formed in the bone marrow and contain hemoglobin.

❑ Oxygen binds with hemoglobin to form oxyhemoglobin, which is then carried by red blood cells throughout the body.

❑ Thrombocytes (also called platelets) are formed in the bone marrow and function in the coagulation of blood.

❑ Leukocytes (also called white blood cells, or WBCs) are formed in the bone marrow and lymphatic tissue and include granulocytes and agranulocytes.

❑ White blood cells provide immunity and protection from infection by phagocytosis (engulfing, digesting, and destroying microorganisms).

❑ Plasma is the liquid portion of the blood; it is composed of water, protein (albumin and globulin), glucose, and electrolytes.

❑ A low-bacteria diet that excludes raw fruits and vegetables would be indicated for a neutropenic client with leukemia.

❑ Multiple myeloma is more common in middle-aged and older clients; mean age at diagnosis is 60 years.

❑ Multiple myeloma is twice as common in blacks as whites, and most often occurs in black men.

❑ Multiple myeloma is characterized by malignant plasma cells that produce an increased amount of immunoglobulin that isn't functional.

❑ As more malignant plasma cells are produced in multiple myeloma, there's less space in the bone marrow for red blood cell production.

❑ In late stages of multiple myeloma, platelets and white blood cell counts are reduced as the bone marrow is infiltrated by malignant plasma cells.

❑ In cell-mediated immunity, T cells respond directly to antigens (foreign substances such as bacteria or toxins that induce antibody formation).

❑ Cell-mediated immunity involves destruction of target cells—such as virus-infected cells and cancer cells—through secretion of lymphokines (lymph proteins).

❑ Examples of cell-mediated immunity are rejection of transplanted organs and delayed immune responses that fight disease.

❑ About 80% of blood cells are T cells.

❑ T cells probably originate from stem cells in the bone marrow; the thymus gland controls their maturity and in the process, a large number of antigen-specific cells are produced.

❑ There are three main types of T cells: killer, helper, and suppressor T cells.

❑ Killer T cells bind to the surface of the invading cell, disrupt the membrane, and destroy it by altering its internal environment.

❑ Helper T cells stimulate B cells to mature into plasma cells, which begin to synthesize and secrete immunoglobulin (proteins with known antibody activity).

❑ Suppressor T cells reduce the humoral response.

❑ B cells act in a different way from T cells to recognize and destroy antigens. B cells are responsible for humoral or immunoglobulin-mediated immunity.

❑ B cells originate in the bone marrow and mature into plasma cells that produce antibodies (immunoglobulin molecules that interact with a specific antigen).

❑ Antibodies destroy bacteria and viruses, thereby preventing them from entering host cells.

❑ Five major classes of immunoglobulin exist: immunoglobulin G, immunoglobulin M, immunoglobulin A, immunoglobulin D, and immunoglobulin E.

❑ Immunoglobulin G makes up about 80% of plasma antibodies, appears in all body fluids, and is the major antibacterial and antiviral antibody.

❑ Immunoglobulin M is the first immunoglobulin produced during an immune response, is too large to easily cross membranes, and is usually present only in the vascular system.

❑ Immunoglobulin A is found mainly in body secretions, such as saliva, sweat, tears, mucus, bile, and colostrums, and defends against pathogens on body surfaces, especially those that enter the respiratory and GI tracts.

❑ Immunoglobulin D is present in plasma, is easily broken down, is the predominant antibody on the surface of B cells, and is mainly an antigen receptor.

❑ Immunoglobulin E is the antibody involved in immediate hypersensitivity reactions, or allergic reactions that develop within minutes of exposure to an antigen.

❑ Immune function declines with age.

❑ Diminished immune function in the elderly can interfere with the ability to fight infection.

❑ Inflammation and increased body temperature are normal immune responses to detected antigens.

❑ Allergies are heightened responses to antigens.

❑ Autoimmune response is one in which the immune system forms antibodies against the body's own tissues, resulting in disease.

❑ Antibodies are produced by B cells.

❑ Genetics and environment haven't been shown to be factors in acquired immune deficiency.

❑ A negative human immunodeficiency virus (HIV) antibody test means that HIV antibodies weren't in the client's blood at the time the test was performed; if antibodies to HIV are present, the test result is positive.

❑ Antibodies to human immunodeficiency virus (HIV) may take 3 weeks to 6 months or longer to develop.

❑ Incidence rate is the rapidity with which individuals without a disease contract it.

❑ Survival is the proportion of individuals affected by a disease who live for a particular length of time.

❑ Risk is the proportion of individuals without a disease who develop the disease within a particular time period.

❑ In community health and epidemiologic studies, the definition of disease prevalence is the number of individuals affected by a particular disease at a specific time.

❑ The American Association of Blood Banks recommends that blood or blood components should be transfused within 4 hours.

❑ Standard precautions stipulate that a health care worker who anticipates coming into contact with a client's blood or body fluids must wear gloves.

❑ In aplastic anemia, the diagnostic findings are decreased levels of all the cellular elements of the blood (pancytopenia).

❑ Reed-Sternberg cells and lymph node enlargement occur with Hodgkin's disease.

❑ Decreased levels of white blood cells, red blood cells, and platelets are consistent in the diagnosis of a client with aplastic anemia.

❑ Two people with the beta-thalassemia trait have a 25% chance of having a child with thalassemia major, a potentially life-threatening disease.

❑ Thalassemia occurs primarily in people of Italian, Greek, African, Asian, Middle Eastern, East Indian, and Caribbean descent.

❑ A client with severe abdominal pain and a history of sickle cell disease may be in a sickle cell crisis.

❑ Acute abdominal pain in sickle cell crisis is caused by sickling in the mesenteric circulation.

❑ Neutropenia occurs when the absolute neutrophil count falls below 1,000/µl, reflecting a severe risk for infection.

❑ Hemophilia A results from a deficiency of factor VIII.

❑ Sickle cell disease is caused by a defective hemoglobin molecule.

❑ Christmas disease is also called hemophilia B and results from a factor IX deficiency.

❑ In disseminated intravascular coagulation, platelets and clotting factors are consumed, resulting in microthrombi and excessive bleeding.

❑ The laboratory finding most consistent with disseminated intravascular coagulation is a low platelet count.

❑ During chemotherapy for leukemia, tumor lysis syndrome may occur as cell destruction releases intracellular components, resulting in hyperuricemia.

❑ People with the D antigen have Rh-positive blood type.

❑ People lacking the D antigen have Rh-negative blood.

❑ It's important that a person with Rh-negative blood receives Rh-negative blood.

❑ If Rh-positive blood is administered to an Rh-negative person, the recipient develops anti-Rh agglutinins.

❑ Subsequent transfusions with Rh-positive blood to an Rh-negative person may cause serious reactions with clumping and hemolysis of red blood cells.

❑ Acute lymphocytic leukemia is most common in young children and in adults age 65 and older; it is more common in Whites than in Blacks or Asians.

## Respiratory system

❑ Pneumococcal or streptococcal pneumonia, caused by *Streptococcus pneumoniae*, is the most common cause of community-acquired pneumonia.

❑ Elderly clients with pneumonia may first appear with only an altered mental status and dehydration due to a blunted immune response.

❑ If the right forearm of a client who had a purified protein derivative (PPD) test for tuberculosis is reddened and raised about 3 mm where the test was given, this test would be classed as negative.

❑ If the site of a purified protein derivative (PPD) test is reddened and raised 10 mm or more, it's considered positive, according to the Centers for Disease Control and Prevention.

❑ The active stage shows the classic symptoms of tuberculosis: fever, hemoptysis, and night sweats.

❑ Some people carry dormant tuberculosis that may develop into active disease.

❑ If there's no active tuberculosis disease, it's called latent or inactive tuberculosis infection.

❑ The tubercle bacilli may remain latent for years and then activate when the client's resistance is lowered, as when a client is being treated for cancer.

❑ The sputum culture for *Mycobacterium tuberculosis* is the only method of confirming the diagnosis of tuberculosis.

❑ A tuberculin converter's skin test will be positive, meaning he has been exposed to and infected with tuberculosis and now has a cell-mediated immune response to the skin test.

❑ Because a tuberculin converter's X-ray is negative, he should be monitored every 6 months to see if he develops changes in his chest X-ray or pulmonary examination.

❑ The treatment regimen for active tuberculosis may last up to 24 months.

❑ It's essential that the client comply with therapy for active tuberculosis during the time prescribed to prevent development of resistance.

❑ The client with active tuberculosis is highly contagious until three consecutive sputum cultures are negative.

❑ Inspiratory and expiratory wheezes are typical findings in asthma.

❑ Nonallergic asthma doesn't have an easily identifiable allergen and can be triggered by the common cold.

❑ A client with acute asthma showing inspiratory and expiratory wheezes and a decreased forced expiratory volume should be treated with bronchodilators.

❑ Clients with chronic obstructive bronchitis appear bloated; they have large barrel chests and peripheral edema, cyanotic nail beds and, at times, circumoral cyanosis.

❑ Because of the large amount of energy it takes to breathe, clients with emphysema are usually cachectic.

❑ In emphysema, the wall integrity of the individual air sacs is damaged, reducing the surface area available for gas exchange.

❑ A client with emphysema should receive only 1 to 3 L/minute of oxygen, if needed, or he may lose his hypoxic drive.

❑ Atelectasis develops when there's interference with the normal negative pressure that promotes lung expansion.

❑ Atelectasis is the most common respiratory disorder to occur in the first 24 to 48 hours after surgery.

❑ Using an incentive spirometer requires the client to take deep breaths and promotes lung expansion, which can reduce or prevent the incidence of atelectasis in a postoperative client.

❑ The upper airways include the nasopharynx (nose), oropharynx (mouth), laryngopharynx, and larynx.

❏ The upper airways warm, filter, and humidify inhaled air.

❏ The lower airways begin with the trachea, or windpipe, which extends from the cricoid cartilage to the carina.

❏ The trachea divides into the right and left mainstem bronchi, which continue to divide all the way down to the alveoli, the gas-exchange units of the lungs.

❏ The larynx houses the vocal cords and is the transition point between the upper and lower airways.

❏ The epiglottis, a flap of tissue that closes over the top of the larynx when the client swallows, protects the client from aspirating food or fluid into the lower airways.

❏ The right lung has three lobes: upper, middle, and lower.

❏ The left lung is smaller and has only an upper and a lower lobe.

❏ The lungs share space in the thoracic cavity with the heart and great vessels, the trachea, the esophagus, and the bronchi.

❏ The space between the lungs is called the mediastinum.

❏ The diaphragm and the external intercostal muscles are the primary muscles used in breathing.

❏ The diaphragm and the external intercostal muscles contract when the client inhales and relax when the client exhales.

❏ Accessory inspiratory muscles include the trapezius, sternocleidomastoid, and scalenes, which combine to elevate the scapulae, clavicles, sternum, and upper ribs.

❏ Men, children, infants, athletes, and singers usually use abdominal, or diaphragmatic, breathing.

❏ Most women usually use chest, or intercostal, breathing.

❏ When checking the client for tactile fremitus, vibrations that feel more intense on one side of the back than the other indicate tissue consolidation on that side.

❏ When checking the client for tactile fremitus, less intense vibrations may indicate emphysema, pneumothorax, or pleural effusion.

❏ When checking the client for tactile fremitus, faint or no vibrations in the upper posterior thorax may indicate bronchial obstruction or a fluid-filled pleural space.

❏ Flat percussion sounds—short, soft, high-pitched, extremely dull sounds—as found over the thigh may indicate consolidation, as in atelectasis and extensive pleural effusion.

❏ Dull percussion sounds—medium in intensity and pitch, moderate length, thudlike sounds—as found over the liver may indicate a solid area, as in lobar pneumonia.

- ❏ Resonant percussion sound—long, loud, low-pitched, hollow sounds—indicate normal lung tissue or bronchitis.

- ❏ Hyperresonant percussion sounds—very loud, lower-pitched sounds—as found over the stomach may indicate a hyperinflated lung, as in emphysema or pneumothorax.

- ❏ Tympanic percussion sounds—loud, high-pitched, moderate length, musical, drumlike sounds—as found over a puffed-out cheek may indicate air collection, as in a large pneumothorax.

- ❏ To distinguish between normal and adventitious breath sounds in the client's lungs, press the diaphragm of the stethoscope firmly against the skin and listen to a full inspiration and a full expiration at each site. Remember to compare sound variations from one side to the other.

- ❏ To elicit bronchophony, ask the client to say "ninety-nine" while you auscultate his chest; over normal lung tissue, the words sound muffled; over consolidated areas, the words sound unusually loud

- ❏ To elicit egophony ask the client to say "E" while you auscultate his chest; over normal lung tissue, the sound is muffled; over consolidated lung tissue, it will sound like the letter "a."

- ❏ To elicit whispered pectoriloquy ask the client to whisper "1, 2, 3" while you auscultate his chest; over normal lung tissue, the numbers will be almost indistinguishable; over consolidated lung tissue, the numbers will be loud and clear.

- ❏ Tracheal breath sounds are harsh, high-pitched sounds and are heard above the supraclavicular notch, over the trachea.

- ❏ Bronchial breath sounds are loud, high-pitched sounds heard just above the clavicles on each side of the sternum, over the manubrium.

- ❏ Bronchovesicular breath sounds are medium in loudness and pitch and can be heard next to the sternum between the scapulae.

- ❏ Vesicular breath sounds are soft low-pitched sounds and are heard in the remainder of lungs.

- ❏ Tachypnea is shallow breathing with increased respiratory rate.

- ❏ Bradypnea is regular breathing at a decreased rate.

- ❏ Apnea is the absence of breathing and may be periodic.

- ❏ Hyperpnea is an increased depth of breathing.

- ❏ Kussmaul's respirations are rapid, deep breathing without pauses that, in adults, result in a rate of more than 20 breaths/minute; breathing usually sounds labored with deep breaths that resemble sighs.

- ❏ Biot's respirations are rapid, deep breathing with abrupt pauses between each breath and an equal depth to each breath.

❑ Decreased breath sounds or inspiratory and expiratory wheezing is associated with asthma.

❑ Positive end-expiratory pressure reduces cardiac output by increasing intrathoracic pressure and reducing the amount of blood delivered to the left side of the heart.

❑ Oxygen toxicity causes direct pulmonary trauma, reduces the amount of alveolar surface area available for gaseous exchange, and can result in increased carbon dioxide levels and decreased oxygen uptake.

❑ Thoracic kyphoscoliosis causes lung compression and restricts lung expansion, resulting in more rapid and shallow respiration.

❑ Spontaneous pneumothorax occurs when the client's lung collapses, causing an acute decrease in the amount of functional lung used in oxygenation.

❑ Pneumonia can produce bronchial breath sounds over the area of consolidation.

❑ The only way to re-expand the lung in right spontaneous pneumothorax is to place a chest tube on the right side so the air in the pleural space can be removed.

❑ A lack of breath sounds in the left upper lobe of a trauma client may indicate pneumothorax.

❑ Rhonchorous breath sounds are present with tuberculosis.

❑ An incentive spirometer is used to encourage deep breathing.

❑ The placement of a chest tube will drain the blood from the space and re-expand the lung in a hemothorax.

❑ Squamous cell carcinoma is a slow-growing cancer, rarely metastasizes, and has the best prognosis of all lung cancer types.

❑ Only surgical biopsy with cytologic examination of the cells can give a definitive diagnosis of cancer and type.

❑ A small area of tissue close to the surface of the lung is removed in a wedge resection.

❑ An entire lung is removed in a pneumonectomy.

❑ A lobe of the lung is removed in a lobectomy.

❑ A segment of the lung is removed in a segmental resection.

❑ In a lobectomy, the remaining lung lobe or lobes overexpand slightly to fill the space previously occupied by the removed tissue.

❑ In a pneumonectomy, serous fluid fills the space and eventually consolidates, preventing extensive mediastinal shift of the heart and remaining lung.

❑ Because the hemidiaphragm is a muscle that doesn't contract when paralyzed, an uncontracted hemidiaphragm remains in an "up" position, which reduces the space left by the pneumonectomy.

❑ During a pneumonectomy, the phrenic nerve on the surgical side is usually cut to cause hemidiaphragm paralysis.

❑ A pulmonary embolism blocks the pulmonary vasculature, preventing bloodflow to the distal region of the lung and interfering with gas exchange.

❑ Blood must perfuse, or flow around each alveolus, for the exchange of carbon dioxide and oxygen to occur across the alveolar-capillary membrane.

❑ When an area of lung is ventilated but not perfused, there is a ventilation-perfusion mismatch.

❑ A mismatch that shows impaired ventilation but normal perfusion indicates a pathologic state in the bronchial tree, such as pneumonia or atelectasis.

❑ In a ventilation-perfusion mismatch that occurs with a pulmonary embolism, the amount of ventilation occurring doesn't equal perfusion.

❑ The inflammatory reaction in the lung with a pulmonary embolism causes chest pain.

❑ Sudden reduction in adequate oxygenation in a client with a pulmonary embolism may cause feelings of apprehension or a sense of "impending doom."

❑ The infarcted area in pulmonary embolism produces alveolar damage that can lead to the production of bloody sputum, sometimes in massive amounts.

❑ The client with a massive pulmonary embolism will have a large region of lung tissue unavailable for perfusion.

❑ Arterial blood gas analysis in a client with a massive pulmonary embolism will reveal respiratory alkalosis.

❑ The $\dot{V}/\dot{Q}$ scan provides information on the extent of occlusion caused by a pulmonary embolism and the amount of lung tissue involved in the area not perfused.

❑ A pulmonary angiogram is used to definitively diagnose a pulmonary embolism.

❑ The goal of oxygen therapy for a client with a pulmonary embolism is to have a $Pao_2$ greater than 60 mm Hg on a fraction of inspired oxygen of 40% or less.

❑ When a pulmonary embolism is suspected, positioning the client on the left side may prevent a clot that has extended through the capillaries and into the pulmonary veins from breaking off.

❑ An umbrella filter breaks the clots into small pieces that won't significantly occlude the pulmonary vasculature.

❑ Surgical removal of pulmonary embolism is rarely done because of the associated high mortality risk.

❑ Pulse oximetry determines the percentage of hemoglobin carrying oxygen.

❑ Hemoglobin carries oxygen to all tissues in the body.

❑ If the hemoglobin level is low, the amount of oxygen-carrying capacity is also low; increasing the hemoglobin level will increase oxygen-carrying capacity and thus increase the total amount of oxygen available in the blood.

❑ If the client has been tachypneic during exertion, or even at rest, because oxygen demand is higher than the available oxygen content, then an increase in hemoglobin may decrease the respiratory rate to normal levels.

❑ Positive end-expiratory pressure (PEEP) delivers positive pressure to the lung at the end of expiration, helps open collapsed alveoli, and helps them stay open so gas exchange can occur in these newly opened alveoli, improving oxygenation.

❑ Gaseous exchange occurs in the alveolar membrane, so if the alveoli collapse, no exchange occurs.

❑ Collapsed alveoli receive oxygen, as well as other nutrients, from the bloodstream.

❑ The continuous positive airway pressure (CPAP) mask provides pressurized oxygen continuously through both inspiration and expiration; the client has less resistance to overcome in taking in his next breath, making it easier to breathe.

❑ Continuous positive airway pressure (CPAP) can be provided through an oxygen mask to improve oxygenation in hypoxic clients.

❑ Bilevel positive airway pressure (BiPAP) delivers both continuous positive airway pressure (CPAP) and positive end-expiratory pressure (PEEP).

❑ Bilevel positive airway pressure (BiPAP) provides the differing pressures throughout the respiratory cycle, attempting to optimize a client's oxygenation and ventilation.

❑ Inspiratory and expiratory pressures are set separately to optimize the client's ventilatory status in bilevel positive airway pressure (BiPAP).

❑ The fraction of inspired oxygen is adjusted to optimize oxygenation in bilevel positive airway pressure (BiPAP).

❑ Pleural fluid normally seeps continually into the pleural space from the capillaries lining the parietal pleura and is reabsorbed by the visceral pleural capillaries and lymphatics.

❑ Thoracentesis is used to remove excess pleural fluid and restore proper lung status.

❑ Transudates found in pleural fluid after thoracentesis are substances that have passed through a membrane and usually occur in clients with low protein.

❑ Exudates are substances found in pleural fluid after thoracentesis that have escaped from blood vessels, contain an accumulation of cells, and have a high specific gravity and a high lactate dehydrogenase level.

❑ Exudates found in the pleural fluid after a thoracentesis usually occur in response to a malignancy, infection, or inflammatory process.

❑ Bubbling in the water-seal chamber of a chest drainage system stems from an air leak.

❑ In pneumothorax, an air leak can occur as air is pulled from the pleural space.

❑ If the client gags or coughs after nasopharyngeal airway placement, the tube may be too long.

❑ Suctioning without a nasopharyngeal airway causes trauma to the natural airway.

❑ To prevent hypoxia, continuous suctioning shouldn't last more than 10 seconds at a time during catheter withdrawal.

❑ Suction shouldn't be applied while the catheter is being advanced.

❑ Normal arterial blood gas values include a pH of 7.35 to 7.45.

❑ Normal $Paco_2$ is 35 to 45 mm Hg.

❑ Normal $Pao_2$ values are 75 to 100 mm Hg.

❑ Normal $HCO_3^-$ levels are 22 to 26 mEq/L.

❑ Below-normal pH, an elevated $Paco_2$, and normal $HCO_3^-$ indicate respiratory acidosis.

❑ With metabolic acidosis, pH and $HCO_3^-$ are low and $Paco_2$ is normal.

❑ In respiratory alkalosis, pH is elevated and $Paco_2$ is low.

❑ In metabolic alkalosis, both pH and $HCO_3^-$ are elevated.

❑ Semi-Fowler's position (with the head of the bed elevated 30 degrees) promotes optimal lung expansion.

❑ A prone position (lying on the abdomen) improves oxygenation in a client with acute respiratory distress syndrome who's receiving mechanical ventilation because it recruits new alveoli in the posterior region of the lung.

❑ A pulse oximetry level above 93% and a normal respiratory rate demonstrate probable lung expansion and normal chest tube functioning.

❑ A client sitting upright and leaning slightly forward suggests that the client has impaired gas exchange because this position increases lung expansion.

❏ Tension pneumothorax causes severe respiratory distress, hypotension, and diminished breath sounds over the affected area.

❏ Tension pneumothorax also causes hyperresonance, distended neck veins, eventual tracheal shift and, possibly, paradoxical chest-wall movement on the injured side.

❏ A ruptured diaphragm leads to hyperresonance on percussion, hypotension, dyspnea, dysphagia, and shifting of heart and bowel sounds in the lower to middle chest.

❏ A massive hemothorax produces signs of shock (such as tachycardia and hypotension) and dullness on percussion on the injured side.

❏ A hemothorax also results in decreased breath sounds on the injured side, respiratory distress and, possibly, mediastinal shift.

❏ Vesicular breath sounds are prolonged on inhalation and shortened on exhalation.

❏ Bronchial breath sounds are discontinuous and are loudest during exhalation.

❏ Tracheal breath sounds are harsh, discontinuous sounds heard over the trachea during inhalation or exhalation.

❏ Bronchovesicular breath sounds are continuous sounds that occur during inhalation or exhalation.

❏ Reduction in vital capacity is a normal physiologic change in the older adult.

❏ Other normal physiologic changes in the older adult include decreased elastic recoil of the lungs, fewer functional capillaries in the alveoli, and an increase in residual volume.

❏ Pneumonia is an acute infection of the lung parenchyma.

❏ If a sputum specimen will be collected by expectoration, the client should be instructed to take several deep abdominal breaths; when he's ready to cough, he should take one more deep abdominal breath, bend forward, and cough into the provided sterile container.

❏ A client should be instructed to drink plenty of fluids the night before a sputum test.

❏ After bronchoscopy, the client is observed for possible complications and can have liquids when the gag reflex returns.

❏ Clients who are allergic to certain cross-reactive foods—including apricots, avocados, bananas, cherries, chestnuts, grapes, kiwis, passion fruit, peaches, and tomatoes— may also be allergic to latex.

❏ The most common etiology of pulmonary embolism is thromboembolism from a distant site, particularly from deep veins of the legs and pelvis (90% to 95%).

❏ Immobility places the client at risk for pneumonia.

❏ Clients with cystic fibrosis may receive chest percussion with a high-frequency chest wall oscillation vest.

❏ Before obtaining an arterial blood sample from a client's radial artery, the Allen's test is performed to assess circulation.

❏ The needle bevel is held at a 30- to 45-degree angle for an arterial blood gas puncture.

❏ A pulmonary embolus occurs when a thrombus lodges in a branch of the pulmonary artery, partially or totally occluding it. Breathing into a paper bag can stop hyperventilation by increasing carbon dioxide levels.

❏ Tuberculosis (TB) infection typically occurs from inhaling infected droplets after a person with TB coughs.

❏ Transmission of tuberculosis infection usually requires close, frequent, prolonged contact.

❏ Human immunodeficiency virus is spread through contact with an infected person's blood.

❏ In pleural effusion, fluid accumulates in the pleural space, impairing transmission of normal breath sounds.

❏ Crackles (short explosive or popping sounds) commonly accompany atel-ectasis, interstitial fibrosis, and left-sided heart failure.

❏ Rhonchi (low-pitched sounds with a snoring quality) suggest secretions in the large airways.

❏ Wheezes (high-pitched, hissing sounds) result from narrowed airways, as in asthma, chronic obstructive pulmonary disease, or bronchitis.

❏ To ensure accurate results, a purified protein derivative (PPD) test must be read 48 to 72 hours after administration.

❏ The nonrebreather mask delivers oxygen concentrations of 80% to 100%.

❏ The nonrebreather mask is reserved for emergency situations.

❏ A partial rebreather mask delivers oxygen concentrations of 60% to 80%.

❏ A nasal cannula delivers oxygen at flow rates of 1 to 6 L/minute.

❏ A flow rate of 4 L/minute delivers an oxygen concentration of 36%.

❏ A flow rate of 6 L/minute delivers an oxygen concentration of 44%.

❏ Immobilizing the cervical spine won't provide the needed oxygenation.

❏ Chest compressions should be delivered only if circulation is absent.

❏ A client with chronic obstructive pulmonary disease should obtain immunizations against pneumococcal pneumonia as well as influenza.

❏ In addition to pleuritic chest pain and dyspnea, a client with a pulmonary embolus may also present with a low-grade fever, tachycardia, and blood-tinged sputum.

❏ Thick green sputum would indicate infection.

❏ Frothy sputum would indicate pulmonary edema.

❏ Respiratory alkalosis is defined by a pH greater than 7.45 and $Paco_2$ less than 35 mm Hg.

❏ Respiratory alkalosis is generally associated with deep, rapid breathing.

❏ Neurologic effects of respiratory alkalosis include light-headedness or dizziness, circumoral and peripheral paresthesia, and carpopedal spasms, twitching, and muscle weakness as it progresses.

❏ Metabolic acidosis is defined as a pH less than 7.3, $Paco_2$ less than or equal to 34 mm Hg depending on respiratory compensation, and $HCO_3^-$ less than 22 mEq/L.

❏ Acute respiratory failure is characterized by a pH less than 3, $Paco_2$ greater than 50 mm Hg, and markedly diminished oxygen saturation levels.

❏ In Cheyne-Stokes respirations, breaths gradually become faster and deeper than normal and then slower during a 30- to 170-second period with intermittent periods of apnea.

## Neurosensory system

❏ Homonymous hemianopia is a type of visual field blindness involving either the two right or the two left halves of the visual fields of both eyes.

❏ Homonymous hemianopia is due to damage to the optic nerves.

❏ Astereognosis is the inability to identify common objects through touch alone.

❏ Oculogyric crisis is a fixed position of the eyeballs that can last for minutes or hours.

❏ Oculogyric crisis occurs in response to antipsychotic medications.

❏ Receptive aphasia is the inability to understand words or word meaning.

❏ Asynchronous atrial contraction that occurs with atrial fibrillation predisposes to mural thrombi, which may embolize, leading to a stroke.

❏ Bradycardia, deep vein thrombosis, or past myocardial infarction won't lead to arterial embolization.

❏ Atrial fibrillation places the client at risk for thromboembolic stroke.

❏ A client with a stroke in evolution may be ordered tissue plasminogen activator, a thrombolytic agent, as treatment.

❏ Because of a potential loss of the gag reflex and potential altered level of consciousness in a client with stroke in evolution, tracheal suction should be available at all times.

❏ Thickening dietary liquids isn't done for a client with stroke in evolution until the gag reflex returns or the stroke has evolved and the deficit can be assessed.

- ❏ Unless heart failure is present in the client with stroke in evolution, restricting fluids isn't indicated.

- ❏ An intact gag reflex shows a properly functioning cranial nerve IX (glossopharyngeal).

- ❏ Speech may be normal while the gag reflex is absent.

- ❏ Cranial nerves III, IV, and VI evaluate eye movement and accommodation.

- ❏ A nurse shouldn't offer food or fluids without assessing for an intact gag reflex.

- ❏ Thickened liquids are easiest to form into a bolus and swallow.

- ❏ Clear and full liquids are amorphous and can't easily form a bolus.

- ❏ A mechanical soft diet may be too hard to chew and too dry to swallow when dysphagia is present.

- ❏ Thickened liquids would be least likely to lead to aspiration in a client who had a stroke with residual dysphagia.

- ❏ In clients with hemiplegia or hemiparesis, loss of muscle contraction decreases venous return and may cause swelling of the affected extremity.

- ❏ Contractures or bony calcifications may occur with a stroke but don't appear with swelling.

- ❏ Deep vein thrombosis may develop in clients with a stroke but is more likely to occur in the lower extremities.

- ❏ Swelling in an extremity after a stroke isn't linked to protein loss.

- ❏ The brain stem contains the medulla and the vital cardiac, vasomotor, and respiratory centers.

- ❏ A brain stem infarction leads to vital sign changes such as bradypnea.

- ❏ Contralateral hemiplegia and numbness or tingling in the face or arm may occur, depending on the level of brain stem injury.

- ❏ Aphasia is associated with lobar strokes in the cerebral hemispheres.

- ❏ Prolonged use of steroidal anti-inflammatory agents is a risk factor for cataracts.

- ❏ The development of cataracts is not linked to a history of frequent streptococcal throat infections, maternal exposure to rubella during pregnancy, or presence of increased intraocular pressure.

- ❏ Pain shouldn't be present after cataract surgery.

- ❏ Pain after cataract surgery may be an indication of hyphema, or clouding in the anterior chamber, and infection.

- ❏ Blurred vision, glare, and itching may be present after cataract surgery.

❏ Clear fluid draining from the ear or nose of a client may mean a cerebrospinal fluid leak, which is common in basilar skull fractures.

❏ The cornea is the nonvascular, transparent fibrous coat where the iris can be seen.

❏ The fovea is the point of central vision.

❏ The sclera is the fibrous tissue that forms the outer protective covering over the eyeball.

❏ Concussion is associated with a brief loss of consciousness.

❏ Cerebral palsy is associated with nonprogressive paralysis present since birth.

❏ Sinus infection is associated with facial pain and pressure, with possible nasal drainage.

❏ Sudden removal of cerebrospinal fluid results in pressures lower in the lumbar area than in the brain and put the client at risk for herniation of the brain.

❏ Lumbar puncture is contraindicated with increased intracranial pressure.

❏ A lumbar puncture is performed if brain imaging is negative or inconclusive in the presence of symptoms that suggest subarachnoid hemorrhage.

❏ Blood in the cerebrospinal fluid is diagnostic for subarachnoid hemorrhage.

❏ Urine output of 300 mL/hour may indicate diabetes insipidus, which is a failure of the pituitary to produce antidiuretic hormone.

❏ Diabetes insipidus may occur with increased intracranial pressure and head trauma.

❏ Diabetes insipidus produces low urine specific gravity, increased serum osmolarity, and dehydration.

❏ Slowing the rate of I.V. fluid would contribute to dehydration when polyuria is present.

❏ Straining when having a bowel movement, sneezing, coughing, and suctioning may lead to increased intracranial pressure (ICP) and should be avoided when potential increased ICP exists.

❏ Stool softeners don't stimulate the bowel and shouldn't be used in combination with osmotic diuretics.

❏ The Valsalva maneuver may lead to bradycardia and reflex tachycardia.

❏ Stool softeners would be given to a client after repair of a cerebral aneurysm to prevent straining, which increases intracranial pressure.

❏ Mannitol promotes osmotic diuresis by increasing the pressure gradient, drawing fluid from intracellular to intravascular spaces.

❑ Mannitol may be ordered for a client with a subdural hematoma who is restless and confused, with dilation of the ipsilateral pupil to promote osmotic diuresis to decrease intracranial pressure.

❑ Mannitol can reduce intraocular pressure, prevent acute tubular necrosis, and draw water into the vascular system to increase blood pressure.

❑ Mannitol promotes osmotic diuresis by increasing the pressure gradient in the renal tubules, thus increasing urine output.

❑ Fixed and dilated pupils are symptoms of increased intracranial pressure or cranial nerve damage.

❑ Carbon dioxide has vasodilating properties.

❑ Lowering $Paco_2$ through hyperventilation in some clients may lower the increased intracranial pressure caused by dilated cerebral vessels.

❑ Oxygenation is evaluated through $Pao_2$ and oxygen saturation.

❑ Alveolar hypoventilation would be reflected in an increased $Paco_2$.

❑ Low-dose heparin therapy and sequential compression boots will prevent deep vein thrombosis.

❑ Although a physical therapy consultation is important before initiating other interventions to prevent footdrop, a nurse may use high-topped sneakers independently.

❑ Frequent swallowing after brain surgery may indicate fluid or blood leaking from the sinuses into the oropharynx.

❑ Blood or fluid draining from the ear may indicate a basilar skull fracture.

❑ Guaiac-positive stools indicate GI bleeding.

❑ Hematuria may result from cystitis or other urologic complications.

❑ A client who had a transsphenoidal hypophysectomy should be watched carefully for hemorrhage.

❑ After hypophysectomy, or removal of the pituitary gland, the body can't synthesize antidiuretic hormone.

❑ The nurse should always reassess the client's airway, breathing, and circulation when the intracranial pressure is elevated.

❑ Normal intracranial pressure is between 0 and 15 mm Hg.

❑ Mean arterial pressure should be maintained at or above 90 mm Hg.

❑ The head of the bed should be elevated between 15 and 30 degrees to facilitate venous drainage in a client with increased intracranial pressure.

❑ External stimulation, such as visitors, should be limited because it may increase intracranial pressure.

❑ In most cases after L4–L5 laminectomy, clients should be out of bed the first postoperative day.

❑ Frequent repositioning, use of a chairlike brace for the lower back when out of bed, and a firm mattress will help minimize complications after L4–L5 laminectomy.

❑ Swelling or pressure on the peripheral nerves controlling micturition, anesthesia, or use of an indwelling urinary catheter may lead to urine retention with frequent overflow of small amounts of urine in the client after lumbar laminectomy.

❑ Frequent voiding of small amounts of urine after a lumbar laminectomy may indicate urine retention.

❑ Strengthening the abdominal muscles after laminectomy will prevent lower back pain.

❑ Radiopaque dyes, used in myelography and cardiac catheterization, are usually iodine-based and may cause a reaction in those clients who are allergic.

❑ Chymopapain, derived from papaya, is an ingredient in meat tenderizers; sensitivity to this substance may preclude the use of chymopapain in chemonucleolysis.

❑ Allergy to shellfish may be a contraindication to tests using iodine-based dyes.

❑ The client may be positioned on his side in a "C" position to allow access to the intervertebral area in chemonucleolysis.

❑ A client may be scheduled for chemonucleolysis with chymopapain to relieve the pain of a herniated disk.

❑ Guillain-Barré syndrome is characterized by ascending paralysis and potential respiratory failure.

❑ Myasthenia gravis, an autoimmune disorder, is caused by the destruction of acetylcholine receptors.

❑ Guillain-Barré syndrome is a postviral illness characterized by ascending paralysis.

❑ Multiple sclerosis is caused by loss of the myelin sheath.

❑ Parkinson disease is caused by the inability of basal ganglia to produce sufficient dopamine.

❑ Ptosis and diplopia are early signs of myasthenia gravis.

❑ Dysphagia and respiratory distress occur in later myasthenia gravis.

❑ Symptoms of myasthenia gravis are typically milder in the morning and may be exacerbated by stress or lack of rest.

❑ Dry mouth and abdominal cramps are adverse effects of increased acetylcholine in the parasympathetic nervous system.

❑ The purpose of plasmapheresis in myasthenia gravis is to separate and remove circulating acetylcholine receptor antibodies from the blood of clients refractory to the usual therapies or clients in crisis.

❑ Stress, including pregnancy, may precipitate crisis in myasthenia gravis.

❑ Plasmapheresis doesn't remove T and B lymphocytes, nor does it deliver acetylcholinesterase inhibitor directly into the bloodstream.

❑ Complaints of halos around lights are a common finding in a client with glaucoma.

❑ Symptoms of glaucoma can include loss of peripheral vision or blind spots, reddened sclera, firm globe, decreased accommodation, halos around lights, and occasional eye pain.

❑ Clients with glaucoma may be asymptomatic.

❑ Normal intraocular pressure is 10 to 21 mm Hg.

❑ Without treatment, glaucoma may progress to irreversible blindness.

❑ Treatment for glaucoma won't restore visual damage, but will halt disease progression.

❑ Blurred or foggy vision is typical in glaucoma.

❑ Central vision loss is typical in glaucoma.

❑ Parkinson disease is characterized by the slowing of voluntary muscle movement, muscular rigidity, and resting tremor.

❑ Diminished distal sensation doesn't occur in Parkinson disease.

❑ The nurse should recognize that a client whose face is expressionless and speech is monotone is showing common symptoms of Parkinson disease.

❑ Parkinson disease is caused by degeneration of the substantia nigra in the basal ganglia of the brain, where dopamine is produced and stored.

❑ Degeneration of the substantia nigra results in motor dysfunction.

❑ Early symptoms Parkinson disease include coarse resting tremors of the fingers and thumb such as pill rolling movements of the hand.

❑ Akinesia and aspiration are late signs of Parkinson disease.

❑ Dementia occurs in only 20% of clients with Parkinson disease.

❑ A clear liquid diet doesn't provide adequate nutrition and may be more difficult to swallow than thickened liquids if dysphagia is present.

❑ Weight loss may occur with Parkinson disease.

❑ The nursing intervention that would best relieve the client's dry mouth is to offer the client ice chips and frequent sips of water, unless contraindicated.

❑ Multiple sclerosis is a chronic autoimmune disease that is more common in women than in men.

❑ Multiple sclerosis is characterized by multiple areas of demyelination and scarring (sclerosis) of the underlying nerve fibers.

❏ There are no known cures for multiple sclerosis, although treatment can help promote remissions and prevent exacerbations.

❏ Early symptoms of multiple sclerosis include slurred speech and diplopia.

❏ Paralysis is a late symptom of multiple sclerosis.

❏ Multiple sclerosis is exacerbated by exposure to stress, fatigue, and heat.

❏ Elevated gamma globulin fraction in cerebrospinal fluid without an elevated level in the blood occurs in multiple sclerosis.

❏ White blood cells or pus in cerebrospinal fluid indicates infection.

❏ Blood may be found in cerebrospinal fluid with trauma or subarachnoid hemorrhage.

❏ Increased glucose concentration in cerebrospinal fluid is a nonspecific finding indicating infection or subarachnoid hemorrhage.

❏ Nystagmus refers to jerking movements of the eye.

❏ Diplopia means double vision.

❏ Exophthalmos refers to bulging eyeballs, as seen in Graves disease.

❏ Oculogyric crisis involves deviation of the eyes.

❏ The priority during and after a seizure is to maintain a patent airway.

❏ Timing the seizure activity and noting the origin of motor dysfunction are important nursing interventions but are not the first priority.

❏ Nothing should be placed in the client's mouth during a seizure because teeth may be dislodged or the tongue pushed back, further obstructing the airway.

❏ An aura (such as a certain smell or a vision such as flashing lights) occurs in some clients as a warning before a seizure.

❏ Atonic seizure, or drop attack, refers to an abrupt loss of muscle tone.

❏ Postictal experience occurs after a seizure, during which the client may be confused, somnolent, and fatigued.

❏ Surgical excision of an epileptic focus is considered when seizures aren't controlled with anticonvulsant therapy.

❏ Incontinence may occur during or after a seizure.

❏ To reduce the risk of injury, the nurse should take an axillary temperature or use a metal thermometer when taking an oral temperature to prevent injury if a seizure occurs.

❏ Status epilepticus (seizures not responsive to usual therapies) occurs with the abrupt cessation of anticonvulsant drugs or ethanol intake.

❏ All clients with a head injury are treated as if a cervical spine injury is present until X-rays confirm their absence.

❑ The airway doesn't need to be opened if the client appears alert and not in respiratory distress.

❑ The head-tilt, chin-lift maneuver wouldn't be used until cervical spine injury is ruled out.

❑ Quadriplegia occurs as a result of cervical spine injuries.

❑ Aphasia refers to difficulty expressing or understanding spoken words.

❑ Hemiparesis describes weakness of one side of the body.

❑ Paraplegia occurs as a result of injury to the thoracic cord and below.

❑ A client with a C6 spinal injury would most likely have quadriplegia.

❑ The hippocampus, amygdala, and fornix make up the limbic system, which regulates emotions.

❑ The hippocampus and associated structures are important for short-term memory.

❑ Coordination is a function of the cerebellum.

❑ The midbrain, pons, medulla oblongata, and reticular formation regulate vital functions.

❑ Nursing care of a client with damage to the hippocampus, amygdala, and fornix should focus on frequent monitoring of vital signs.

❑ After a spinal cord injury, ascending cord edema may cause a higher level of injury.

❑ The diaphragm is innervated at the level of C4, so assessment of adequate oxygenation and ventilation is necessary.

❑ Other assessment parameters for the client with C5 fracture also include bladder distention, neurologic deficit, and the client's feelings about the injury.

❑ A 30-year-old client admitted with a C5 fracture from a motorcycle collision would require assessment of pulse oximetry readings as a priority.

❑ Symptoms of neurogenic shock include hypotension, bradycardia, and warm, dry skin.

❑ Symptoms of neurogenic shock are due to loss of adrenergic stimulation below the level of the lesion.

❑ Hemorrhagic shock is associated with an injury and presents with anxiety, tachycardia, and hypotension.

❑ Pulmonary embolism presents with chest pain, hypotension, hypoxemia, tachycardia, and hemoptysis.

❑ Pulmonary embolism may be a later complication of spinal cord injury due to immobility.

❑ Anxiety, flushing above the level of the lesion, piloerection, hypertension, bradycardia, flushing and sweating of the skin are symptoms of autonomic dysreflexia.

❑ Autonomic dysreflexia is typically caused by such noxious stimuli as a full bladder, fecal impaction, or pressure ulcer.

❑ Putting the client flat will cause the blood pressure to increase more in autonomic dysreflexia.

❑ The indwelling urinary catheter should be assessed immediately after the head of the bed is raised in the client with autonomic dysreflexia.

❑ The Minerva vest will provide significant immobilization, including lateral flexion.

❑ Most soft collars do not limit cervical motion but act as a reminder against excessive motion.

❑ More rigid devices such as the Philadelphia collar provide reasonable immobilization of the midcervical segments for flexion and extension, but not for lateral flexion.

❑ The wrench must be attached at all times to remove the halo vest in case the client needs cardiopulmonary resuscitation.

❑ The halo vest is designed to improve mobility; the client may use a wheelchair.

❑ Peroxide, especially when applied full-strength to halo vest pin sites, can disrupt the healing process and normal flora.

❑ The purpose of the halo vest is to immobilize the neck.

❑ Range-of-motion exercises to the neck are prohibited in the client with a halo vest but should be performed to other areas.

❑ Cauda equina syndrome occurs when there is compression on the nerve roots

❑ Cauda equina syndrome affects areas below the level of the compressed nerve roots.

❑ Cauda equina syndrome is an emergency that requires surgical intervention.

❑ If not treated, cauda equina syndrome may lead to permanent loss of bladder and bowel control and paralysis of the legs.

❑ Inserting a urinary drainage device, increasing the frequency of vital sign measurements, and administering anti-inflammatory medication are interventions that may be needed for the client with cauda equina syndrome.

❑ A client with intervertebral disk prolapse, showing new symptoms of loss of bladder control and paralysis of both legs requires the physician to be notified immediately.

❑ The bladder treatment program for a client in rehabilitation for spinal cord injury should begin early and should include intermittent catheterization every 2 to 4 hours.

❑ When residual volume is less than 400 mL, the catheterization schedule may advance to every 4 to 6 hours.

❑ Indwelling catheters may predispose the client with a spinal cord injury to infection and are removed as soon as possible.

❑ Credé's maneuver is applied after voiding to enhance bladder emptying.

❑ Symptoms of back pain and neurologic deficits may be symptoms of metastasis in a client with breast cancer.

❑ The physician should be notified if the client with breast cancer is experiencing back pain and neurologic deficits.

❑ Repositioning the client, encouraging physical therapy, or giving acetaminophen may help the client with back pain but may delay evaluation and treatment.

❑ Ménière disease results in dizziness, so the client should be protected from falling.

❑ Ménière disease doesn't alter cerebral tissue perfusion or directly affect nutrition.

❑ Ménière disease may cause hearing loss, leading to impaired social interaction.

❑ The client who has had a stapedectomy should be positioned on the unaffected side with the operative ear up.

❑ Tinnitus, dizziness, and vertigo occur in Ménière disease.

❑ Epistaxis may occur with a variety of blood dyscrasias or local lesions.

❑ Facial pain may occur with trigeminal neuralgia.

❑ Ptosis occurs with a variety of conditions, including myasthenia gravis.

❑ One or both eyes may be patched to prevent pain with extraocular movement or accommodation when the client has a foreign body protruding from the eye.

❑ Chemicals or small foreign bodies in the eye may be irrigated.

❑ Assessment of visual acuity isn't a priority in an emergency, although it may be done after treatment.

❑ Protruding objects in the eye aren't removed by the nurse because the vitreous body may rupture.

❑ Corneal damage may occur with the prolonged use of topical anesthetics.

❑ Hearing loss in an elderly client typically involves the upper ranges.

❑ Lowering the pitch of your voice and facing the client are essential to enable the client with hearing loss to use other means of understanding, such as lip reading, mood, and so on.

❑ An ear wick is used to allow medications to enter the ear canal.

❑ Shouting is typically in the upper ranges and could cause anxiety to an already anxious client with hearing impairment.

❑ Alternative means of communication such as writing may also be used to assess chest pain while waiting for the family to bring the hearing aid from home.

❑ The palpebral fissures are in the eye.

❑ After cataract surgery, there's no need to restrict sodium.

❑ Using makeup, bending, straining, lifting, vomiting, and sleeping on the affected side may increase intraocular pressure and put strain on the sutures after cataract surgery.

❑ The earliest symptom of increased intracranial pressure is a change in mental status.

❑ Bradycardia, widened pulse pressure, and bradypnea occur later with increased intracranial pressure.

❑ The client may void large amounts of very dilute urine if the posterior pituitary has been damaged.

❑ Epidural hematoma or extradural hematoma is usually caused by laceration of the middle meningeal artery.

❑ An embolic stroke is a thromboembolism from a carotid artery that ruptures.

❑ Venous bleeding from the arachnoid space is usually observed with subdural hematoma.

❑ Clear liquid from the nose (rhinorrhea) or ear (otorrhea) can be determined to be cerebrospinal fluid or mucus by the presence of glucose.

❑ Placing the client flat in bed may increase intracranial pressure and promote pulmonary aspiration.

❑ The nose shouldn't be suctioned if the client is suspected to be draining cerebrospinal fluid nasally because of the risk of suctioning brain tissue through the sinuses.

❑ Nothing is inserted into the ears or nose of a client with a skull fracture because of the risk of infection.

❑ A lucid interval is described as a brief period of unconsciousness followed by alertness; after several hours, the client again loses consciousness.

❑ Garbled speech is known as dysarthria.

❑ An interval in which the client is alert but can't recall recent events is known as amnesia.

❑ Warning symptoms or auras typically occur before seizures.

❑ When suctioning the trachea, suction should be applied for 10 to 15 seconds at a time.

❑ Suction is regulated to 80 to 120 cm $H_2O$ when suctioning the trachea.

❑ Suction should be applied only during withdrawal of the catheter from the trachea.

❑ When suctioning the trachea, the catheter is inserted 4" to 6" (10 to 15 cm) or until resistance is felt.

❑ Uncontrolled hypertension is the major cause of hemorrhagic stroke.

❑ Both diabetes and heart disease increase the probability of stroke by hastening atherosclerosis.

❑ Nutrition may be delivered by tube when dysphagia exists.

❑ Autonomic dysreflexia refers to uninhibited sympathetic outflow in clients with spinal cord injuries, most commonly above the level of T6.

❑ Clients with brain injury, herniated nucleus pulposus, or stroke aren't prone to dysreflexia.

❑ Spasticity, the return of reflexes, is a sign of resolving shock.

❑ Spinal or neurogenic shock is characterized by hypotension, bradycardia, dry skin, flaccid paralysis, and the absence of reflexes below the level of injury.

❑ The absence of pain sensation in the chest doesn't apply to spinal shock.

❑ Spinal shock descends from the injury, and respiratory difficulties occur at C4 and above.

❑ Slight muscle contraction at the bulbocavernosus reflex occurs in a client with C7 quadriplegia and spinal shock, but not enough for urinary continence to occur.

❑ Lifting more than 10 lb (4.5 kg) for several weeks after laminectomy surgery is contraindicated.

❑ Advise the client being discharged from the hospital after a laminectomy that he will need to sleep on a firm mattress.

❑ Progressive neurologic deficits at L4–L5, including worsening muscle weakness, paresthesia, and loss of bowel and bladder control, are symptoms of spinal cord compression.

❑ Lower back pain, pain radiating across the buttocks, and positive Kernig's sign usually occur in clients with herniated nucleus pulposus without spinal cord compression.

❑ Autonomic dysreflexia is most commonly seen with injuries at T6 or above.

❏ Putting the client in high Fowler's position will decrease cerebral blood flow, decreasing hypertension during an episode of autonomic dysreflexia.

❏ Elevating the client's legs, putting the client flat in bed, or putting the bed in Trendelenburg's position places the client in positions that improve cerebral blood flow, worsening hypertension in autonomic dysreflexia.

❏ Gardner-Wells tongs are used to reduce dislocations, subluxations, pain, and spasm in cervical spinal cord injuries.

❏ Gardner-Wells tongs aren't used to reduce intracranial pressure, prevent deep vein thrombosis, or improve neurologic outcome.

❏ Loss of sympathetic control and unopposed vagal stimulation below the level of the injury typically cause hypotension, bradycardia, pallor, flaccid paralysis, and warm, dry skin in the client in neurogenic shock.

❏ Hypervolemia is indicated by a rapid and bounding pulse and edema.

❏ Autonomic dysreflexia occurs after neurogenic shock abates.

❏ Signs of sepsis would include elevated temperature, increased heart rate, and increased respiratory rate.

❏ The diaphragm is stimulated by the phrenic nerve, which arises from C3, C4, and C5 nerve roots.

❏ Initially, a client with a cervical spine injury at the level of C5 may need mechanical ventilation due to cord edema, which may resolve in time.

❏ Absent corneal reflexes, decerebrate posturing, and hemiplegia occur with brain injuries rather than spinal cord injuries.

❏ Clients with quadriplegia have paralysis or weakness of the diaphragm, abdominal muscles, or intercostal muscles.

❏ In clients with quadriplegia, maintenance of airway and breathing take top priority.

❏ Hypertension, bradycardia, anxiety, blurred vision, and flushing above the lesion occur with autonomic dysreflexia due to uninhibited sympathetic nervous system discharge.

❏ Symptoms of a transient ischemic attack result from a transient lack of oxygen to the brain and usually resolve within 24 hours; the average time to resolution is less than 30 minutes.

❏ Hemorrhage into the brain has the worst neurologic outcome and isn't associated with a transient ischemic attack.

❏ Due to the weight of the flaccid extremity, the shoulder of a client with a stroke may disarticulate.

❏ A sling will support the flaccid extremity of a client with a stroke.

❑ Intermittent catheterization may be performed chronically with clean technique, using soap and water to clean the urinary meatus.

❑ The meatus is always cleaned from front to back in a woman, or in expanding circles working outward from the meatus in a man.

❑ It isn't necessary to measure the urine of a paraplegic client with intermittent catheterization.

❑ Accommodation refers to convergence and constriction of the pupil while following a near object.

❑ Touching the cornea lightly with a wisp of cotton describes assessment of the corneal reflex.

❑ Having the client follow an object upward, downward, obliquely, and horizontally tests the cardinal fields of gaze.

❑ Night blindness (nyctalopia) may be caused by a vitamin A deficiency or dysfunctional rod receptors.

❑ When using a Snellen alphabet chart, describing a client's visual acuity as 20/40 indicates that the client can see at 20 feet what the person with normal vision sees at 40 feet.

❑ Legal blindness refers to visual acuity of 20/150 or less.

❑ Alterations in near vision may be due to loss of accommodation caused by the aging process (presbyopia) or farsightedness.

❑ A tonometer is a device used in glaucoma screening to record intraocular pressure.

❑ An ophthalmoscope examines the interior of the eye, especially the retina.

❑ A slit lamp evaluates structures in the anterior chamber of the eye.

❑ Driving may be contraindicated after instillation of atropine eyedrops due to blurred vision.

❑ Maintaining nothing-by-mouth status for at least 8 hours before surgical procedures to the eye prevents vomiting and aspiration.

❑ There's no need to patch an eye before most surgeries or to clip the eyelashes unless specifically ordered by the physician.

❑ The physician is responsible for obtaining informed consent for eye surgery; the nurse validates that the consent is obtained.

❑ Lifting, usually involving the Valsalva maneuver, increases intraocular pressure and strain on the surgical site after cataract surgery.

❑ Preventing nausea and subsequent vomiting will prevent increased intraocular pressure, as will avoiding bending or placing the head in a dependent position.

❑ Aphakia means "without lens."

❑ A keyhole pupil results from iridectomy.

❑ Loss of accommodation is a normal response to aging.

❑ A retinal detachment is usually associated with retinal holes created by vitreous traction.

❑ Open-angle glaucoma causes a painless increase in intraocular pressure with loss of peripheral vision.

❑ Individuals older than age 40 should be screened for glaucoma.

❑ Signs and symptoms of retinal detachment include abrupt flashing lights, floaters, loss of peripheral vision, and a sudden shadow or curtain in the vision.

❑ If any part of the retina is lifted or pulled from its normal position, it is considered detached and will cause some vision loss.

❑ Enucleation of the eye refers to surgical removal of the entire eye; therefore, the client needs instructions about the prosthesis.

❑ There are no activity restrictions or need for eyedrops with enucleation surgery.

❑ Irrigation of the ear canal is contraindicated with perforation of the tympanic membrane.

❑ Irrigation solution entering the inner ear may cause dizziness, nausea, vomiting, and infection.

❑ Ear pain, hearing loss, and otitis externa aren't contraindications to irrigation of the ear canal.

❑ The ear drops may be warmed to prevent pain or dizziness, but this action isn't essential.

❑ The client should be placed in the lateral position, not semi-Fowler's position, to prevent the ear drops from draining out for 5 minutes.

❑ The client with Ménière disease shouldn't drive because he may reflexively turn the wheel to correct for vertigo.

❑ Changes in level of consciousness may indicate expanding lesions such as subdural hematoma.

❑ Orientation and level of consciousness are assessed frequently for 24 hours after a head injury.

❑ Profuse or projectile vomiting is a symptom of increased intracranial pressure and should be reported immediately.

❑ A slight headache may last for several days after concussion; severe or worsening headaches should be reported.

❑ Motor movement is regulated by the basal ganglia.

❑ The basal ganglia consists of the caudate nucleus, putamen, and globus pallidus.

❑ Several cranial nerves are responsible for various forms of eye movement.

❑ Modulation of sounds occurs from the occipital lobe.

❑ The cerebellum regulates muscle synergy.

❑ Damage to the thalamus may result in thalamic syndrome.

❑ Thalamic syndrome is characterized by pain, burning, or an aching sensation over one half of the body.

❑ Thalamic syndrome is often accompanied by mood swings.

❑ Problems initiating movement are associated with the basal ganglia and memory problems with the hippocampus.

❑ When communicating with a client with second-stage Alzheimer disease, listening and deciphering word substitutions are the most helpful, because the client may have difficulty expressing thoughts.

❑ Sentences should be repeated as often as needed with second-stage Alzheimer disease clients.

❑ In questioning the client with second-stage Alzheimer disease, yes-or-no and multiple choice questions are very helpful.

❑ Sentences should be short and literal for clients with second-stage Alzheimer disease, following the subject-verb-object format.

❑ The parietal lobe regulates sensory function, which would include the ability to sense hot or cold objects.

❑ The frontal lobe regulates thinking, planning, and judgment.

❑ The occipital lobe is primarily responsible for vision function.

❑ The temporal lobe regulates memory.

❑ Cranial nerve III, the oculomotor nerve, controls pupil constriction.

❑ Cranial nerve II, the optic nerve, controls vision.

❑ Cranial nerve IV, the trochlear nerve, coordinates eye movement.

❑ Cranial nerve V, the trigeminal nerve, innervates the muscles of chewing.

❑ An EEG measures the electrical activity of the brain.

❑ The extent of intracranial bleeding and location of the injury are determined by computed tomography or magnetic resonance imaging.

❑ The percentage of functional brain tissue is determined by a series of tests.

❑ The eating problems associated with Parkinson disease include dysphagia, risk of choking, drooling, aspiration, and constipation.

❑ In plasmapheresis, antibodies are removed from the client's plasma.

❑ In some clients with multiple sclerosis, plasmapheresis diminishes symptoms.

❏ To assess the motor function of cranial nerve VII, the nurse should ask the client to frown, smile, and raise his eyebrows.

❏ If facial expressions are symmetrical, motor function is intact.

❏ Jaw clenching is a test for cranial nerve V function.

❏ Testing the gag reflex by placing an applicator against the pharynx and assessing swallowing ability are ways to evaluate cranial nerve IX function.

❏ Testing the gag reflex also helps assess cranial nerve X function.

❏ Ineffective airway clearance related to the inability to expectorate takes priority in an unconscious client.

❏ In an unconscious client, airway, breathing, and circulation are the priority over other client needs.

❏ In the client with increasing intracranial pressure (ICP), the nurse should first attempt repositioning the client to avoid neck flexion, which increases venous return and lowers ICP.

❏ An epidural hematoma occurs when blood collects between the skull and dura mater.

❏ In a subdural hematoma, venous blood collects between the dura mater and arachnoid mater.

❏ In a subarachnoid hemorrhage, blood collects between the pia mater and arachnoid membrane.

❏ A contusion is a bruise on the brain's surface.

❏ A client with a spinal cord injury at levels from C5 to C6 has quadriplegia with gross arm movement and diaphragmatic breathing.

❏ Injuries at levels between C1 and C4 lead to quadriplegia with total loss of respiratory function.

❏ Paraplegia with intercostal muscle loss occurs with injuries at levels between T1 and L2.

❏ Injuries below L2 cause paraplegia and loss of bowel and bladder control.

❏ If the client has a suspected cervical spine injury, the jaw-thrust maneuver should be used to open the airway.

❏ If the tongue or relaxed throat muscles are obstructing the airway, a nasopharyngeal or oropharyngeal airway can be inserted.

❏ The head-tilt, chin-lift maneuver requires neck hyperextension, which can worsen a cervical spine injury.

❏ Expressive (Broca's) aphasia results from damage to Broca's area, located in the frontal lobe of the brain's dominant hemisphere.

❏ Typically, the client with expressive aphasia has difficulty expressing himself and his speech is slow, nonfluent, and labored.

❑ Comprehension of written and verbal communication is intact in the client with expressive aphasia.

❑ With receptive (Wernicke's) aphasia (which results from injury to Wernicke's area), the client can't comprehend written or verbal communication.

❑ With receptive (Wernicke's) aphasia the client's speech is normal but he conveys information poorly.

❑ The Wernicke's area is located in the temporal lobe of the dominant hemisphere.

❑ With global aphasia most of the brain's communication system is damaged.

❑ Global aphasia results from extensive damage to Broca's and Wernicke's areas.

❑ Global aphasia is a combination of receptive and expressive aphasia.

❑ Vertigo is the most frequent complication of stapedectomy.

❑ After stapedectomy, the client should move slowly to avoid triggering or worsening vertigo and should ask for assistance with ambulation.

❑ Ringing in the ears (tinnitus) rarely follows stapedectomy and should be reported to the physician.

❑ Hearing typically decreases after stapedectomy because of ear packing and tissue swelling, but commonly returns over the next 2 to 6 weeks.

❑ Usually, postoperative drainage and pain are minimal with stapedectomy; excessive drainage should be reported.

❑ Risk for injury related to peripheral vision loss takes priority because open-angle glaucoma limits peripheral vision.

❑ The client with open-angle glaucoma risks injury from stumbling over peripheral objects that he can't see.

❑ Angle-closure glaucoma—not open-angle glaucoma—commonly causes acute pain.

❑ Primary open-angle glaucoma is an incurable disease that requires life-long treatment.

❑ Adverse effects of medications to treat open-angle glaucoma are common.

❑ To test for Babinski's reflex, use a tongue blade to slowly stroke the lateral side of the underside of the foot.

❑ When testing for Babinski's reflex start at the heel and move toward the great toe.

❑ The normal Babinski's reflex response in an adult is plantar flexion of the toes.

❑ Upward movement of the great toe and fanning of the little toes, called the Babinski reflex, is abnormal.

❑ To test the biceps reflex, the client's elbow is flexed at a 45-degree angle.

❑ To test the biceps reflex, place your thumb or index finger over the biceps tendon and strike the digit with the pointed end of the reflex hammer, watching and feeling for the contraction of the biceps muscle and flexion of the forearm.

## Musculoskeletal system

❑ The primary complication of osteoporosis is fractures.

❑ With osteoporosis, bones soften, and there's a decrease in bone matrix and remineralization.

❑ Relieving pain and making the client more comfortable should have the highest priority in care of the client with osteoporosis.

❑ Hormonal imbalance, faulty metabolism, and poor dietary intake of calcium cause primary osteoporosis.

❑ Alcoholism, malnutrition, osteogenesis imperfecta, rheumatoid arthritis, liver disease, scurvy, lactose intolerance, hyperthyroidism, and trauma cause secondary osteoporosis.

❑ Menopause at any age puts women at risk for osteoporosis because of the associated hormonal imbalance.

❑ With her ovaries removed, the client with osteoporosis is no longer producing hormones.

❑ Primary prevention of osteoporosis includes maintaining optimal calcium intake.

❑ Placing items within reach of the client, using a professional alert system in the home, and installing bars in bathrooms are all secondary and tertiary prevention methods to prevent falls.

❑ Nursing actions appropriate in the care of the client with acute gout include forcing fluids, instructing the client on relaxation techniques, and encouraging bed rest.

❑ The usual pattern of gout involves painful attacks with pain-free periods.

❑ Chronic gout may lead to frequent attacks with persistently painful joints.

❑ Bananas and dried fruits are high in potassium.

❑ Milk, ice cream, and yogurt are rich in calcium.

❑ Wine, cheese, preserved fruits, meats, and vegetables contain tyramine.

❑ Weight loss will decrease uric acid levels and decrease stress on joints.

❑ X-rays are normal in the early stages of gout and can be valuable in the diagnosis of gout.

❑ Fluids promote the excretion of uric acid.

❑ The most common symptom of osteoarthritis is joint pain after exercise or weight-bearing, usually relieved by rest.

❑ Symmetrical swelling of the joints of both hands, morning stiffness lasting longer than 30 minutes, and fever are all symptoms of rheumatoid arthritis.

❑ Osteoarthritis is the most common form of arthritis and can be extremely debilitating.

❑ Osteoarthritis can afflict people of any age, although most clients with osteoarthritis are elderly.

❑ Primary osteoarthritis may be caused by the overuse of joints, aging, or obesity.

❑ Congenital abnormalities and diabetes mellitus can cause secondary osteoarthritis.

❑ A client with osteoarthritis has joint stiffness that may be partially relieved by a warm shower on arising in the morning.

❑ Splints are usually used by clients with rheumatoid arthritis.

❑ Because the problem with osteoarthritis is continued stress on the joint, the client may want to try an exercise that puts less strain on the joint, such as swimming.

❑ Many elderly people already have diminished hearing, and salicylate use can lead to further or total hearing loss.

❑ A bedridden client with osteoarthritis needs to be turned every 2 hours, provided adequate nutrition, and encouraged to cough and deep breathe.

❑ Hydration, active and passive range-of-motion exercises, and adequate pain medication are also appropriate nursing measures for the client with osteoarthritis.

❑ To prevent contractures, the client with osteoarthritis should increase his fluid intake and move around as much as possible.

❑ Clients have dislocations and subluxations in both osteoarthritis and rheumatoid arthritis.

❑ Asymmetrical joint involvement is present in osteoarthritis.

❑ Elevated sedimentation rate is present in rheumatoid arthritis.

❑ Multiple subcutaneous nodules, as well as such signs and symptoms of inflammation as heat, fever, and malaise, are present in rheumatoid arthritis.

❑ Primary prevention of injury from osteoarthritis includes warming up before exercise and avoiding repetitive tasks.

❑ Osteoarthritis is a noninflammatory joint disease, with degeneration and loss of articular cartilage in synovial joints.

❑ Rheumatoid arthritis is a systemic inflammatory joint disease.

❑ Arthrodesis is fusion of the joints.

❑ The nurse's goal for the client with osteoarthritis should be to allow him to maintain his self-care abilities with help as needed but not to perform the care for him.

❑ In the late stages of osteoarthritis, the client often describes joint pain as grating.

❑ As osteoarthritis progresses, the cartilage covering the ends of bones is destroyed and bones rub against each other.

❑ Osteophytes, or bone spurs, may also form on the ends of bones in osteoarthritis.

❑ A dull ache and deep aching pain with or without relief with rest is often seen in the earlier stages of osteoarthritis.

❑ A client with osteoarthritis should be encouraged to ambulate with a cane, walker, or other assistive device as needed.

❑ The use of assistive devices takes weight and stress off of joints.

❑ A client with osteoarthritis should pace his activities and avoid overexertion.

❑ The client with osteoarthritis shouldn't become sedentary because this will increase his risk of pneumonia and contractures.

❑ With a herniated nucleus pulposus, or herniated disk, the nucleus of the disk puts pressure on the annulus, causing pressure on the nerve root.

❑ Compression of nerves by the herniated nucleus pulposus causes back pain that radiates into the leg, with numbness and weakness of the leg.

❑ Parkinson disease is characterized by progressive muscle rigidity and tremors.

❑ Osteoarthritis causes deep, aching joint pain.

❑ Conservative treatment of a herniated nucleus pulposus may include bed rest, pain medication, and physiotherapy.

❑ Aggressive treatment for herniated nucleus pulposus may include surgery such as a bone fusion.

❑ Closed spine surgery uses endoscopy to fix a herniated disk.

❑ Closed spine surgery is less risky than open surgery and has a shorter recovery time.

❑ Physical therapy may be less intensive or not needed at all in closed spine surgery.

❑ The client should bend at the knees, not the waist, to maintain proper body mechanics.

❑ Pelvic tilt exercises are recommended to strengthen back muscles.

❑ Increasing fiber and fluid intake helps soften stool, thereby preventing straining, which increases intraspinal pressure.

❑ Any extra weight carried by the client increases back strain.

❑ Application of a cold pack to a sprained ankle causes the blood vessels to constrict, which reduces the leakage of fluid into the tissues and prevents swelling.

❑ Application of a cold pack may have an effect on muscle spasms.

❑ Cold therapy may reduce pain by numbing the nerves and tissues.

❑ The most common areas of herniation are L4–L5 and L5–S1.

❑ Tests used to diagnose a herniated nucleus pulposus include myelography, magnetic resonance imaging, and computed tomography scan.

❑ Sleeping on the side and carrying objects close to the body produce less strain on the back.

❑ Tell the client to change position slowly to avoid dizziness when taking skeletal muscle relaxants.

❑ With compartment syndrome, the client can't perform active movement, and pain occurs with passive movement.

❑ Osteoporosis brings a bodywide decrease in bone mass.

❑ Severe pain, numbness, and tingling are symptoms of impaired circulation due to compartment syndrome.

❑ Compartment syndrome is a medical emergency.

❑ In compartment syndrome, lowering the affected arm below the level of the heart and applying heat will decrease venous outflow and impair the circulation even more.

❑ The hemorrhage in compartment syndrome causes edema, increased venous pressure, and decreased venous and arterial circulation.

❑ After development of compartment syndrome, there is an increase in pressure within the affected compartment that compromises circulation to the muscle tissue and to nerves.

❑ Compartment syndrome may lead to the death of tissues within 2 to 4 hours.

❑ Treatment of compartment syndrome includes fasciotomy.

❑ Fasciotomy involves cutting the fascia over the affected area to permit muscle expansion.

❑ The purpose of the brace for a fracture is to act as a splint, maintain immobility, and prevent direct contact.

❑ Paresthesia is described as numbness and tingling.

❑ Initial treatment of obvious and suspected fractures includes immobilizing and splinting the limb.

❏ Any attempt to realign or rest the fracture at the stem may cause further injury and complications.

❏ The fractured leg may be elevated only after immobilization.

❏ Paresthesia is the earliest sign of compartment syndrome.

❏ Pain, heat, and swelling are also signs of compartment syndrome but occur after paresthesia.

❏ Signs of a fracture may include redness, warmth, numbness or loss of sensation, and a new site of pain.

❏ A correct neurovascular assessment should include examination for capillary refill, movement, pulses, and warmth.

❏ The correct method for measuring calf circumference is to place a measuring tape at the level where the calf circumference is largest; measure at the same place each time.

❏ If pulses aren't palpable, verify the assessment with Doppler ultrasonography.

❏ If pulses can't be found with Doppler ultrasonography, immediately notify the physician.

❏ A foul odor from a cast may be a sign of infection.

❏ The nurse needs to assess for infection, which can include fever, malaise and, possibly, an elevation in white blood cells.

❏ Signs of neurovascular compromise include decreased pulses, coolness, and paresthesia.

❏ To reduce the roughness of the cast, petal the edges.

❏ Elevating the limb will prevent swelling.

❏ Distributing pressure evenly will prevent pressure ulcers on a casted extremity.

❏ To reduce swelling, place the limb with the cast above the level of the heart.

❏ A plaster cast that becomes wet will weaken or be destroyed.

❏ Fiberglass casts do not lose integrity or strength when wet or damp.

❏ Fracture pain is sharp and is related to movement.

❏ A client who complains of severe leg pain in skeletal traction may need realignment to ease some pressure on the fracture site.

❏ If realignment of the client in skeletal traction is ineffective, then the physician may need to be notified.

❏ The weights ordered in skeletal traction may be too heavy, but the nurse can't remove them without a physician's order.

❏ Russell's traction must not be disturbed, to maintain correct alignment.

❑ The client can have back care as long as he uses the trapeze and doesn't disturb the alignment of Russell's traction.

❑ The weight shouldn't be moved without a physician's order with Russell's traction.

❑ Weights of Russell's traction should hang freely without touching anything.

❑ Classic fractures that occur with trauma are those of the humerus and clavicle.

❑ A transverse fracture commonly occurs with such bone diseases as osteomalacia and Paget disease.

❑ Linear, longitudinal, and oblique fractures generally occur with trauma.

❑ Spiral fractures are commonly seen in the upper extremities and are related to physical abuse.

❑ Longitudinal and oblique fractures generally occur with trauma.

❑ Neurovascular checks are most important because they're used to determine if any impairment exists after cast application and reduction of the fracture.

❑ Femoral shaft fractures may cause hemorrhage, with as much as 1,000 to 1,500 mL of blood loss.

❑ A serious complication of long-bone fractures is the development of fat emboli, in which the fat molecules enter the venous circulation and travel to the lung, obstructing pulmonary circulation.

❑ Bone or platelet emboli are rare occurrences and are infrequently associated with long-bone fractures.

❑ Signs and symptoms of fat emboli include tachypnea, tachycardia, shortness of breath, and a petechial rash on the chest and neck.

❑ High-protein intake promotes cell growth and bone union.

❑ In Buck's traction, the weights should hang freely without touching the bed or floor.

❑ Lifting the weights would break the traction.

❑ The client should be moved up in bed, allowing the weight to move freely along with the client.

❑ The leg should be kept in straight alignment with traction.

❑ Performing ankle rotation exercises could cause the leg to go out of alignment when using traction.

❑ The client with a right total hip replacement should be turned at least every 2 hours and always from the unaffected side to the back.

❑ The client with a total hip replacement should never be placed on the affected side.

❑ Turning the client every 4 to 6 hours places her at greater risk for skin breakdown.

❑ Vitamin D increases the absorption and use of calcium and phosphorus.

❑ After surgical repair of the hip, the legs and hips should be placed in abduction.

❑ Adduction, prone, or subluxated positions don't keep the prosthesis within the acetabulum.

❑ After a hip replacement, the client's activity is usually ordered as limited weight bearing.

❑ The client is allowed to move with restrictions for approximately 2 to 3 months after a hip replacement.

❑ The hip shouldn't be flexed more than 90 degrees after a hip replacement.

❑ Abduction past the midline of the body is prohibited after a hip replacement.

❑ Progressive weight bearing reduces the complications of immobility after a hip replacement.

❑ To prevent deep vein thrombosis after hip surgery, subcutaneous heparin and pneumatic compression boots are used.

❑ Discharge instructions for a client after surgery for repair of a hip fracture should include not crossing the legs and getting help to put on shoes.

❑ Restrictions, such as not flexing the hip more than 90 degrees, prevent dislocation of the new prosthesis in a client after surgery for repair of a hip fracture.

❑ To avoid damage to the brachial plexus nerves in the axilla, the palms of the hands should bear the client's weight on crutches.

❑ Minimal weight should be placed on the affected leg when using crutches.

❑ Unilateral leg pain and edema with a positive Homans' sign (not always present) might be symptoms of deep vein thrombosis.

❑ Symptoms of fat emboli include restlessness, tachypnea, and tachycardia and are more common in long-bone injuries.

❑ Tachycardia, chest pain, and shortness of breath may be symptoms of a pulmonary embolism.

❑ For a client in traction, give range-of-motion exercises every shift to all joints, except those immediately proximal and distal to the fracture.

❑ After helping the physician apply a cast, support it with the palms of the hands; don't rest the cast on a hard or sharp surface.

❑ Normally, as the cast dries, a client may complain of heat from the cast.

❑ To prevent foot drop in a leg with a cast, the foot should be supported with 90 degrees of flexion.

❑ A client with a hip-spica cast should avoid gas-forming foods to prevent abdominal distention.

❏ After cast removal, the dry, peeling skin will heal in a few days with normal cleaning; therefore, lotions are unnecessary.

❏ Touchdown weight bearing involves no weight on the extremity, but the client may touch the floor with the affected extremity.

❏ Full weight bearing allows for full weight to be put on the affected extremity.

❏ Partial weight bearing allows for 30% to 50% weight bearing on the affected extremity.

❏ Non-weight bearing is no weight on the extremity.

❏ Pacing activity, building strength, and using moderate intensity are prevention measures to avoid injury.

❏ The operative leg must be kept abducted to prevent dislocation of the hip after internal fixation of a left femoral neck fracture.

❏ Acute flexion of the operated hip may cause dislocation.

❏ The head of the bed may be raised 35 to 49 degrees after undergoing internal fixation of a left femoral neck fracture.

❏ Muscle spasms in the left thigh are a neuromuscular response of the local muscle around the femoral fracture.

❏ Open reduction means that the tissue must be surgically opened and the fractured bones realigned.

❏ To maintain proper alignment, a screw, plate, nail, or wire is inserted to prevent the bones from separating.

❏ Although traction may have been used before surgery, it won't be needed any longer once the fracture is reduced.

❏ A cast or crutches may be used after open reduction surgery of a fractured femur.

❏ A dislocated hip will create problems with walking, and pain is often due to a pinched nerve in the joint.

❏ The leg is usually adducted and shortened with a dislocated hip.

❏ Bone has very poor blood circulation, making it difficult to treat an infection in the bone.

❏ Degenerative joint disease is due to noninflammatory wear and tear on joints and is often seen in athletes.

❏ The kidney excretes uric acid, an end product of metabolism.

❏ Hyperbaric oxygen therapy has been used to treat refractory osteomyelitis.

❏ High-protein intake promotes cell growth and bone union.

❏ Cold causes the blood vessels to constrict, which reduces the leakage of fluid into the tissues and prevents swelling and muscle spasms.

❑ Heat therapy promotes circulation, enhances flexibility, reduces muscle spasms, and also provides analgesia.

❑ Fever, foul odor, and warmth over a specific area of the cast after it is dry may be signs of infection.

❑ The casted extremity should be elevated for 24 to 48 hours.

❑ Because people with diabetes commonly have microvascular compromise and delayed wound healing, clients who are in traction need careful monitoring for early signs of skin breakdown due to risk for traction-related complications.

❑ Acute wrist flexion places pressure on the inflamed median nerve, causing the pain and numbness of carpal tunnel syndrome (Phalen's sign).

❑ Tapping gently over the median nerve tests for Tinel's sign, another sign of carpal tunnel syndrome.

❑ Placing the wrists in extension against resistance tests strength.

❑ Callus formation is a normal stage of bone repair.

❑ Callus formation is characterized by an overgrowth of bone that's reabsorbed gradually during the remodeling stage.

❑ Misalignment and malunion typically cause pain.

❑ Swelling and bruising should not be present 6 weeks after a fracture.

❑ Phantom limb pain is common after limb amputation and may be more severe with traumatic injury.

❑ If the limb was severed traumatically rather than removed because of poor circulation, peripheral circulation should be adequate.

❑ The risk of shock is relatively low on the fourth postoperative day after an amputation.

❑ Tender, painful, stiff joints characterize acute rheumatoid arthritis.

❑ Osteoarthritis signs can include flexion and deviation deformities, such as radial deviation of the distal phalanges.

❑ Nodules on the proximal interphalangeal joints in osteoarthritis are called Bouchard nodes.

❑ Dark green, leafy vegetables are the best nondairy sources of calcium.

❑ Bananas and avocados are good sources of vitamin K.

❑ Beef liver and broccoli supply iron.

❑ Lack of sunlight exposure decreases absorption of vitamin D, which must be present for calcium to be absorbed from the small intestine.

❑ Immobility results in a loss of bone density.

❑ The best time to teach about postoperative care is preoperatively.

❑ Straight-leg raising and quadriceps-setting exercises help maintain the strength of the affected extremity in a client with a torn meniscus.

❑ The physician, not the nurse, should explain the surgical procedure.

❑ Weight bearing may begin as soon as the day of surgery in a client with a torn meniscus.

❑ Mild to moderate pain is normal after arthroscopic knee surgery and can be relieved by oral narcotic analgesics.

❑ To minimize swelling after arthroscopic knee surgery, the client should ice and elevate the extremity for at least 24 hours after surgery.

❑ Swelling and coolness of the joint and limb may indicate complications from tourniquet use during arthroscopic knee surgery.

❑ Adequate calcium and vitamin D intake are an important part of an overall prevention program in osteoporosis.

❑ Studies show that estrogen in hormone replacement therapy may influence the development of breast and uterine cancers.

❑ For a client diagnosed with Ewing sarcoma, a bone scan is most useful in determining the extent of metastasis.

❑ In chronic rheumatoid arthritis, the fingers may show hyperextension of the proximal interphalangeal joints with fixed flexion of the distal interphalangeal joints, referred to as swan neck deformities.

❑ Flattened thenar eminence characterizes thenar atrophy, a condition which suggests an ulnar nerve disorder.

❑ The first sign of a Dupuytren contracture is a thickened plaque overlying the flexor tendon of the ring finger and possibly the little finger at the level of the distal palmar crease.

❑ Ganglia are cystic, round, usually nontender swellings located along tendon sheaths or joint capsules and frequently involve the dorsum of the wrist.

❑ Gibbus deformity is an angular deformity of collapsed vertebra and is frequently caused by metastatic cancer or tuberculosis of the spine.

❑ A rounded thoracic convexity, kyphosis, is common in aging, especially in women.

❑ Gentle curves of the normal spine include concavities in the cervical and lumbar regions and a convexity of the thorax.

❑ An accentuation of the normal lumbar curve, called lordosis, frequently develops to compensate for the protuberant abdomen of pregnancy or marked obesity.

❑ Serous drainage around the pin insertion site is a normal finding.

❑ A pale extremity may indicate arterial compromise for the client in skeletal traction.

❑ Erythema and swelling signal infection for the client in skeletal traction.

❑ Severe muscle spasms may indicate improper alignment of the body or traction.

❑ The client with diabetes mellitus has a significant risk of osteomyelitis secondary to the skeletal pin due to impaired wound healing.

❑ Relaxation and imagery are effective adjuncts to pharmacologic pain management that the nurse can implement without a physician's order.

❑ Heberden nodes appear on the distal interphalangeal joints.

❑ Heberden nodes are bony and cartilaginous enlargements that are usually hard and painless and typically occur in middle-aged and elderly clients with osteoarthritis.

❑ Clients with gout should avoid foods that are high in purines, such as liver, cod, and sardines.

❑ Clients with gout should avoid anchovies, sweetbreads, lentils, and alcoholic beverages, especially beer and wine.

❑ In a hip fracture, the affected leg is shorter, adducted, and externally rotated.

## Gastrointestinal system

❑ A hiatal hernia is caused by weakness of the diaphragmatic muscle and increased intra-abdominal—not intrathoracic—pressure.

❑ This weakness in the diaphragmatic muscle allows the stomach to slide into the esophagus.

❑ The esophageal supports weaken, but esophageal muscle weakness or increased esophageal muscle pressure isn't a factor in hiatal hernia.

❑ Obesity may cause increased abdominal pressure that pushes the lower portion of the stomach into the thorax.

❑ A volvulus is a type of intestinal obstruction.

❑ Esophageal reflux is a common symptom of hiatal hernia.

❑ Esophageal reflux seems to be associated with chronic exposure of the lower esophageal sphincter to the lower pressure of the thorax, making the sphincter less effective.

❑ Abdominal cramping can be caused by intestinal infection.

❑ A barium swallow with fluoroscopy shows the position of the stomach in relation to the diaphragm.

❑ A colonoscopy and a lower GI series show disorders of the intestine.

❑ An abdominal X-ray series will show structural defects but not necessarily a hiatal hernia, unless it's sliding or rolling at the time of the X-ray.

❑ The client with right lower quadrant pain, anorexia, nausea, low-grade fever, and elevated white blood cell count is experiencing appendicitis.

❑ A fecalith is a fecal calculus, or stone, that occludes the lumen of the appendix and is the most common cause of appendicitis.

❑ Bowel wall swelling, kinking of the appendix, and external occlusion of the bowel by adhesions can also be causes of appendicitis.

❑ The pain with appendicitis begins in the epigastrium or periumbilical region, then shifts to the right lower quadrant and becomes steady.

❑ The pain in appendicitis may be moderate to severe.

❑ Lying still with the legs drawn up toward the chest helps relieve tension on the abdominal muscles, which helps to reduce the amount of discomfort felt in appendicitis.

❑ Lying flat or sitting may increase the amount of pain experienced in appendicitis.

❑ The focus of care for the client with appendicitis is to assess for peritonitis.

❑ Peritonitis is an inflammation of the peritoneal cavity.

❑ Peritonitis is most commonly caused by appendix rupture and invasion of bacteria, which could be lethal.

❑ In the acute phase of appendicitis, management should focus on minimizing preoperative complications and recognizing when they may be occurring.

❑ Gastritis is an inflammation of the gastric mucosa that may be acute, often resulting from exposure to local irritants.

❑ Gastritis may be chronic, associated with autoimmune infections or atrophic disorders of the stomach.

❑ Inflammation of a diverticulum is called diverticulitis.

❑ Reflux of stomach acid is known as gastroesophageal reflux disease.

❑ Esophageal reflux is a common symptom of hiatal hernia. The client who has had a gastric resection should be monitored closely for signs and symptoms of hemorrhage.

❑ Signs of gastric hemorrhage may include bright red blood in the nasogastric tube suction, tachycardia, or a drop in blood pressure.

❑ Bowel sounds may not return for up to 72 hours postoperatively after a gastric resection.

❑ Reducing the amount of stress and reducing or eliminating oral intake until the symptoms of gastritis are gone are important in the recovery phase.

❏ A gastric resection is only an option when serious erosion has occurred.

❏ *Helicobacter pylori* infection can lead to chronic atrophic gastritis.

❏ Chronic gastritis can occur at any age but is more common in older adults and may be caused by conditions that allow reflux of bile acids into the stomach.

❏ With gastritis, the stomach lining becomes thin and atrophic, decreasing stomach acid secretion.

❏ Stomach acid secretion is the source of intrinsic factor.

❏ Decreased intrinsic factor causes a reduction in the absorption of vitamin $B_{12}$, leading to pernicious anemia.

❏ Inability to absorb vitamin $B_{12}$ associates chronic gastritis with pernicious anemia.

❏ As clients age, the incidence of diverticulosis increases.

❏ Almost two-thirds of the population is diagnosed with diverticulosis by age 85.

❏ Low-fiber diets have been implicated in the development of diverticula.

❏ Low-fiber diets decrease the bulk in the stool and predispose the person to the development of constipation.

❏ Undigested food can block a diverticulum, decreasing blood supply to the area and predisposing the area to bacterial invasion.

❏ Chronic laxative use is a common problem in elderly clients, but it doesn't cause diverticulitis.

❏ Herniation of the intestinal mucosa causes an intestinal perforation.

❏ Change in bowel habits, anorexia, low-grade fever, and episodic, dull or steady midabdominal pain are signs and symptoms of diverticulitis.

❏ A barium enema will cause diverticula to fill with barium and be easily seen on an X-ray.

❏ An abdominal ultrasound can tell more about other structures, such as the gallbladder, liver, and spleen, than the intestine.

❏ A barium swallow and gastroscopy view upper GI structures.

❏ Antibiotics are used to reduce the inflammation with acute diverticulitis.

❏ Parenteral fluids are given until the client with acute diverticulitis feels better; then it's recommended that the client drink eight 8-oz glasses of water per day and gradually increase fiber in the diet to improve intestinal motility.

❏ During the acute phase, activities that increase intra-abdominal pressure in the client with acute diverticulitis should be avoided to decrease pain and the chance of intestinal obstruction.

❏ Crohn disease commonly involves any segment of the small intestine, the colon, or both, and affects the entire thickness of the bowel.

❏ Crohn disease can affect the digestive system anywhere from the mouth to the anus.

❏ Ulcerative colitis can affect the entire length of the large colon through the layers of mucosa and submucosa.

❏ Studies have shown that the terminal ileum is the most common site for recurrence in clients with Crohn disease.

❏ The ascending colon, descending colon, and sigmoid colon may be involved in Crohn disease, but aren't as common as the terminal ileum.

❏ Although the definitive cause of Crohn disease is unknown, it's thought that Crohn disease is associated with infectious, immune, or psychological factors.

❏ Because Crohn disease has a higher incidence in siblings, it may have a genetic cause.

❏ Several theories exist regarding the cause of ulcerative colitis.

❏ One theory of ulcerative colitis suggests that it is caused by an altered immune system, based on the extraintestinal characteristics of the disease, such as peripheral arthritis and cholangitis.

❏ As the disease progresses, the lesions of Crohn disease become transmural; that is, they involve all thicknesses of the bowel.

❏ The lesions of Crohn disease may perforate the bowel wall, forming fistulas with adjacent structures.

❏ Fistulas don't develop in diverticulitis or diverticulosis.

❏ The ulcers in the submucosal and mucosal layers of the intestine in ulcerative colitis usually don't progress to fistula formation, as in Crohn disease.

❏ Signs and symptoms of dehydration that can occur with excessive diarrhea include poor skin turgor, increased heart rate, concentrated urine, and decreased blood pressure.

❏ Other signs of dehydration are dry skin and mouth, sunken eyes, and lethargy.

❏ Toxic megacolon is extreme dilation of a segment of the diseased colon caused by paralysis of the colon, resulting in complete obstruction.

❏ Toxic megacolon is associated with both Crohn disease and ulcerative colitis.

❏ Gallstones, hydronephrosis, and nephrolithiasis are commonly associated with Crohn disease.

❏ Because of the transmural nature of Crohn disease lesions, malabsorption may occur with Crohn disease.

❏ Although ankylosing spondylitis and colon cancer are more commonly associated with ulcerative colitis, they may be seen in clients with Crohn disease.

❏ Lactase deficiency is caused by a congenital defect.

❏ A priority in the care of a client with Crohn disease experiencing fever, weight loss, leg cramping, diarrhea, frequent premature ventricular contractions, and abdominal pain is evaluation of the potassium level.

❏ Clients with ulcerative colitis should follow a low-residue, high-protein diet.

❏ High-residue food, such as grains and nuts, should be avoided in clients with ulcerative colitis.

❏ A colonoscopy with biopsy can be performed to determine the state of the colon's mucosal layers, presence of ulcerations, and level of cytologic involvement.

❏ In a client with irritable bowel syndrome, an abdominal X-ray, or a computed tomography scan wouldn't provide the cytologic information necessary to diagnose Crohn disease or ulcerative colitis.

❏ Management of Crohn disease may include long-term steroid therapy to reduce the extensive inflammation associated with the deeper layers of the bowel wall.

❏ Other steps in the management of Crohn disease focus on bowel rest (not increasing oral intake) and reducing diarrhea with medications (not giving laxatives).

❏ Promoting bowel rest is the priority during an acute exacerbation of Crohn disease.

❏ Bowel rest is accomplished by decreasing activity and initially putting the client on nothing-by-mouth status.

❏ Bowel perforation, obstruction, hemorrhage, and toxic megacolon are common complications of ulcerative colitis that may require surgery.

❏ Gastritis and herniation aren't associated with irritable bowel diseases.

❏ Outpouching of the bowel wall is diverticulosis.

❏ Being able to safely manage the ostomy is crucial for the client before discharge.

❏ Chronic ulcerative colitis, granulomas, and familial polyposis seem to increase a person's chance of developing colon cancer.

❏ Surface blood vessels of polyps and cancers are fragile and often bleed with the passage of stools, so a fecal occult blood test should be performed annually.

❏ A colonoscopy can help to locate a tumor as well as polyps, but is only recommended every 10 years.

❏ The most common complaint of the client with colon cancer is a change in bowel habits.

❑ The client with colon cancer may have anorexia, secondary abdominal distention, or weight loss.

❑ Bowel spillage could occur during surgery for colon cancer, resulting in peritonitis.

❑ Complete or partial intestinal obstruction may occur before bowel resection.

❑ The client with suspected gastric cancer may report a feeling of fullness in the stomach, but not enough to cause him to seek medical care.

❑ Anorexia and weight loss are common symptoms of gastric cancer.

❑ An endoscopy will allow direct visualization of the tumor in gastric cancer.

❑ A colonoscopy or a barium enema would help to diagnose colon cancer.

❑ Clients with gastric cancer commonly have nutritional deficits and may be cachectic.

❑ After gastric resection, a client may require total parenteral nutrition or jejunostomy tube feedings to maintain adequate nutritional status, which promotes healing.

❑ Dumping syndrome is a problem that occurs postprandially after gastric resection.

❑ In dumping syndrome, ingested food rapidly enters the jejunum without proper mixing and without the normal duodenal digestive processing.

❑ A client with adenomatous polyps has a higher risk for developing rectal cancer than others do.

❑ Clients with diverticulitis are more likely to develop colon cancer.

❑ Clients with peptic ulcer disease have a higher incidence of gastric cancer.

❑ Portal hypertension and other conditions associated with persistently high intra-abdominal pressure, such as pregnancy, can lead to hemorrhoids.

❑ Rectal bleeding can be a symptom of hemorrhoids.

❑ Digital rectal examination is important to assess for internal hemorrhoids and to determine if other causes for the pain and bleeding are present.

❑ A vagotomy is performed to eliminate the acid-secreting stimulus to gastric cells.

❑ Repair of hiatal hernia (fundoplication) prevents the stomach from sliding through the diaphragm.

❑ The most common cause of peritonitis is a perforated ulcer, which can pour contaminants into the peritoneal cavity, causing inflammation and infection within the cavity.

❑ If cholelithiasis leads to rupture of the gall bladder, peritonitis may develop.

❑ If gastritis leads to erosion of the stomach wall, peritonitis may develop.

- ❏ Incarcerated hernia leading to rupture of the intestines may result in peritonitis.

- ❏ Abdominal pain causing rigidity of the abdominal muscles is characteristic of peritonitis.

- ❏ Right upper quadrant pain is characteristic of cholecystitis or hepatitis.

- ❏ I.V. fluids are given to maintain hydration and hemodynamic stability and to replace electrolytes in peritonitis.

- ❏ Peritonitis can advance to shock and circulatory failure, so fluid and electrolyte balance is the priority focus of nursing management.

- ❏ Gastric irrigation may be needed periodically to ensure patency of the nasogastric tube.

- ❏ Focusing on fluid and electrolyte balance will maintain hemodynamic stability.

- ❏ Alcohol abuse is the major cause of acute pancreatitis in males.

- ❏ Gallbladder disease is more commonly implicated in women as a cause of acute pancreatitis.

- ❏ Hypercalcemia, hyperlipidemia, and pancreatic duct obstruction are also causes of pancreatitis but occur less frequently.

- ❏ Reflux of bile into the pancreatic duct and clogging of the pancreatic duct may occur before autodigestion of the pancreas occurs in pancreatitis.

- ❏ Amylase is an enzyme secreted by the pancreas and when elevated, is useful in diagnosing pancreatitis.

- ❏ Cullen sign is bluish discoloration of the periumbilical area from subcutaneous intraperitoneal hemorrhagic pancreatitis.

- ❏ Pain with movement is a common finding with peritonitis.

- ❏ Turner sign is the bluish discoloration of the left flank area, which can be present in peritonitis.

- ❏ In a client with acute pancreatitis, it is essential to minimize discomfort and restlessness, which may further stimulate pancreatic secretion.

- ❏ The client with acute pancreatitis may exhibit hypocalcemia due to the deposit of calcium in areas of fat necrosis.

- ❏ Hyperglycemia, not hypoglycemia, may occur with acute pancreatitis due to reduced insulin production caused by islet of Langerhans involvement.

- ❏ Hypokalemia and hyponatremia may occur with acute pancreatitis because potassium is lost in emesis.

- ❏ The client with gastric ulcer perforation should be treated with antibiotics as well as fluid, electrolyte, and blood replacement.

❑ A client presenting with abdominal pain, weight loss, steatorrhea, and a random glucose of 417 mg/dL correlates with chronic pancreatitis.

❑ The nurse should expect ultrasound of the abdomen to be performed on a client with suspected chronic pancreatitis.

❑ Lying in a supine position usually aggravates pancreatic pain because it stretches the abdominal muscles.

❑ Taking aspirin can cause bleeding in hemorrhagic pancreatitis.

❑ High bilirubin levels irritate peripheral nerves, causing an intense itching sensation in cirrhosis.

❑ Chronic biliary inflammation or obstruction causes biliary cirrhosis.

❑ Acute viral hepatitis can cause postnecrotic cirrhosis.

❑ Alcohol hepatotoxicity is Laënnec cirrhosis.

❑ The client with cirrhosis has a liver that is enlarged (hepatomegaly), fibrotic, and nodular, which makes it palpable.

❑ The client with cirrhosis may develop dry skin, pruritus, and peripheral edema, but these symptoms may have other causes.

❑ A liver biopsy can reveal the exact cause of the hepatomegaly.

❑ In a client with esophageal varices, nursing care should focus on assessing for variceal rupture or hemorrhage, as the client could succumb to this quickly as a result of blood loss.

❑ Controlling blood pressure in the client with esophageal varices is also important because it helps reduce the risk of variceal rupture.

❑ It's important to teach the client with esophageal varices what foods he should avoid, such as spicy foods, and what varices are.

❑ Hepatitis A is transmitted via the fecal-oral route due to poor hand hygiene practices and poor sanitation.

❑ Hepatitis A can be caused by contact with contaminated feces and may be transmitted through infected water, milk, or food, especially shellfish from contaminated waters.

❑ Arthralgia is common in clients with viral hepatitis.

❑ Other symptoms of viral hepatitis include lethargy, flulike symptoms, anorexia, nausea and vomiting, abdominal pain, diarrhea, constipation, and fever.

❑ Asterixis, also known as liver flap, is commonly present in clients with hepatic encephalopathy.

❑ To elicit asterixis have the client extend his arms, dorsiflex his wrists, and spread his fingers and observe for the characteristic flapping motion of the hands.

❏ Lack of concentration, fatigue, and introversion are also symptoms of encephalopathy.

❏ The results of a computed tomography scan are much more definitive in liver cancer than the findings of an ultrasound or X-ray.

❏ Liver enzyme levels and white blood cell count should also be monitored in clients with liver disorders.

❏ Because the most common adverse effect of a liver biopsy is bleeding, the nurse should provide relevant information regarding the potential for hemorrhage.

❏ Chemotherapy and radiation therapy may also be used to reduce the chance of cancerous hepatocytes from regrowing.

❏ Obesity is a known cause of cholecystitis.

❏ Excessive consumption of cholesterol is associated with the development of gallstones in many people.

❏ Liquid protein and low-calorie diets (with rapid weight loss of more than 5 lb [2.3 kg] per week) are implicated as the cause of some cases of cholecystitis.

❏ Reducing stress may reduce bile production, which may also indirectly decrease the chances of developing cholecystitis.

❏ Murphy's sign, elicited when the client reacts to pain and stops breathing in response to palpation in the area of the gallbladder, is a common finding in clients with cholecystitis.

❏ Rebound tenderness is pain on deep palpation and release.

❏ An abdominal ultrasound can show if the gallbladder is enlarged, if gallstones are present, if the gallbladder wall is thickened, or if distention of the gallbladder lumen is present.

❏ A barium swallow looks at the stomach and the duodenum.

❏ Endoscopy looks at the esophagus, stomach, and duodenum.

❏ The client with acute cholecystitis should first be monitored for such complications as perforation, fever, abscess, fistula, and sepsis.

❏ Surgery is usually done after the acute infection has subsided in acute cholecystitis.

❏ Conservative therapy for chronic cholecystitis includes weight reduction by increasing physical activity and following a low-fat diet.

❏ The client with a duodenal ulcer may have bleeding at the ulcer site, which shows up as melena.

❏ Hematemesis, malnourishment, and pain with eating are consistent with a gastric ulcer.

❑ To reduce the occurrences of the dumping syndrome after gastric bypass surgery, clients should be told to lie down for 30 minutes after eating.

❑ Taking fluids only between meals and none with meals, as well as eating smaller amounts more frequently in a semi-recumbent position, can reduce occurrences of dumping syndrome.

❑ Eating a low-carbohydrate diet, with high-protein and moderate-fat foods, and avoiding sweets also reduces dumping syndrome.

❑ Pain of a duodenal ulcer on an empty stomach is relieved by eating or taking antacids.

❑ Early satiety, pain on eating, and dull upper epigastric pain are signs of a gastric ulcer.

❑ In clients with peptic ulcers, an esophagogastroduodenoscopy can visualize the entire upper GI tract and allow for tissue specimens and electrocautery if needed.

❑ A barium swallow can locate a gastric ulcer and may be an initial test performed.

❑ A computed tomography scan and an abdominal X-ray aren't useful in the diagnosis of an ulcer.

❑ The inflammation in pancreatitis also causes a blockage of the ducts from the pancreas to the GI tract; therefore, pancreatic enzymes are released into the blood, resulting in an elevation of amylase and lipase levels.

❑ Carbohydrate metabolism is impaired secondary to damage to the pancreatic beta cells in pancreatitis.

❑ Impairment of pancreatic beta cells causes the client to become hyperglycemic.

❑ In pancreatitis, as in many other disease processes, serum calcium level decreases because of the saponification of calcium by fatty acids in the area of the inflamed pancreas.

❑ A client with pancreatitis must avoid foods or beverages that can cause a relapse of the disease.

❑ Caffeine must be avoided with pancreatitis because it's a stimulant that will further irritate the pancreas.

❑ The client with pancreatitis must avoid all alcohol because chronic alcohol use is one of the causes of pancreatitis.

❑ The diet for the client with pancreatitis should be low in fat and high in calories, especially carbohydrates.

❑ Having the client lie on his right side with the bed flat will splint the liver biopsy site and minimize bleeding.

❑ Left side-lying position with the bed flat or in semi-Fowler's position or right side-lying position with the bed in semi-Fowler's position may cause increased bleeding at the liver biopsy site or internally.

❑ The client with irritable bowel syndrome needs to be on a diet that contains at least 25 grams of fiber per day.

❑ Fatty foods are to be avoided with irritable bowel syndrome because they may precipitate symptoms.

❑ Gastric acid contains large amounts of potassium, chloride, and hydrogen ions.

❑ To further prevent reflux, the client should remain upright for 2 to 3 hours after eating and avoid eating for 2 to 3 hours before bedtime.

❑ Avoiding drinking large fluid volumes with meals, and eating small, frequent meals to help reduce gastric acid secretion can help prevent reflux.

❑ Although adding bran to cereal helps prevent constipation by increasing dietary fiber, the client should start with a small amount of bran and gradually increase the amount as tolerated to a maximum of 2 grams daily.

❑ Firm skin turgor would be one indication of successful fluid resuscitation.

❑ Other indications of successful fluid resuscitation include moist mucous membranes and urine output of at least 30 ml/hour.

❑ Passage of formed stools at regular intervals and a decrease in stool frequency and liquidity indicate successful resolution of diarrhea.

❑ To help prevent colon cancer, fats should account for no more than 25% of total daily calories and the diet should include 25 to 30 grams of fiber per day.

❑ For colorectal cancer screening, the American Cancer Society advises clients over age 50 to have a flexible sigmoidoscopy every 5 years.

❑ Yearly fecal occult blood tests are recommended for colorectal cancer screening.

❑ A double-contrast barium enema every 5 years, or a colonoscopy every 10 years, is recommended for colorectal cancer screening.

❑ To manage gluten-induced enteropathy, the client must eliminate gluten. In initial disease management of gluten-induced enteropathy, clients eat a high-calorie, high-protein diet with mineral and vitamin supplements to help normalize the nutritional status.

❑ Lactose intolerance is sometimes an associated problem with gluten-induced enteropathy, so milk and dairy products are limited until improvement occurs.

❑ For a paracentesis, the nurse should document the date and time of the procedure, the physician's name, pertinent information about the procedure (including tests done on the specimen obtained), the client's response, and client teaching.

❑ To prevent aspiration of stomach contents in the client with a percutaneous endoscopic gastrostomy tube, the nurse should place the client in semi-Fowler's position for feeding.

❑ The supine and reverse Trendelenburg positions may cause aspiration with a percutaneous endoscopic gastrostomy.

❑ Enemas are contraindicated in an acute abdominal condition of unknown origin (such as suspected appendicitis) and after recent colon or rectal surgery.

❑ A client with a lower GI bleed may receive packed red blood cells to raise the hemoglobin level.

❑ The nurse can palpate the liver by standing at the client's right side and placing her right hand on the client's abdomen, to the right of midline.

❑ The nurse should point the fingers of her right hand toward the client's head, just under the right rib margin, when palpating the liver.

## Genitourinary system

❑ It's important to empty the bowel before treatment with intracavitary radiation for cancer of the cervix because pressure changes in the pelvis associated with bowel movements can alter the position of the applicator and the radiation source.

❑ Chlamydia is a common cause of pelvic inflammatory disease and infertility.

❑ Chlamydia can cause conjunctivitis and respiratory infection in neonates exposed to infected cervicovaginal secretions during delivery.

❑ Cool, wet compresses can be used to soothe the itch caused by genital herpes.

❑ Clients with ovarian cancer are at increased risk for breast cancer.

❑ Breast self-examination supports early detection and treatment of breast cancer and is very important.

❑ Human papilloma virus causes genital warts, which are associated with an increased incidence of cervical cancer.

❑ Candidiasis is rare before menarche and after menopause.

❑ The discharge associated with infection caused by *Trichomonas* organisms is homogenous, greenish gray, watery, and frothy or purulent.

❑ The discharge associated with candidiasis is thick and white and resembles cottage cheese in appearance.

❑ Infection due to *Gardnerella vaginalis* produces a thin and grayish white discharge, with a marked fishy odor.

❑ After intracavitary radiation, some vaginal bleeding occurs for 1 to 3 months.

❑ Intermittent painless vaginal bleeding is a classic symptom of cervical cancer.

❑ By removing water from the body in the form of urine, the kidneys also help regulate blood pressure.

❑ Urine is formed when blood from the renal artery is filtered across the glomerular capillary membrane in Bowman's capsule; formed filtrate (composition similar to blood plasma without proteins) moves through the tubules of the nephron, which reabsorb and secrete electrolytes, water, glucose, amino acids, ammonia, and bicarbonate; what's left is excreted as urine.

❑ In urine formation antidiuretic hormone and aldosterone control the reabsorption of water and electrolytes.

❑ Blood from renal artery filtration requires adequate intravascular volume and adequate cardiac output.

❑ The kidneys have four main components: cortex, medulla, renal pelvis, and nephron.

❑ The cortex of the kidney makes up the outer layer and contains the glomeruli, the proximal tubules of the nephron, and the distal tubules of the nephron.

❑ The medulla of the kidney makes up the inner layer and contains the loops of Henle and the collecting tubules.

❑ The renal pelvis of the kidney collects urine from the calyces.

❑ The nephron of the kidney makes up the functional unit and contains Bowman's capsule, the glomerulus, and the renal tubule, which consists of the proximal convoluted tubule and collecting segments.

❑ Regulation of fluid volume by the kidneys affects blood pressure.

❑ The renin-angiotensin system is activated by decreased blood pressure and can be altered by renal disease.

❑ The ureter, which transports urine from the kidney to the bladder, is a tubule that extends from the renal pelvis to the bladder floor.

❑ The bladder, a muscular, distendable sac, can contain up to 1 L of urine at a single time.

❑ The urethra, extending from the bladder to the urinary meatus, transports urine from the bladder to the exterior of the body.

❑ The prostate gland surrounds the male urethra and contains ducts that secrete the alkaline portion of seminal fluid.

❑ The bulbourethral glands (or Cowper's glands) are two pea-sized glands opening into the posterior portion of the urethra.

❑ The bulbourethral glands (or Cowper's glands) secrete a thick alkaline fluid that neutralizes acidic secretions in the female reproductive tract, thus prolonging spermatozoa survival.

❑ The prostate gland, located just below the bladder, is considered homologous to Skene's glands in females.

❑ The epididymides serve as the initial section of the testes' excretory duct system and store spermatozoa as they mature and become motile.

❑ The vas deferens, which connects the epididymal lumen and the prostatic urethra, serves as a conduit for spermatozoa.

❑ The ejaculatory ducts—located between the seminal vesicles and the urethra—serve as passageways for semen and seminal fluid.

❑ The urethra, which extends from the bladder through the penis to the external urethral opening, serves as the excretory duct for urine and semen.

❑ The seminal vesicles are two pouchlike structures between the bladder and the rectum that secrete a viscous fluid that aids in spermatozoa motility and metabolism.

❑ Urinalysis involves an examination of urine for color, appearance, pH, urine specific gravity, protein, glucose, ketones, red blood cells, white blood cells, and casts.

❑ External male genitalia include the penis and scrotum.

❑ The penis, consisting of the body (shaft) and glans, has three layers of erectile tissue: two corpora cavernosa and one corpus spongiosum.

❑ The penis deposits spermatozoa in the female reproductive tract and provides sexual pleasure.

❑ The scrotum is a pouchlike structure composed of skin, fascial connective tissue, and smooth-muscle fibers that houses the testes and protects spermatozoa from high body temperature.

❑ Internal male genitalia produce and transport semen and seminal fluid.

❑ The testes, or testicles, two oval-shaped glandular organs inside the scrotum, function to produce spermatozoa and testosterone.

❑ The fallopian tubes are about 4½" (12 cm) long and consist of four layers: peritoneal, subserous, muscular, and mucous.

❑ The fallopian tubes are divided into four portions: interstitial, isthmus, ampulla, and fimbria.

❑ The fallopian tubes transport ovum from the ovary to the uterus, provide a nourishing environment for zygotes, and serve as the site of fertilization.

❑ The ovaries are two almond-shaped glandular structures resting below and behind the fallopian tubes on either side of the uterus.

❏ The ovaries produce sex hormones (estrogen, progesterone, androgen) and serve as the site of ovulation.

❏ The breasts consist of glandular, fibrous, and adipose tissue.

❏ Stimulated by secretions from the hypothalamus, anterior pituitary, and ovaries, the breasts provide nourishment to an infant, transfer maternal antibodies during breast-feeding, and enhance sexual pleasure.

❏ The female urethral meatus is located $\frac{3}{8}$" to 1" (1 to 2.5 cm) below the clitoris.

❏ The paraurethral glands (Skene's glands) are located on both sides of the urethral opening and produce mucus.

❏ Internal female genitalia include the vagina, uterus, fallopian tubes, and ovaries.

❏ The vagina is a vascularized musculomembranous tube extending from the external genitals to the uterus.

❏ Hollow and pear-shaped, the uterus is a muscular organ divided by a slight constriction (isthmus) into an upper portion (body or corpus) and a lower portion (cervix).

❏ The body, or corpus, of the uterus has three layers: perimetrium, myometrium, and endometrium.

❏ The uterus receives support from broad, round, uterosacral ligaments and provides an environment for fetal growth and development.

❏ The vaginal vestibule extends from the clitoris to the posterior fourchette and consists of the vaginal orifice, the hymen, the fossa navicularis, and Bartholin's glands.

❏ The hymen is a thin, vascularized mucous membrane at the vaginal orifice.

❏ The fossa navicularis is a depressed area between the hymen and fourchette.

❏ Bartholin's glands are two bean-shaped glands on either side of the vagina that secrete mucus during sexual stimulation.

❏ The perineal body (the area between the vagina and the anus) is the site where an episiotomy may be performed during childbirth.

❏ External female genitalia include the mons pubis, labia, clitoris, vaginal vestibule, perineal body, urethral meatus, and paraurethral glands.

❏ The mons pubis provides an adipose cushion over the anterior symphysis pubis, protects the pelvic bones, and contributes to the rounded contour of the female body.

❏ The labia majora are two folds that converge at the mons pubis and extend to the posterior commissure.

❑ The labia majora consist of connective tissue, elastic fibers, veins, and sebaceous glands, and they protect components of the vulval cleft.

❑ The labia minora are within the labia majora and consist of connective tissue, sebaceous and sweat glands, nonstriated muscle fibers, nerve endings, and blood vessels.

❑ The labia minora unite to form the fourchette, the vaginal vestibule, and serve to lubricate the vulva, which adds to sexual enjoyment and fights bacteria.

❑ The clitoris—located in the anterior portion of the vulva above the urethral opening—is made up of erectile tissue, nerves, and blood vessels and, homologous to the penis, provides sexual pleasure.

❑ The clitoris consists of the glans, the body, and two crura.

❑ In cystoscopy, a cytoscope is used to directly visualize the bladder.

❑ During a cystoscopy the bladder is usually distended with fluid to enhance visualization.

❑ Renal angiography provides a radiographic examination of the renal arterial supply by injecting dye into the vascular system.

❑ A renal scan involves injecting a radioisotope to allow visual imaging of blood flow distribution to the kidneys.

❑ Elevation of the affected arm after mastectomy promotes venous and lymphatic return from the extremity.

❑ Blood pressure measurements in the affected arm also should be avoided after mastectomy.

❑ Priapism is a condition in which the penis is persistently erect and painful and is a urologic emergency because gangrene secondary to ischemia can result if venous drainage of the corpora cavernosa doesn't occur.

❑ The cause of toxic shock syndrome is a toxin produced by *Staphylococcus aureus* bacteria.

❑ Toxic shock syndrome occurs most commonly in menstruating women using tampons.

❑ Tampons, particularly when left in place for more than 8 hours (such as overnight), are believed to provide a good environment for growth of the bacteria, which then enter the bloodstream through breaks in the vaginal mucosa.

❑ Strenuous work, which can result in increased bleeding after a dilatation and curettage procedure, should be avoided for 2 weeks to allow time for healing.

❑ Sexual intercourse should also be avoided for 2 weeks after a dilatation and curettage procedure to allow healing and thus decrease the risk of infection.

- ❏ Tampons and tub baths should be avoided for 1 week after a dilatation and curettage procedure.
- ❏ Androgens are responsible for the development of the male genitalia and secondary male sex characteristics.
- ❏ Sperm continues to be produced despite the age-related degenerative changes that occur in the male reproductive system.
- ❏ Normal age-related changes in the male are decreased size and increased firmness of the testes, a decrease in sexual potency, and decreased production of testosterone and progesterone.
- ❏ Ejaculation can aid in the treatment of chronic prostatitis by decreasing the retention of prostatic fluid.
- ❏ Coffee should be eliminated from the diet in the client with prostatitis because it can increase prostate secretion.
- ❏ Warm sitz baths and not sitting for too long at a time promote comfort for chronic prostatitis.
- ❏ Prostatitis can cause prostate pain, which is felt as perineal discomfort.
- ❏ Endometriosis can cause pain low in the abdomen, deep in the pelvis, or in the rectal or sacrococcygeal area, depending on the location of the ectopic tissue.
- ❏ Azotemia, a buildup of nitrogenous waste products in the blood, indicates impaired renal function.
- ❏ Breast enlargement, decrease in prostate size, and flushing are expected effects of finasteride.
- ❏ Douching is generally avoided for 2 weeks, as is the use of tampons, in the client with cervical polyps who has been treated with cryosurgery.
- ❏ Clients receiving intracavitary radiation therapy are placed on strict bed rest, with the head of the bed elevated no more than 15 degrees to avoid displacing the radiation source.
- ❏ Chlamydia is a common sexually transmitted disease requiring the treatment of all current sexual partners to prevent reinfection.
- ❏ Bartholinitis results from obstruction of a duct of the Bartholin gland.
- ❏ Sexual partners may become infected with chlamydia, although men can usually be treated with over-the-counter products.
- ❏ Candidiasis is a yeast infection that typically occurs as a result of antibiotic use.
- ❏ Endometriosis occurs when endometrial cells are seeded throughout the pelvis and isn't a sexually transmitted disease.
- ❏ After vasectomy, the client remains fertile for several weeks until sperm stored distal to the severed vas are evacuated.

❑ After vasectomy, sperm are still produced but they don't enter the ejaculate and are absorbed by the body.

❑ A vasectomy can be reversed, but the success rate is low.

❑ After vasectomy, the client will have to limit usual activities for about 1 week.

❑ Proper cleaning of the preputial area to remove secretions is critical to the prevention of noncongenital phimosis.

❑ Regular ejaculation can decrease the symptoms of chronic prostatitis, but it has no effect on the development of phimosis.

❑ Testicular self-examination is important in the early detection and treatment of testicular cancer.

❑ Alpha-fetoprotein is a tumor marker elevated in nonseminomatous malignancies of the testicle.

❑ A persistent elevation of alpha-fetoprotein after orchiectomy indicates presence of a tumor someplace outside the testicle that was removed.

❑ Small blood clots or pieces of tissue commonly are passed in the urine for up to 2 weeks postoperatively after prostatectomy.

❑ Tub baths are prohibited after prostatectomy because they cause dilation of pelvic blood vessels.

❑ Sexual intercourse and driving are usually prohibited for about 3 weeks after prostatectomy.

❑ Exercising and returning to work are usually prohibited for about 6 weeks after prostatectomy.

❑ Difficulty urinating suggests urethral obstruction after biopsy of the prostate.

❑ Mild pain is expected for 1 to 3 days after biopsy of the prostate.

❑ Semen may be discolored for up to a month after biopsy of the prostate.

❑ Temperature higher than 101° F (38.3° C) after a biopsy of the prostate should be reported because it suggests infection.

❑ After a transrectal prostatic biopsy, blood in the stool is expected for a number of days.

❑ Pruritus and paresthesia as well as redness of the genital area are prodromal symptoms of recurrent herpes infection.

❑ Vaginal and urethral discharge are also signs of primary genital herpes infection.

❑ Dysuria and lymphadenopathy are local symptoms of primary genital herpes infection that may also occur with recurrent infection.

❑ Stress, anxiety, and emotional upset seem to predispose to recurrent outbreaks of genital herpes.

❑ Because a relationship has been found between genital herpes and cervical cancer, a Pap test is recommended every 6 months for the client who tests positive for genital herpes.

❑ Breast self-examination requires palpation of all breast tissue, including the area above the breast up to the collarbone and all the way over to the shoulder as well as the area between the breast and the underarm, including the underarm itself.

❑ Prerenal failure refers to renal failure due to an interference with renal perfusion.

❑ Decreased cardiac output causes a decrease in renal perfusion, which leads to a lower glomerular filtration rate.

❑ In acute pyelonephritis, the client may complain of pain on the affected side because the kidney is enlarged and might have formed an abscess.

❑ Hypertension is associated with chronic pyelonephritis.

❑ Pyelonephritis typically recurs as a relapse or new infection and frequently recurs within 2 weeks of completing therapy.

❑ Fluid intake of 3 to 4 qt (3 to 4 L)/day is encouraged to flush the urinary tract and prevent further calculi formation.

❑ Ambulation is encouraged to help pass the calculi through gravity.

❑ Cystitis is the most common adverse reaction of clients undergoing radiation therapy.

❑ Cystitis symptoms include dysuria, frequency, urgency, and nocturia.

❑ Urine of clients with radiation implants for bladder cancer should be sent to the radioisotopes laboratory for monitoring.

❑ It's recommended that fluid intake be increased in a client receiving a radiation implant for the treatment of bladder cancer.

❑ A client who has undergone a radical cystectomy may have an ileal conduit for the treatment of bladder cancer.

❑ The stoma of an ileal conduit should be red and moist, indicating adequate blood flow; a dusky or cyanotic stoma indicates insufficient blood supply and is an emergency needing prompt intervention.

❑ Urine output of less than 30 ml/hour or no urine output for more than 15 minutes from an ileal conduit should be reported.

❑ Cotton underwear prevents cystitis infection because it allows for air to flow to the perineum.

❑ Women should shower instead of taking a tub bath to prevent cystitis infection.

❑ The urinary drainage bag shouldn't be placed alongside the client or on the floor because of the increased risk of infection caused by microorganisms.

- ❏ The urinary drainage bag should hang on the bed in a dependent position.
- ❏ The kidneys are responsible for excreting potassium.
- ❏ In renal failure, the kidneys are no longer able to excrete potassium, resulting in hyperkalemia.
- ❏ The kidneys are responsible for regulating the acid-base balance.
- ❏ Generally, hyponatremia would be seen in chronic renal failure because of the dilutional effect of water retention.
- ❏ Hypokalemia is generally seen in clients undergoing diuresis.
- ❏ A client with a history of chronic renal failure can develop pulmonary edema after missing a dialysis treatment.
- ❏ Acute renal failure can result in hyperkalemia, which can manifest in widening of the PR interval and QRS complex on the ECG.
- ❏ Urine specific gravity, mental status, and blood pressure are monitored in the client with acute renal failure.
- ❏ Fever, a flushed feeling, or lethargy suggests infection, which is the major complication to watch for in clients on cyclosporine therapy.
- ❏ A client who has received a renal transplant may be started cyclosporine (an immunosuppressive drug) therapy to prevent graft rejection.
- ❏ In a client with acute renal graft rejection, evidence of deteriorating renal function (elevated blood urea nitrogen and creatinine levels) is expected.
- ❏ The nurse would see fever and elevated white blood cell counts with acute renal graft rejection because the body is recognizing the graft as foreign and is attempting to fight it.
- ❏ Before renal transplantation, the client is most likely anuric or oliguric.
- ❏ Postoperatively after renal transplantation, the client will require close monitoring of urine output to make sure the transplanted kidney is functioning optimally.
- ❏ Don't give the next scheduled exchange with peritoneal dialysis until the dialysate is drained because abdominal distention will occur, unless the output is within the parameters set by the physician.
- ❏ The client with renal failure can develop pulmonary edema from fluid overload; he will need to undergo dialysis and fluid restriction.
- ❏ The first intervention in a client with renal failure who develops pulmonary edema should be aimed at the immediate treatment of hypoxia.
- ❏ Blood urea nitrogen and creatinine levels should be monitored closely in the client with renal insufficiency receiving nephrotoxic antibiotics.
- ❏ A client with a transurethral prostatectomy for benign prostatic hypertrophy may be treated with continuous bladder irrigation.

❑ Vital signs should initially be taken every 30 minutes for the first 4 hours and then every 2 hours with postobstructive diuresis.

❑ Urine output needs to be assessed hourly with postobstructive diuresis.

❑ No blood pressures or venipunctures should be taken in the arm with the arteriovenous fistula.

❑ Renal calculi are commonly composed of calcium.

❑ Pain during or after voiding indicates a bladder problem, usually infection.

❑ Problems of the urethra would cause pain at the external orifice that's commonly felt at the start of voiding.

❑ Urine retention is usually a temporary problem that requires insertion of a straight catheter.

❑ An indwelling urinary catheter is used for longer-term bladder problems.

❑ Benign prostatic hypertrophy (BPH) typically results in urine retention, frequency, dribbling, and difficulty starting the urine stream.

❑ The laboratory results indicating an elevated serum creatinine may reflect dehydration.

❑ Normal serum creatinine ranges are from 0.7 to 1.5 mg/dL.

❑ Volume depletion or dehydration is a risk factor for developing acute renal failure due to decreased perfusion of the kidneys.

❑ A client injected with radiographic contrast medium who immediately shows signs of dyspnea, flushing, and pruritus is showing symptoms of an allergy to the iodine in the contrast medium.

❑ Bladder biopsies shouldn't be done when an active urinary tract infection is present because sepsis may result.

❑ The bladder needs to be emptied frequently after cystoscopy, and output should be measured to make sure the bladder is emptying.

❑ Blood in the urine isn't normal after cystoscopy except for small amounts during the first 24 hours after the procedure.

❑ Kegel exercises begin with tightening and relaxing the vagina, rectum, and urethra 4 or 5 times during each session, gradually increasing to 25 times for each session.

❑ Kegel exercises are used to gain control of bladder function in women with stress incontinence and in some men after prostate surgery.

❑ Chronic pyelonephritis can be a long-term condition requiring antibiotic treatment for several weeks or months as well as close monitoring to prevent permanent damage to the kidneys.

❑ Continuous bladder irrigation shouldn't be stopped as long as the catheter is draining because clots will form.

❑ Clients with diabetes are prone to renal insufficiency and renal failure.

❑ The contrast media used for heart catheterization must be eliminated by the kidneys, which further stresses them and may produce acute renal failure.

❑ The absence of a thrill or bruit should be reported promptly to the physician because it indicates an occlusion in an arteriovenous fistula and is not a normal finding.

❑ Signs and symptoms of acute rejection of a transplanted kidney include pain at the graft site and decreased urine output.

❑ Signs of acute rejection of a transplanted kidney include hypertension, elevated white blood cell count, fever, and elevated creatinine level.

❑ High urine specific gravity indicates dehydration.

❑ In females, the urethra and rectum are in close proximity, posing a greater risk for urethral contamination with feces after a bowel movement.

❑ In secondary syphilis, a maculopapular, nonpruritic rash appears on the palms of the hands and soles of the feet.

❑ During the second stage of syphilis, nontender lymphadenopathy occurs.

❑ Personality changes occur during the late stage of syphilis.

❑ Incontinence and diarrhea don't result in obstruction of the urinary system or bowel, respectively.

❑ Hemolytic streptococci are common in throat infections and can cause an immune reaction that causes glomerular damage.

❑ Straining all urine helps identify renal calculi that have passed through the urine.

❑ To control uric acid calculi, the client should avoid high-purine foods such as organ meats.

❑ When the glomeruli are damaged, as in nephrotic syndrome, the kidneys are excessively permeable to plasma protein.

❑ In nephrotic syndrome, proteinuria and hypoalbuminemia occur.

❑ Proteinuria and hypoalbuminemia lead to a decreased oncotic pressure, which results in anasarca (massive generalized edema).

❑ The nurse subtracts the amount of infused bladder irrigation from the total volume in the drainage bag to determine urine output.

## Endocrine system

❑ A client with diaphoresis, palpitations, jitters, and tachycardia approximately 1½ hours after taking his regular morning insulin is experiencing symptoms of hypoglycemia.

❑ Retinopathy is a chronic complication of diabetes mellitus.

❑ Exercise decreases insulin resistance.

❑ Insulin lipodystrophy produces fatty masses at injection sites, causing unpredictable absorption of insulin injected into these sites.

❑ Insulin edema is sometimes seen after normal blood glucose levels are established in a client with prolonged hyperglycemia.

❑ Insulin resistance occurs mostly in overweight clients and is due to insulin binding with antibodies, decreasing the amount of absorption.

❑ Results of a urine glucose test correlate poorly with blood glucose levels.

❑ Weight gain, lethargy, and slow pulse rate along with decreased $T_3$ and $T_4$ levels indicate hypothyroidism.

❑ $T_3$ and $T_4$ are thyroid hormones that affect growth and development as well as metabolic rate.

❑ Tetany is related to low calcium levels.

❑ To palpate the thyroid gland, ask the client to swallow; as he does so, palpate the gland for enlargement as the tissue rises and falls.

❑ Measurement of glycosylated hemoglobin (Hb $A_{1c}$) is used to assess hyperglycemia.

❑ Coarsening of facial features and extremity enlargement are symptoms of acromegaly.

❑ The medulla of the adrenal gland releases two hormones: epinephrine and norepinephrine.

❑ Thyroxine ($T_4$), triiodothyronine ($T_3$), and calcitonin are secreted by the thyroid gland.

❑ The islet cells of the pancreas secrete insulin, glucagon, and somatostatin.

❑ The client with diabetes insipidus is at risk for developing hypovolemic shock because of increased urine output.

❑ In clients with diabetes insipidus, urine specific gravity should be monitored for low osmolality (generally less than 1.005) due to the body's inability to concentrate urine.

❑ The fluid deprivation test involves withholding water for 4 to 18 hours and checking urine osmolarity periodically.

❑ A client with diabetes insipidus will have an increased serum osmolarity (less than 300 mOsm/kg).

❑ Lethargy and depression are early symptoms of Addison disease.

❑ Daily weight is an objective way to monitor fluid balance in Addison disease.

❑ Rapid variations in weight in Addison disease reflect changes in fluid volume and the need for more glucocorticoids.

❑ The best indicator for determining if a client with Addison disease is receiving the correct amount of glucocorticoid replacement is by daily weight.

❑ In addisonian crisis the uncontrolled loss of sodium and impaired mineralocorticoid function result in loss of extracellular fluid and low blood volume and possible irreversible shock.

❑ With hyperthyroidism, the client has high levels of $T_3$ and $T_4$.

❑ A definitive diagnosis of Addison disease must reflect low levels of adrenocortical hormones.

❑ Clients with Addison disease experience fatigue related to decreased metabolic energy production and altered body chemistry.

❑ Clients with Addison disease experience fluid volume deficit secondary to decreased mineralocorticoid secretion.

❑ Stress can precipitate a hypotensive crisis in clients with Addison disease.

❑ Clients with Addison disease must monitor salt intake.

❑ Overproduction of adrenocortical hormone results in growth arrest and obesity.

❑ Thin extremities, an obese truncal area, presence of a "buffalo hump" at the shoulder area, weakness, and disturbed sleep are symptoms of Cushing syndrome.

❑ Increased mineralocorticoid activity resulting in sodium and water retention in a client with Cushing syndrome commonly contributes to hypertension and heart failure.

❑ Hypoglycemia and dehydration are uncommon in a client with Cushing syndrome.

❑ Test results in Cushing syndrome include high serum sodium and glucose levels, low potassium level, reduction of eosinophils, and disappearance of lymphoid tissue.

❑ A low-dose dexamethasone suppression test can diagnose Cushing syndrome.

❑ A fluid deprivation test is used to diagnose diabetes insipidus.

❑ Removing a major source of adrenal hormones may cause a state of temporary adrenal insufficiency, requiring short-term replacement therapy.

❑ When both adrenal glands are removed, the client requires lifelong hormone replacement.

❑ Clients with Cushing syndrome have an increased susceptibility to injury or infection, secondary to the immunosuppression caused by excessive cortisol.

❑ Clients with Addison disease must increase sodium intake and fluid intake in times of stress to prevent hypotension.

❑ Diabetic ketoacidosis is caused by inadequate amounts of insulin or absence of insulin, and leads to a series of biochemical disorders.

❑ Diabetes insipidus is caused by a deficiency of vasopressin.

❑ Hyperaldosteronism is an excess in aldosterone production, causing sodium and fluid excesses and hypertension.

❑ Hyperosmolar hyperglycemic nonketotic syndrome is a coma state in which hyperglycemia and hyperosmolarity dominate.

❑ A client with chronic pancreatitis may develop diabetes secondary to the pancreatitis.

❑ A client with syndrome of inappropriate antidiuretic hormone secretion is unable to excrete dilute urine, causing hyponatremia.

❑ Amylase, lipase, and trypsin are enzymes produced by the pancreas that aid in digestion.

❑ The pituitary gland secretes vasopressin and oxytocin.

❑ By secretion of thyroid-stimulating hormone, the pituitary gland controls the rate of thyroid hormone released.

❑ The parathyroid gland secretes parathyroid hormones, depending on the levels of calcium and phosphorus in the blood.

❑ The thyroid gland secretes thyroid hormone, but doesn't control how much is released.

❑ Irradiation, involving administration of iodine 131 ($^{131}$I), destroys the thyroid gland and thereby treats hyperthyroidism.

❑ The pancreas is an accessory gland of digestion.

❑ In its exocrine function, the pancreas secretes digestive enzymes (amylase, lipase, and trypsin).

❑ Amylase breaks down starches into smaller carbohydrate molecules.

❑ Lipase breaks down fats into fatty acids and glycerol.

❑ Trypsin breaks down proteins.

❑ The pancreas secretes enzymes into the duodenum through the pancreatic duct.

❑ In its endocrine function, the pancreas secretes hormones from the islets of Langerhans (insulin, glucagon, and somatostatin).

❑ Insulin regulates fat, protein, and carbohydrate metabolism and lowers blood glucose levels by promoting glucose transport into cells.

❑ Glucagon increases blood glucose levels by promoting hepatic glyconeogenesis.

❑ Somatostatin inhibits the release of insulin, glucagon, and somatotropin.

❑ Endocrine glands discharge secretions into the blood or lymph.

❑ The Whipple procedure is a surgical treatment for pancreatic cancer.

❑ Most elderly clients with hyperthyroidism present with depression, apathy, and weight loss.

❑ Cold intolerance, weight gain, and thinning hair are some of the signs of hypothyroidism.

❑ Numbness, tingling, and cramping of extremities are symptoms of hypocalcemia, which may be a symptom of hypoparathyroidism.

❑ Thyroid storm is a form of severe hyperthyroidism that can be precipitated by stress, injury, or infection.

❑ Myxedema coma is a rare disorder characterized by hypoventilation, hypotension, hypoglycemia, and hypothyroidism.

❑ Hyperthyroidism is known as Graves disease.

❑ Hyperparathyroidism is overproduction of parathyroid hormone and is characterized by bone calcification or renal calculi.

❑ Signs and symptoms of hyperthyroidism include nervousness, palpitations, irritability, bulging eyes, heat intolerance, weight loss, and weakness.

❑ Hyperparathyroidism is characterized by weakness and anorexia.

❑ Signs and symptoms of hypothyroidism include fatigue, cool skin, and sensitivity to cold.

❑ The adrenal glands are composed of the adrenal cortex and the adrenal medulla.

❑ The adrenal cortex secretes three major types of hormones: glucocorticoids, mineralocorticoids, and sex hormones.

❑ Glucocorticoids (cortisol, cortisone, and corticosterone) mediate the stress response, promote sodium and water retention and potassium secretion, and suppress corticotropin secretion.

❑ Mineralocorticoids (aldosterone and deoxycorticosterone) promote sodium and water retention and potassium secretion.

❑ Sex hormones (androgens, estrogens, and progesterone) develop and maintain secondary sex characteristics and libido.

❑ The parathyroid gland secretes parathyroid hormone (parathormone), which regulates calcium and phosphorus levels and promotes the resorption of calcium from bones.

❑ The pituitary gland is composed of anterior and posterior lobes; together these lobes produce various hormones that affect the body.

❑ The anterior lobe of the pituitary secretes follicle-stimulating hormone, luteinizing hormone, corticotropin, thyroid-stimulating hormone, and growth hormone.

❑ Follicle-stimulating hormone stimulates graafian follicle growth and estrogen secretion in women and sperm maturation in men.

❑ Luteinizing hormone induces ovulation and the development of the corpus luteum in women and stimulates testosterone secretion in men.

❑ Corticotropin stimulates secretion of hormones from the adrenal cortex.

❑ Thyroid-stimulating hormone regulates the secretory activity of the thyroid gland.

❑ Growth hormone is an insulin antagonist that stimulates the growth of cells, bones, muscle, and soft tissue.

❑ The posterior lobe of the pituitary secretes vasopressin and oxytocin.

❑ Vasopressin (antidiuretic hormone, also called ADH), helps the body retain water.

❑ Oxytocin stimulates uterine contractions during labor and milk secretion in lactating women. Norepinephrine regulates generalized vasoconstriction.

❑ Epinephrine regulates instantaneous stress reaction and increases metabolism, blood glucose levels, and cardiac output.

❑ Amenorrhea is a sign of decreased levels of follicle-stimulating hormone, which is one of the anterior pituitary hormones.

❑ Weight gain is associated with Cushing syndrome, which is associated with the adrenal cortex.

❑ Urine output is related to posterior pituitary function.

❑ Two leading causes of diabetes insipidus are hypothalamic or pituitary tumors and closed-head injuries.

❑ Normal sodium levels are 135 to 145 mEq/dL.

❑ Clients with Kussmaul's respirations, abdominal discomfort, lethargy, and serum glucose levels above 300 mg/dL could be diagnosed with diabetic ketoacidosis.

❑ Serum ketones would aid in confirming the diagnosis of diabetic ketoacidosis.

❑ Insulin forces potassium out of the plasma, back into the cells, causing hypokalemia.

❑ Diabetic clients are especially prone to infections.

❑ Normal calcium levels are 8.5 to 10.5 mg/dL.

❑ Symptoms of hypoparathyroidism include hyperphosphatemia and hypocalcemia.

❑ Excessive thyroid hormone levels indicate Graves disease (hyperthyroidism).

❑ Low thyroid hormone levels indicate hypothyroidism.

❏ Clients with hyperthyroidism are typically anxious, diaphoretic, nervous, and fatigued and need a calm, restful environment in which to relax and get adequate rest.

❏ A client with hypoparathyroidism has a decreased calcium level.

❏ Graves disease causes bulging of the eyes, weight loss, and heat intolerance.

❏ Pheochromocytoma is a tumor of the adrenal gland that causes hypertension.

❏ Tumors that affect the pituitary gland would lead to acromegaly, Cushing syndrome, and hypopituitarism.

❏ Tumors of the adrenal gland would cause symptoms such as hypertension.

❏ The hypothalamus secretes corticotropin-releasing factor, which stimulates the anterior pituitary to secrete corticotropin.

❏ Chvostek's sign is positive when a sharp tapping over the facial nerve, in front of the parotid gland and anterior to the ear, causes the mouth, nose, and eye to twitch.

❏ Immediate treatment for a client who develops hypocalcemia and tetany after thyroidectomy is calcium gluconate.

❏ Hypophysectomy is the surgical removal of the pituitary gland.

❏ Pheochromocytoma is a tumor of the adrenal gland and doesn't cause abdominal or back symptoms.

❏ Spicy foods, caffeine, and alcohol should be avoided in pancreatitis.

❏ A high-calorie, high-protein diet is appropriate for clients with hyperthyroidism.

❏ During periods of infection or illness, insulin-dependent clients may need even more insulin to compensate for increased blood glucose levels.

❏ Based on the American Diabetes Association guidelines, fasting blood glucose of 126 mg/dl or more on at least two occasions is indicative of diabetes mellitus.

❏ Tests that help determine a definitive diagnosis of diabetes mellitus include random blood glucose levels, glucose tolerance tests, and measurement of glycosylated hemoglobin (Hb $A_{1c}$).

❏ A pheochromocytoma is usually a benign tumor of the adrenal medulla.

❏ A pheochromocytoma secretes epinephrine and norepinephrine, resulting in hypertension and paroxysmal tachycardia.

❏ An endemic goiter is an iodine-deficient enlargement of the thyroid gland.

❏ Tumors of the adrenal medulla usually produce hypertension because they release excessive amounts of epinephrine and norepinephrine.

- ❏ The endocrine system consists of chemical transmitters called hormones and specialized cell clusters called glands.

- ❏ The hypothalamus controls temperature, respiration, blood pressure, thirst, hunger, and water balance.

- ❏ The functions of the hypothalamus affect the client's emotional states.

- ❏ The hypothalamus also produces hypothalamic-stimulating hormones, which affect the inhibition and release of pituitary hormones.

- ❏ Carpopedal spasm occurs as a result of hypocalcemia.

- ❏ Hyperglycemia is a result of low insulin levels.

- ❏ Clients with Cushing syndrome usually have a "moonface."

- ❏ A major adverse effect of corticosteroid therapy is a slowing of metabolism.

- ❏ Thyroidectomy may lead to hypoparathyroidism if the parathyroid is also removed during surgery.

- ❏ Hyperparathyroidism may cause serum calcium levels to rise.

- ❏ Steroid use induces calcium to leave bone, suppressing parathyroid hormone.

- ❏ A client with Addison disease needs more steroids than the body produces.

- ❏ A client being treated for adrenal crisis (addisonian crisis) should have serum sodium and potassium values monitored.

- ❏ Elevated serum glucose levels contribute to long-term effects of diabetes mellitus, such as coronary artery disease, hypertension, and peripheral vascular disease.

- ❏ Failure to maintain levothyroxine therapy can lead to a low body temperature.

- ❏ Balancing diet, exercise, and medication is essential to diabetes control in type 1, type 2, or gestational diabetes mellitus.

- ❏ Hypothyroidism slows the metabolic rate and mental responses, causing edema, decreased body temperature, and slower respiratory and heart rates.

- ❏ The predominant feature of syndrome of inappropriate antidiuretic hormone secretion is water retention with oliguria, edema, and weight gain.

## Integumentary system

- ❏ A burn injury causes a hypermetabolic state resulting in protein and lipid catabolism that affects wound healing.

- ❏ A deep partial-thickness burn causes necrosis of the epidermal and dermal layers.

- ❏ Necrotic, painful rashes are associated with the bite of a brown recluse spider.

- ❏ A bull's eye rash located primarily at the site of the bite is a classic sign of Lyme disease.

❑ Diffuse pruritic wheals are associated with an allergic reaction.

❑ The varicella-zoster virus causes herpes zoster.

❑ The papulovesicular lesions of varicella are distributed over the trunk, face, and scalp and don't follow a dermatome.

❑ A client with small, red, pruritic dots between his fingers and toes most likely has scabies.

❑ Petechiae are small macular lesions 1 to 3 mm in diameter.

❑ Ecchymosis is a purple-to brown bruise, macular or papular, and varied in size.

❑ Purpura are purple macular lesions larger than 1 cm.

❑ A diffuse rash usually has widely distributed scattered lesions.

❑ An annular rash is ring-shaped.

❑ The skin, hair, and nails make up the integumentary system, which serves as protection for the body's inner organs.

❑ The integumentary system helps regulate body temperature through the sweat glands.

❑ The integumentary system contains three types of glands: sebaceous, eccrine, and apocrine.

❑ Sebaceous, or oil, glands lubricate the hair and the epidermis and are stimulated by sex hormones.

❑ Eccrine sweat glands regulate body temperature through water secretion.

❑ Apocrine sweat glands are located in the axilla, nipple, anal, and pubic areas and secrete odorless fluid.

❑ The skin provides the first line of defense against microorganisms.

❑ The skin is composed of three layers: epidermis, dermis, and hypodermis.

❑ The epidermis, or outer layer of the skin, contains keratinocytes and melanocytes and acts as a protective barrier against the environment.

❑ The dermis, or middle layer of the skin, is a collagen layer that supports the epidermis, contains nerves and blood vessels, and is the origin of hair, nails, sebaceous glands, eccrine sweat glands, and apocrine sweat glands.

❑ The hypodermis, or third layer of the skin, is composed of loose connective tissue filled with fatty cells; it provides heat, insulation, and shock absorption and acts as a nutritional reservoir.

❑ The hypodermis, or third layer of the skin, is also known as subcutaneous tissue.

❑ Herpes zoster lesions are unilaterally clustered skin vesicles along peripheral sensory nerves on the trunk, thorax, or face that produce severe, deep pain.

❑ Hair is formed from keratin produced by matrix cells in the dermal layer of the skin.

❑ Nails are formed when epidermal cells are converted into hard plates of keratin.

❑ Dermatomal lesions form a line or an arch and follow a dermatome.

❑ A pustule is a small, pus-filled lesion (called a follicular pustule if it contains a hair).

❑ A cyst is a closed sac in or under the skin that contains fluid or semisolid material.

❑ A papule is a solid, raised lesion that's usually less than 1 cm in diameter.

❑ A vesicle is a small, fluid-filled blister that's usually 1 cm or less in diameter.

❑ A bulla is a large, fluid-filled blister that's usually 1 cm or more in diameter.

❑ An ulcer is a craterlike lesion of the skin that usually extends at least into the dermis.

❑ A macule is a small, discolored spot or patch on the skin.

❑ A wheal is a raised, reddish area that's commonly itchy and lasts 24 hours or less.

❑ A nodule is a raised lesion detectable by touch that's usually 1 cm or more in diameter.

❑ A fissure is a painful, cracklike lesion of the skin that extends at least into the dermis.

❑ Contact dermatitis is an inflammatory disorder that results from contact with an irritant.

❑ Tinea corporis, or ringworm, is characterized by round, red, scaly lesions that are accompanied by intense itching; lesions have slightly raised, red borders consisting of tiny vesicles.

❑ Pressure ulcers are localized areas of skin breakdown that occur as a result of prolonged pressure.

❑ In pressure ulcers, necrotic tissue develops because the vascular supply to the area is diminished.

❑ An unstageable pressure ulcer involves full-thickness tissue loss, with the base of the ulcer covered by slough and yellow, tan, gray, green, or brown eschar.

❑ A stage IV pressure ulcer involves full-thickness skin loss, with exposed muscle, bone, and tendon.

❑ A stage IV pressure ulcer may be accompanied by eschar, slough, undermining, and tunneling.

❑ A stage III pressure ulcer is a full-thickness wound with tissue loss and possibly visible subcutaneous tissue, but no exposed muscle, tendon, or bone.

❏ A stage III pressure ulcer may have slough, but not enough to hide the depth of tissue loss and may be accompanied by undermining and tunneling.

❏ A stage II pressure ulcer is a superficial partial-thickness wound that presents as a shallow, open ulcer without slough and with a red and pink wound bed.

❏ A stage I pressure ulcer involves intact skin that doesn't blanch and may differ in color from the surrounding area in people with darkly pigmented skin.

❏ A stage I pressure ulcer is usually found over a bony prominence and may be painful, firm or soft, and warmer or cooler than surrounding tissue.

❏ A suspected deep tissue injury involves maroon or purple intact skin or a blood-filled blister.

❏ A suspected deep tissue injury may be painful; mushy, firm, or boggy; and warmer or cooler than other tissue before discoloration occurs.

❏ Splinter hemorrhages are reddish brown narrow streaks under the nails that run in the same direction as nail growth and are caused by minor trauma but can also occur in clients with bacterial endocarditis.

❏ Muehrcke's lines, or leukonychia striata, are longitudinal white lines that can indicate trauma but may also be associated with metabolic stress, which impairs the body from using protein.

❏ A burn is the destruction of skin that causes loss of intracellular fluid and electrolytes.

❏ A burn is characterized by the extent (area) and depth of the burn.

❏ Most burns are a combination of thicknesses.

❏ A superficial partial-thickness burn (previously known as a first-degree burn) involves only the epidermal layer.

❏ A deep dermal partial-thickness burn (previously known as a second-degree burn) involves the epidermal and dermal layers.

❏ A full-thickness burn (previously known as third- and fourth-degree burns) involves epidermal, dermal, and subcutaneous layers, and nerve endings, muscle, and bone.

❏ Confluent lesions are touching or adjacent to each other.

❏ Linear rashes are lesions arranged in a line.

❏ Seborrhea is a chronic inflammatory dermatitis.

❏ Atopic dermatitis is a hereditary disorder associated with a family history of asthma, allergic rhinitis, or atopic dermatitis.

❑ Venereal warts appear on the genital mucosa and are confluent papules with rough surfaces.

❑ Candidiasis is a fungal infection of the skin or mucous membranes and is commonly found in the oral, vaginal, and intestinal mucosal tissue.

❑ Molluscum contagiosum is a viral skin infection with small, red, papular lesions.

❑ Tinea pedis is a superficial fungal infection on the feet, commonly called athlete's foot, that causes itching, sweating, and a foul odor.

❑ Psoriasis is characterized by thick, discolored nails with splintered hemorrhages that easily separate from the nail bed.

❑ Psoriasis also shows "ice pick" pits and ridges of the nail bed.

❑ A paronychia is a bacterial infection of the nail bed.

❑ Seborrhea is a chronic inflammatory dermatitis known as cradle cap.

❑ Scabies are mites that burrow under the skin, generally between the webbing of the fingers and toes.

❑ Cherry-red skin indicates exposure to high levels of carbon monoxide.

❑ Tinea capitis is a fungal infection of the scalp.

❑ Tinea corporis describes fungal infections of the body.

❑ Tinea cruris describes fungal infections of the inner thigh and inguinal creases.

❑ Escharotomy is a surgical incision used to relieve pressure from edema and is needed with circumferential burns that prevent chest expansion or cause circulatory compromise.

❑ During the first 48 hours after a burn, capillary permeability increases, allowing fluids to shift from the plasma to the interstitial spaces.

❑ Potassium also leaks from the cells into the plasma after a burn, causing hyperkalemia.

❑ The correct way to culture a wound is to roll the swab from the center of the wound outward.

❑ Irrigating the wound washes away drainage, debris, and many of the microorganisms colonizing or infecting the wound.

❑ When moving a client, lift, rather than slide, the client to avoid shearing.

❑ A client in bed for prolonged periods should be turned every 1 to 2 hours.

❑ The sun is the best-known and most common cause of basal cell epithelioma.

❑ Overhydration causes the skin to appear edematous and spongy.

❑ Normal skin turgor is dry and firm.

❏ Dehydration causes inelastic skin with tenting.

❏ Cold, moist towels help stop the burning process.

❏ According to the Rule of Nines, the posterior trunk, anterior trunk, and legs are each 18% of the total body surface.

❏ The head, neck, and arms are each 9% of total body surface according to the Rule of Nines.

❏ The perineum is 1% of total body surface according to the Rule of Nines.

❏ Burns in the adult client receiving burns to his back (18%) and one arm (9%) would total 27% of his body.

❏ Wounds should be cleaned from the most contaminated area to the least contaminated area; for example, from the center outward.

❏ Rings or donuts shouldn't be used for the wheelchair- or bed-bound client because they restrict circulation.

❏ In early burn care, the client's greatest need is fluid resuscitation because of large-volume fluid loss through the damaged skin.

❏ Fluid management is a priority in the early phase of burn care.

❏ Melanomas have an irregular shape, lack uniformity in color, and may appear brown or black with red, white, or blue areas.

❏ A shave biopsy removes only the first or second layer of skin, causing a superficial wound with no suture line and minimal scarring.

❏ For healing to occur, necrotic (dead) tissue must be removed from the wound; usually, this is done by debridement.

❏ Wound incision and drainage and wound culturing are done when infection is present or suspected.

❏ A keloid results from a defect in the healing process in which excess collagen develops at the healing site.

❏ Erosion refers to loss of part or the entire skin surface, usually from infection or pressure.

❏ Urticaria is commonly accompanied by a transient, elevated, solid, firm, irregularly shaped area of cutaneous edema, with a variable diameter.

❏ To maintain asepsis of a blistered area, the nurse should clean the area with normal saline solution and cover it with a dressing.

❏ Removing the raised skin of a blistered area would cause further skin damage.

❏ Cryosurgery leaves a wound resembling a burn, with swelling, blistering, and tenderness.

❏ Oozing and pain after cryosurgery suggest an infection.

# Maternal-Neonatal care

## Antepartum

❏ Antepartum care refers to care of a mother before childbirth.

❏ On bimanual examination, if the lower uterine segment is tapped sharply by the lower examining hand, the fetus can be felt to bounce (ballot) or rise in the amniotic fluid up against the top examining hand.

❏ Braxton Hicks contractions are painless uterine contractions that occur throughout pregnancy.

❏ Chadwick's sign, a probable sign of pregnancy, refers to the color of the vaginal walls, which change from normal light pink to deep violet.

❏ Goodell's sign, a probable sign of pregnancy, is softening of the cervix.

❏ Hegar's sign, a probable sign of pregnancy, is softening of the lower uterine segment, which may be present at 6 to 8 weeks' gestation.

❏ Intrauterine development of the fetus begins with gametogenesis, the production of specialized sex cells called gametes.

❏ The male gamete (spermatozoon) is produced in the seminiferous tubules of the testes during spermatogenesis.

❏ The female gamete (ovum) is produced in the graafian follicle of the ovary during oogenesis.

❏ As gametes mature, the number of chromosomes they contain is halved (through meiosis) from 46 to 23.

❏ Conception, or fertilization, occurs with the fusion of a spermatozoon and an ovum (oocyte) in the ampulla of the fallopian tube.

❏ The fertilized egg is called a zygote.

❏ The diploid number of chromosomes (a pair of each chromosome; 44 autosomes and 2 sex chromosomes) is restored when the zygote is formed.

❏ A male zygote is formed if the ovum is fertilized by a spermatozoon carrying a Y chromosome.

❏ A female zygote is formed if the ovum is fertilized by a spermatozoon carrying an X chromosome.

❏ Implantation occurs when the cellular wall of the blastocyst (trophoblast) implants itself in the endometrium of the anterior or posterior fundal region, about 7 to 9 days after fertilization.

❏ After implantation, the endometrium is called the decidua.

❏ The umbilical cord serves as the lifeline from the embryo to the placenta.

❑ At term, the umbilical cord measures from 20″ to 22″ (51 to 56 cm) in length and about ¾″ (2 cm) in diameter.

❑ The umbilical cord contains two arteries, one vein, and Wharton's jelly (which prevents kinking of the cord in utero).

❑ Blood flows through the umbilical cord at about 400 mL/minute.

❑ The fetal membranes include the chorion and the amnion.

❑ The chorion is the fetal membrane closest to the uterine wall; it gives rise to the placenta.

❑ The amnion is the thin, tough, inner fetal membrane that lines the amniotic sac.

❑ The embryonic germ layers include the ectoderm, endoderm, and mesoderm; they generate fetal tissue.

❑ The ectoderm generates the epidermis, nervous system, pituitary gland, salivary glands, optic lens, lining of the lower portion of the anal canal, hair, and tooth enamel.

❑ The endoderm generates the epithelial lining of the larynx, trachea, bladder, urethra, prostate gland, auditory canal, liver, pancreas, and alimentary canal.

❑ The mesoderm generates the connective and supporting tissues; the blood and vascular system; the musculature; teeth (except enamel); mesothelial lining of the pericardial, pleural, and peritoneal cavities; and kidneys and ureters.

❑ As the enlarging uterus increases pressure on the inferior vena cava, it compromises venous return, which can cause dizziness, light-headedness, and pallor when the client is supine.

❑ The nurse can relieve symptoms of dizziness, light-headedness, and pallor in the supine maternity client by turning the client on her left side, which relieves pressure on the vena cava and restores venous return.

❑ The amniotic fluid prevents heat loss, preserves constant fetal body temperature, cushions the fetus, and facilitates fetal growth and development.

❑ Amniotic fluid is replaced every 3 hours.

❑ When the fetus is in the breech position, fetal heart tones are best heard at or above the level of the umbilicus.

❑ Leopold's maneuvers can determine the fetal position.

❑ In twin-to-twin transfusion syndrome, the arterial circulation of one twin is in communication with the venous circulation of the other twin.

❑ In twin-to-twin transfusion syndrome, the recipient twin has polyhydramnios, becomes polycythemic, and often has heart failure due to circulatory overload while the donor becomes anemic.

❑ The recipient twin in twin-to-twin transfusion syndrome is usually large, whereas the donor twin is often small.

- ❏ A marginal placenta previa is characterized by implantation of the placenta in the margin of the cervical os, not covering the os.

- ❏ A low-lying placenta is implanted in the lower uterine segment but doesn't reach the cervical os.

- ❏ Placenta previa occurs when the placenta is implanted in the lower uterine segment.

- ❏ In a partial placenta previa, the placenta partially occludes the cervical os.

- ❏ In a total placenta previa, the internal cervical os is completely covered by the placenta.

- ❏ In clients with placenta previa, fetal surveillance through ultrasound examination every 2 to 3 weeks is indicated to evaluate fetal growth, amniotic fluid, and placental location.

- ❏ Antenatal steroids may be given to clients between 26 and 32 weeks' gestation to enhance fetal lung maturity.

- ❏ Ultrasound is the technique of choice in diagnosing a hydatidiform mole.

- ❏ As pregnancy advances, the apical pulse may be found slightly higher than the fourth intercostal space because uterine displacement of the diaphragm causes transverse and leftward rotation of the heart.

- ❏ The chorionic villi of a molar pregnancy resemble a "snowstorm" pattern on ultrasound.

- ❏ Bleeding with a hydatidiform mole is often dark brown and may occur erratically for weeks or months.

- ❏ Ectopic pregnancies must be considered in any sexually active woman of childbearing age who complains of menstrual irregularity, cramping, abdominal pain, and mild vaginal bleeding.

- ❏ A molar pregnancy generally would be detected before 34 weeks' gestation; no fetal heart sounds would be present.

- ❏ Human chorionic gonadotropin is a glycoprotein hormone produced in pregnancy that is made by the developing embryo after conception and later by the syncytiotrophoblast (part of the placenta).

- ❏ Human chorionic gonadotropin increases in a woman's blood and urine to fairly large concentrations until the 15th week of pregnancy.

- ❏ A pregnant woman breathes deeper, which increases the tidal volume of gas moved in and out of the respiratory tract with each breath.

- ❏ The expiratory volume and residual volume decrease as the pregnancy progresses.

- ❏ The inspiratory capacity increases during pregnancy.

- ❏ The oxygen consumption in the pregnant woman is 15% to 20% greater than in the nonpregnant state.

❑ Before amniocentesis, the client should void to empty the bladder, reducing the risk of bladder perforation.

❑ The client doesn't need to drink fluids before amniocentesis, nor does she need to fast.

❑ The client should be placed in a supine position for amniocentesis.

❑ Dizygotic twinning is influenced by age, increased maternal age, increased parity, and the use of fertility drugs, especially ovulation-inducing drugs.

❑ Hemoglobin and hematocrit values decrease during pregnancy as the increase in plasma volume exceeds the increase in red blood cell production.

❑ Clients with gestational diabetes are usually managed by diet alone to control their glucose intolerance.

❑ Long-acting insulin usually isn't needed for blood glucose control in the client with gestational diabetes.

❑ Oral hypoglycemic drugs are contraindicated in pregnancy.

❑ Glucagon raises blood glucose levels and is used to treat hypoglycemic reactions.

❑ The anticonvulsant mechanism of magnesium is believed to depress seizure foci in the brain and peripheral neuromuscular blockade; magnesium may be administered to pregnant clients with preeclampsia to prevent seizures.

❑ A contraction stress test measures the fetal response to uterine contractions.

❑ A sickle cell crisis during pregnancy is usually managed by exchange transfusion, oxygen, and I.V. fluids.

❑ Systolic murmurs are heard in up to 90% of pregnant clients; the murmur disappears soon after delivery.

❑ Despite the increases in intravascular volume and workload of the heart associated with pregnancy, heart failure isn't normal in pregnancy.

❑ The incidence of gestational trophoblastic disease (hydatidiform mole) is higher in women who are older than age 35 years, have low protein intake, or are of Asian heritage.

❑ Gestational trophoblastic disease (hydatidiform mole) should be suspected in clients who have bleeding during the first half of pregnancy, hyperemesis, hypertension disorders of pregnancy, absent fetal heart tones, and enlarged uterus for the time of pregnancy.

❑ A magnesium serum level of 8 to 10 mEq/L may cause absent reflexes, serum levels of 10 to 12 mEq/L may cause respiratory depression, and a serum level of greater than 15 mEq/L may result in respiratory paralysis. Decreased urine output may occur in clients receiving I.V. magnesium and should be monitored closely to keep urine output at greater than 30 ml/hour because magnesium is excreted through the kidneys and can easily accumulate to toxic levels.

❏ $Rh_o(D)$ immune globulin is given to women with Rh-negative blood to prevent antibody formation from Rh-positive conceptions.

❏ A positive purified protein derivative (PPD) result is an indurated wheal more than 10 mm in diameter that appears in 48 to 72 hours.

❏ Complaints of fever, nausea, vomiting, malaise, unilateral flank pain, and costovertebral angle tenderness indicate acute pyelonephritis.

❏ Acute pyelonephritis is a serious condition in a pregnant client.

❏ Clients with placenta previa or a prior classical cesarean delivery shouldn't be given a trial of labor due to the risk of uterine rupture or severe bleeding.

❏ When assessing a pregnant client, remember that, although the mother and fetus have separate and distinct needs, they have an interdependent relationship; factors that influence the mother's health can also affect the fetus, and changes in fetal well-being can influence the mother's physical and emotional health.

❏ Use Leopold's maneuvers to determine fetal position, presentation, and attitude.

❏ To perform the first of Leopold's maneuvers, place your hands over the patient's abdomen and curl your fingers around the fundus.

❏ When the fetus is in the vertex position (head first), the buttocks should feel irregularly shaped and firm.

❏ When the fetus is in the breech position, the head should feel hard, round, and completely moveable.

❏ To perform the second of Leopold's maneuvers, move your hands down the side of the abdomen, applying gentle pressure.

❏ If the fetus is in the vertex position, you'll feel a smooth, hard surface on one side—the fetal back—and on the opposite side, you'll feel lumps and knobs—the knees, hands, feet, and elbows.

❏ If the fetus is in the breech position, you may not feel the back at all.

❏ To perform the third of Leopold's maneuvers, spread your thumb and fingers of one hand and place them just above the patient's symphysis pubis and then bring your fingers together.

❏ If the fetus is in the vertex position and hasn't descended, you'll feel the head.

❏ If the fetus is in the vertex position and has descended, you'll feel a less distinct mass.

❏ If the fetus is in the breech position, you'll feel a less distinct mass, which could be the feet or knees.

❑ The fourth of Leopold's maneuvers will help you to determine flexion or extension of the fetal head and neck.

❑ To perform the fourth of Leopold's maneuvers, place your hands on both sides of the lower abdomen and gently apply pressure with your fingers as you slide downward toward the symphysis pubis.

❑ If the head is the presenting part, one of your hands will be stopped by the cephalic prominence.

❑ If the fetus is in the vertex position, you'll feel the cephalic prominence on the same side as the back.

❑ Rh isoimmunization occurs when Rh-positive fetal blood cells cross into the maternal circulation and stimulate maternal antibody production.

❑ In subsequent pregnancies with Rh-positive fetuses, maternal antibodies may cross back into the fetal circulation and destroy the fetal blood cells in Rh isoimmunization.

❑ Gravida refers to the number of times a woman has been pregnant.

❑ Para refers to the number of viable children born after 20 weeks' gestation.

❑ A woman with a history of diabetes has an increased risk for perinatal complications, including hypertension, preeclampsia, and neonatal hypoglycemia.

❑ Tocolytics are used to stop labor contractions.

❑ The most common adverse effect associated with the use of tocolytics is pulmonary edema.

❑ Oxytocin is the hormone responsible for stimulating uterine contractions.

❑ The weight of the pregnant uterus is sufficiently heavy to compress the vena cava, which could impair blood flow to the uterus, possibly decreasing oxygen to the fetus.

❑ The side-lying position prevents compression of the vena cava.

❑ Eating small, frequent meals will place less pressure on the esophageal sphincter, reducing the likelihood of the regurgitation of stomach contents into the lower esophagus.

❑ The incidence of preeclampsia in obese clients is about seven times greater than that in nonobese pregnant clients.

❑ A nonstress test is based on the theory that a healthy fetus will have transient fetal heart rate accelerations with fetal movement.

❑ Serial ultrasounds will detect intrauterine growth retardation and oligohydramnios in a fetus.

❑ Recommended fasting blood sugar levels in pregnant clients with diabetes are 60 to 90 mg/dl.

❏ The nonstress test is the preferred antepartum heart rate screening test for pregnant clients with diabetes.

❏ A reactive nonstress test is two or more fetal heart rate accelerations that exceed the baseline by at least 15 beats/minute and that last longer than 15 seconds within a 20-minute period.

❏ Fluttering in the abdomen, also called quickening, begins between 16 and 22 weeks' gestation and is caused by fetal movement.

❏ The dilated arterioles that occur during pregnancy are due to the elevated level of circulating estrogen and are called telangiectasias.

❏ The linea nigra is a pigmented line extending from the symphysis pubis to the top of the fundus during pregnancy.

❏ Striae gravidarum, or stretch marks, are slightly depressed streaks that commonly occur over the abdomen, breast, and thighs during the second half of pregnancy.

❏ The calcium requirement for pregnancy is 1300 mg/day; over-the-counter supplements aren't always safe and should be specifically recommended by the health care practitioner.

❏ During pregnancy there is a slight increase (2 breaths/minute) in respiratory rate.

❏ Heart rate may increase up to 15 beats/minute by the end of pregnancy.

❏ Systolic and diastolic pressures may decrease by 5 to 10 mm Hg by the end of pregnancy.

❏ The transverse diameter, also known as the ischial tuberosity diameter, is the distance between the ischial tuberosities.

❏ The transverse diameter is the one diameter that commonly leads to problems with delivery.

❏ A gynecoid pelvis is ideal for childbirth.

❏ A gynecoid pelvis is characterized by well-rounded inlets and wide forward and backward diameters and pubic arch.

❏ An android pelvis is characterized by extremely narrow lower dimensions of the pelvis (the pelvic arch forms an acute triangle).

❏ An android pelvis is most common in males but can occur in females and may cause difficulty delivering a fetus because of the narrow shape.

❏ An anthropoid pelvis, also known as an apelike pelvis, is characterized by a narrow transverse diameter and a larger-than-normal inlet and anteroposterior diameter.

❏ An anthropoid pelvis doesn't accommodate the fetal head well because the transverse diameter is narrow.

❑ A platypelloid pelvis, also known as a flattened pelvis, has an oval, smoothly curved inlet but shallow anteroposterior diameter.

❑ A platypelloid pelvis can cause problems during childbirth with rotation of the fetal head.

❑ Fetal presentation refers to the relationship of the fetus to the cervix.

❑ Fetal presentation is assessed through vaginal examination, abdominal inspection and palpation, sonography, or auscultation of fetal heart tones.

❑ Fetal presentation indicates which part of the fetus will pass through the cervix first during birth.

❑ Cephalic fetal présentations include vertex, brow, sinciput, and mentum.

❑ Fetal position is the relationship of the presenting part of the fetus to a specific quadrant of the mother's pelvis.

❑ Fetal position influences the progression of labor and helps determine whether surgical intervention is needed.

❑ Fetal position is defined using three or four letters.

❑ The first letter used to define fetal position designates whether the presenting part is facing the mother's right (R) or left (L) side.

❑ The middle letter(s) refers to the presenting part of the fetus: the occiput (O), mentum (M), sacrum (Sa), or scapula or acromion process (A).

❑ The last letter designates whether the presenting part is pointing to the anterior (A), posterior (P), or transverse (T) section of the mother's pelvis.

❑ Narrowing of the birth canal at the inlet, midpelvis, or outlet causes a disproportion between the size of the fetal head and the pelvic diameters, or cephalopelvic disproportion.

❑ Cephalopelvic disproportion results in failure of labor to progress.

❑ With a twin or other multiple pregnancy, the fetuses can be in several presentation combinations; both vertex, both breech, one vertex and one in transverse lie, or one vertex and one breech.

❑ The white blood cell count rises in pregnancy and may range from 10,000 to 12,000/µl.

❑ Gestational diabetes is diagnosed if, on a 3-hour glucose tolerance test, the 1-hour glucose level is 140 mg/dL or greater, the 2-hour glucose level is 165 mg/dL or greater, or the 3-hour glucose level is 145 mg/dL or greater.

❑ In the GTPAL system, T indicates the number of term neonates born at 37 weeks' gestation or after; P, the number of preterm neonates born before 37 weeks' gestation; A, the number of pregnancies ending with spontaneous or therapeutic abortion; and L, the number of children currently living.

❑ A history of hypertension predisposes the client for developing abruptio placentae.

❑ The blood pressure, urine, and weight and fundal height are monitored during prenatal visits.

❑ When findings suggest that the client is experiencing abruptio placentae, fetal heart tones should immediately be assessed to determine fetal well-being.

❑ Leg cramps, ankle edema, and shortness of breath are normal during the second and third trimesters.

❑ Nausea and vomiting should subside by the end of the first trimester; if they don't, the nurse should suspect an undiagnosed problem, such as hyperemesis gravidarum or emotional factors that may be exacerbating the nausea and vomiting.

❑ Increased vaginal discharge generally occurs during the first trimester and decreases at the end of this period.

❑ At 20 weeks' gestation, fundal height should be at about the umbilicus.

❑ Fundal height should be measured from the symphysis pubis to the top of the uterus.

❑ Serial measurements of the fundus assess fetal growth over the course of the pregnancy.

❑ Between weeks 18 and 34, the fundal height as measured in centimeters correlates roughly with the week of gestation.

## Intrapartum

❑ Intrapartum care refers to care of the client during labor.

❑ Fetal attitude refers to the relationship of the fetal parts (such as the chest, chin, or arms) to one another during the passage through the birth canal.

❑ The fetal head may be in a flexed (chin-to-chest) or extended (head-to-back) position.

❑ Pressure exerted by the maternal pelvis and birth canal during labor and delivery causes the sutures of the skull to allow the cranial bones to shift, resulting in molding of the fetal head.

❑ During labor, cervical dilation and effacement occur.

❑ Cervical dilation is the increasing of the size of the cervical os from 0 to 10 cm.

❑ Cervical effacement is cervical thinning and shortening, which is measured from 0% (thick) to 100% (paper thin).

❑ Fetal station is the relationship of the fetal presenting part to the pelvic ischial spines; 0 station when the presenting part is even with the ischial spines; −3, −2, or −1 when the presenting part is above the ischial spines; and +3, +2, or +1 when the presenting part is below the ischial spines.

❑ Phases of uterine contractions include increment (buildup and longest phase), acme (peak of the contraction), and decrement (letting-down phase).

❑ Contractions are measured by duration, frequency, and intensity.

❑ Contraction duration is measured from the beginning of the increment of the contraction to the end of the decrement of the contraction and averages 30 seconds early in labor and 60 seconds later in labor.

❑ Contraction frequency is measured from the beginning of one contraction to the beginning of the next and averages 5 to 30 minutes apart early in labor, and 2 to 3 minutes apart later in labor.

❑ Contraction intensity is assessed during the acme phase and can be measured with an intrauterine catheter or by palpation.

❑ The first stage of labor is measured from the onset of true labor to complete dilation of the cervix, which lasts from 6 to 18 hours in a primiparous client and from 2 to 10 hours in a multiparous client.

❑ There are three phases of the first stage of labor: latent, active, and transitional.

❑ During the latent phase of the first stage of labor, the cervix is dilated 0 to 3 cm, contractions are irregular, and cervical effacement is almost complete.

❑ During the latent phase of the first stage of labor, the client may experience anticipation, excitement, or apprehension.

❑ During the active phase of the first stage of labor, the cervix is dilated 4 to 7 cm, cervical effacement is complete, and contractions are about 5 to 8 minutes apart and last 45 to 60 seconds with moderate to strong intensity.

❑ During the transitional phase of the first stage of labor, the cervix is dilated 8 to 10 cm, and contractions are about 1 to 2 minutes apart and last 60 to 90 seconds with strong intensity.

❑ The second stage of labor extends from complete dilation to delivery and lasts an average of 40 minutes (20 contractions) for the primiparous client and 20 minutes (10 contractions) for the multiparous client.

❑ The fetus's head is considered to be engaged when the biparietal diameter passes the pelvic inlet.

❑ The movement of the fetal presenting part through the pelvis is called descent.

❑ The third stage of labor extends from birth of the neonate to expulsion of the placenta and lasts from 5 to 30 minutes.

❑ The fourth stage of labor is 1 to 4 hours after birth.

❑ As the fetus moves through the birth canal, it goes through position changes to ensure that the smallest diameter of fetal head presents to the smallest diameter of the birth canal.

❑ Termed the cardinal mechanisms or movements of labor, these position changes occur in the following sequence: descent, flexion, internal rotation, extension, external rotation, and expulsion.

❑ Meconium in a breech presentation may be caused by compression of the fetus's intestinal tract during descent.

❑ Meconium in the amniotic fluid is a sign of fetal distress in a cephalic presentation and isn't a normal finding, even during a prolonged delivery.

❑ Yellow-stained amniotic fluid is a sign of a possible blood incompatibility between fetus and mother and is due to bilirubin from the breakdown of red blood cells.

❑ Fetal tachycardia and excessive fetal activity are the first signs of fetal hypoxia.

❑ During a vaginal examination of a client in labor, if the nurse palpates the fetus's larger, diamond-shaped fontanel toward the anterior portion of the patient's pelvis, the fetal position is occiput posterior.

❑ Occiput posterior position of the fetus commonly produces intense back pain during labor.

❑ Positioning the client on her side can facilitate the rotation to occiput anterior position.

❑ The client should be placed on her left side or sitting upright, with her shoulders parallel and legs slightly flexed, for an epidural block.

❑ The patient's back shouldn't be flexed for an epidural block because this position increases the possibility that the dura may be punctured and the anesthetic will accidentally be given as spinal, not epidural, anesthesia.

❑ Dehydration is indicated by dry mucous membranes and decreased skin turgor.

❑ A normal fetal heart rate is 120 to 160 beats/minute.

❑ A vertex presentation (flexion of the fetal head) is the optimal presentation for passage through the birth canal.

❑ A frank breech presentation occurs when the buttocks present first.

❑ Posterior positioning of the fetal head can make it difficult for the head to pass under the maternal symphysis pubis bone.

❑ Approximately 40% of a woman's cardiac output is delivered to the uterus; therefore, blood loss can occur quite rapidly in the event of uncontrolled bleeding.

❑ Accelerations in the fetal heart rate strip indicate good oxygenation, whereas decelerations in the fetal heart rate sometimes indicate poor fetal oxygenation.

❑ Labor progress can be directly assessed only through cervical examination.

❑ One of the major adverse effects of epidural administration is hypotension.

❑ Placenta accreta is the abnormal attachment of the placenta to the myometrium of the uterus.

❑ Placenta percreta occurs when the villi of the placenta penetrate the myometrium to the serosa level.

❑ Confirmation of ruptured amniotic membranes is done with nitrazine paper and a positive ferning test.

❑ With premature rupture of membranes in a client under 37 weeks' gestation, cervical examinations are contraindicated to reduce the incidence of infection.

❑ True contractions begin irregularly but become regular and predictable, increasing in frequency and intensity, causing cervical effacement and dilation.

❑ True contractions are felt initially in the lower back and radiate to the abdomen in a wavelike motion.

❑ As part of the history, asking about the patient's most recent blood glucose levels will indicate how well her diabetes has been controlled.

❑ When the umbilical cord precedes the fetal presenting part, it's known as a prolapsed cord.

❑ The client with a prolapsed cord should not push with the next contraction because it would force the presenting part against the cord, causing severe bradycardia and possible fetal demise.

❑ Performing a cervical examination in a possible placenta previa or abruptio placentae is contraindicated because any agitation of the cervix can result in hemorrhage and death for the mother or fetus.

❑ A complaint of rectal pressure usually indicates a low presenting fetal part, signaling imminent delivery.

❑ The nurse's priority when an amniotomy is performed on a client in labor is to assess fetal heart tones.

❑ When the amniotic membrane is ruptured, the umbilical cord may enter the birth canal with the gush of fluid and the presenting part may cause cord compression.

❑ After amniotomy, contractions may intensify.

❑ When the placenta covers the cervical os, it's called placenta previa.

❑ Premature rupture of membranes is the rupture of membranes beyond 37 weeks' gestation but before the onset of labor.

❑ Late fetal heart rate decelerations are due to uteroplacental insufficiency from decreased blood flow during uterine contractions.

❑ Variable decelerations are an indication of cord compression.

❑ A variable fetal heart rate deceleration is an abrupt decrease of 15 beats per minute or greater, lasting 15 seconds or more, and less than 2 minutes in duration.

❑ Baseline fetal heart rate (FHR) variability refers to fluctuations in the baseline FHR that are irregular in amplitude and frequency.

❑ Baseline fetal heart rate variability that is absent means the amplitude range is undetectable.

❑ Baseline fetal heart rate variability that is minimal means the amplitude range is detectable by 5 beats/minute or fewer.

❑ A baseline fetal heart rate variability that is moderate, or normal, means the amplitude range is 6 to 25 beats/minute.

❑ A baseline fetal heart rate variability that is marked means the amplitude range is greater than 25 beats/minute.

❑ A prolonged deceleration of the fetal heart rate is a visually apparent decrease from the baseline that is 15 beats/minute or more, lasting 2 minutes or more but less than 10 minutes.

❑ Baseline fetal tachycardia is a fetal heart rate greater than 160 beats/minute.

❑ Baseline fetal bradycardia is a fetal heart rate less than 110 beats/minute.

❑ Women with severe preeclampsia may develop HELLP syndrome (H = hemolysis; EL = elevated liver enzymes; LP = low platelet count).

❑ Gestational hypertension refers to elevated blood pressure without proteinuria in a woman after 20 weeks' gestation; blood pressure levels return to normal in these clients postpartum.

❑ Preeclampsia is a syndrome defined by hypertension and proteinuria that may be associated with other signs and symptoms, such as edema, visual disturbances, headache, and epigastric pain.

❑ Criteria for diagnosing preeclampsia include a blood pressure of 140 mm Hg systolic or higher or 90 mm Hg diastolic or higher that occurs after 20 weeks' gestation in a woman with previously normal blood pressure, as well as the presence of proteinuria, defined as urinary excretion of 0.3 g of protein or higher in a 24-hour urine specimen.

❑ If a fetal heart rate deceleration lasts longer than 10 minutes, it is considered a baseline change.

❑ A late deceleration is a visually apparent, usually symmetrical gradual decrease and return of the fetal heart rate associated with a uterine contraction lasting 30 seconds or more.

❑ In umbilical prolapse, the protruding umbilical cord should never be pushed back into the uterus because this could damage the cord, obstruct the flow of blood through the cord to the fetus, or introduce infection into the uterus.

❑ With Nägele's rule, after determining the first day of the last menstrual period, subtract 3 months and add 7 days to calculate the estimated date of birth.

❑ Heart rate, respiratory effort, muscle tone, reflex irritability, and color of the neonate are assessed to measure the Apgar score.

❑ Each of the signs in the Apgar score is assigned a score of 0, 1, or 2 with the highest possible total score being a 10.

❑ The relationship of the long axis of the fetus to the long axis of the mother refers to fetal lie.

❑ There are three possible fetal lies: longitudinal, transverse, and oblique.

❑ During pregnancy of a diabetic patient, the fetus secretes high levels of insulin to counteract the high maternal glucose levels, resulting in severe hypoglycemia after birth.

❑ In a right occiput anterior position, the fetus' occiput points to the maternal right posterior quadrant.

❑ Oligohydramnios (less than the normal amount of amniotic fluid) may be associated with variable decelerations.

❑ Hydramnios (excessive amniotic fluid) may be associated with uterine rupture.

## Postpartum

❑ Prolactin is the hormone responsible for milk production.

❑ Postpartum women are at increased risk of deep vein thrombosis because of changes in clotting mechanisms to control bleeding at delivery.

❑ Kegel exercises result in increased blood flow, which brings oxygen and other nutrients to the perineal area to aid in healing.

❑ Twelve hours after delivery, the fundus should be 1 cm above or at the level of the umbilicus.

❑ When the placenta invades the myometrium, it's called placenta increta.

❑ The breasts normally produce colostrum for the first few days after delivery.

❑ Milk production begins 1 to 3 days postpartum.

❑ By the third day postpartum, the fundus should be 3 cm below the umbilicus.

❑ The fundus will continue to descend about 1 cm/day until it isn't palpable above the symphysis pubis (about 9 days after delivery).

❑ The uterus shrinks to its prepregnancy size by 5 to 6 weeks after delivery.

❑ A firm uterus helps control postpartum hemorrhage by clamping down on uterine blood vessels.

❑ Lochia is the discharge from the sloughing of the uterine decidua.

❑ Lochia rubra is the vaginal discharge that occurs for the first 2 to 3 days after delivery; it has a fleshy odor and is bloody with small clots.

❑ Lochia serosa refers to the vaginal discharge that occurs during days 3 through 9 postpartum; it is pinkish or brown with a serosanguineous consistency and fleshy odor.

❑ Lochia alba is a yellow to white discharge that usually begins about 10 days after delivery; it may last from 2 to 6 weeks.

❑ A full bladder may displace the uterine fundus to the left or right side of the abdomen.

❑ Because human immunodeficiency virus (HIV) can be transmitted to the baby through breast milk, the HIV-positive client shouldn't breast-feed. The client with postpartum hemorrhage should be placed in Trendelenburg's position to prevent or control hypovolemic shock.

❑ For the client with postpartum hemorrhage, vital signs should be monitored continuously or at least every 10 to 15 minutes, until the client's condition stabilizes.

❑ The client with type 1 diabetes mellitus whose delivery was complicated by polyhydramnios and macrosomia is at risk for a postpartum hemorrhage from the overdistention of the uterus.

❑ The diabetic mother usually has decreased insulin needs for the first few days postpartum.

❑ Mastitis is an infection of the breast characterized by flulike symptoms, along with redness and tenderness in the breast.

❑ Measures that the client with mastitis should follow include breast-feeding on the affected side first, drinking plenty of fluids, and completely emptying the affected breast with each feeding, expressing milk by hand or using a pump, if necessary.

❑ Postpartum hemorrhage involves blood loss in excess of 500 ml.

❑ Most delayed postpartum hemorrhages occur between the fourth and ninth days postpartum.

❑ The most frequent causes of a delayed postpartum hemorrhage include retained placental fragments, intrauterine infection, and fibroids.

❑ A focused physical assessment should be performed every 15 minutes for the first 1 to 2 hours postpartum, including assessment of the fundus, lochia, perineum, blood pressure, pulse, and bladder function.

❑ Postpartum insulin requirements are usually significantly lower than prepregnancy requirements; occasionally, diabetic clients may require little to no insulin during the first 24 to 48 hours postpartum.

❑ Bleeding is considered heavy when a woman saturates a sanitary pad in 1 hour.

❑ Excessive bleeding occurs when a postpartum woman saturates a pad in 15 minutes.

❑ Moderate bleeding occurs when the bleeding saturates less than 6 inches (15 cm) of a pad in 1 hour.

❑ A positive Coombs' test means that the Rh-negative woman is now producing antibodies to the Rh-positive blood of the neonate.

❑ The most common cause of mastitis is *Staphylococcus aureus*, transmitted from the neonate's mouth.

❑ Group beta-hemolytic streptococci, or GBS infection, is associated with neonatal sepsis and death.

❑ During the taking-hold phase, which usually lasts from days 3 to 10 postpartum, the mother strives for independence and autonomy; she also becomes curious and interested in the care of the baby and is most ready to learn.

❑ During the taking-in phase, which usually lasts 2 to 3 days, the mother is passive and dependent and expresses her own needs rather than the neonate's needs.

❑ During this taking-in phase, the client may ask the nurse to help her with self-care, wants to talk about the birth experience, and lets others make decisions for her.

❑ A mother experiencing postpartum blues may say she feels empty now that the infant is no longer in her uterus.

❑ A mother experiencing postpartum blues may verbalize that she feels unprotected now.

❑ Continuous seepage of blood may be due to cervical or vaginal lacerations if the uterus is firm and contracting.

❑ Retained placental fragments and uterine atony may cause subinvolution of the uterus, making it soft, boggy, and larger than expected.

❑ Shortness of breath in the client on anticoagulant therapy for deep vein thrombosis should be reported immediately because it may be a symptom of pulmonary embolism.

❑ TORCH is an acronym for a group of diseases that cause congenital conditions if a fetus is exposed to them when in the uterus and include: Toxoplasmosis; Others, such as gonorrhea, syphilis, varicella, hepatitis, and human immunodeficiency virus; Rubella; Cytomegalovirus; and Herpes simplex virus.

❑ When a nurse is assessing the fundus of a postpartum client and finds that the fundus is boggy, the nurse should first massage the uterus to stimulate it to contract.

❑ When breast-feeding after a cesarean birth, the client should be encouraged to use the football hold to avoid incisional discomfort.

❑ Breast-feeding should be initiated as soon after birth as possible.

❑ The mother should be encouraged to breast-feed her infant every 2 to 3 hours throughout the night as well as during the day to increase the milk supply.

❑ The nipples should be allowed to air dry after breast-feeding to keep them dry and prevent irritation.

❑ Only water should be used to wash the nipples because soap removes natural oils and dries out the nipples.

❏ When breast-feeding, the baby should grasp both the nipple and areola with his mouth.

❏ Postpartum depression occurs in approximately 10% to 15% of all postpartum women.

❏ Postpartum depression is characterized by disabling feelings of inadequacy and an inability to cope that can last up to 3 years.

❏ The client is often tearful and despondent with postpartum depression.

❏ The client with postpartum blues experiences crying and sadness, generally between 3 to 5 days postpartum, but this condition resolves itself quickly.

❏ Postpartum neurosis includes neurotic behavior during the initial 6 weeks after birth.

❏ Postpartum psychosis includes hallucinations, delusions, and phobias.

❏ Cervical or perineal lacerations can cause an immediate postpartum hemorrhage.

❏ A client with a clotting deficiency may have an immediate postpartum hemorrhage if the deficiency isn't corrected at the time of delivery.

❏ The rubella virus isn't transmitted into breast milk, so the client may continue to breast-feed after vaccination.

❏ Because magnesium sulfate relaxes smooth muscle and can increase the risk of postpartum hemorrhage, the uterus should be assessed for uterine atony in a client who experienced preeclampsia.

❏ Ice should only be applied to the perineum for the first 24 hours after delivery.

❏ The client should cleanse the perineal area after urinating or a bowel movement using a spray or peri-bottle.

❏ The client should wipe from front to back after urination or a bowel movement to avoid contaminating the perineal area.

❏ Perineal pads should be changed when they are soiled to keep the perineum clean.

❏ Multiparous women often experience a loss of uterine tone due to frequent distention of the uterus from past pregnancies and are at a higher risk for postpartum hemorrhage.

❏ During the taking-in phase, the mother is concerned with her own needs and requires support from staff and relatives.

❏ The letting-go phase begins several weeks later, when the mother incorporates the new infant into the family unit.

❏ The taking-hold phase occurs when the mother is ready to take responsibility for her own care as well as her infant's.

❏ Women who deliver twins are at a higher risk for postpartum hemorrhage due to overdistention of the uterus, which causes uterine atony.

❑ In the early postpartum period, the glomerular filtration rate rises and progesterone levels drop, resulting in rapid diuresis.

❑ Urine retention causes a distended bladder to displace the uterus above the umbilicus and to the side, which prevents the uterus from contracting.

❑ "Postpartum blues"—a transient mood alteration that arises during the first 3 weeks postpartum and is typically self-limiting— affects 50% to 80% of postpartum clients.

❑ A more severe mood alteration, seen in approximately 20% of clients, involves changes that occur within a few days after delivery and may last for a few days to more than 1 year.

❑ Administering $Rh_o(D)$ immune globulin to the client within 72 hours of delivery prevents antibodies from forming that can destroy fetal blood cells in the next pregnancy.

❑ $Rh_o(D)$ immune globulin isn't given to the baby.

❑ The breast-feeding client should consume an additional 500 calories/day, increase protein intake, and eat foods high in vitamins and minerals.

❑ Retained placental fragments, which prevent the uterus from contracting properly, increase postpartum blood loss.

❑ Sitz baths help decrease inflammation and tension in the perineal area.

❑ The uterus should be felt at the level of the umbilicus from 1 hour after birth and for about the next 24 hours.

❑ Sudden dyspnea, along with diaphoresis and confusion, are classic symptoms that develop when a thrombus (stationary blood clot) from a varicose vein becomes an embolus (moving clot) that lodges in the pulmonary circulation.

❑ Talking, cooing, and cuddling are positive signs of mother-infant attachment.

❑ Eye contact, touching, and speaking help establish attachment with a neonate.

❑ Feeding a neonate is an important role of a new mother and facilitates attachment.

❑ Encouraging the father to hold the neonate will facilitate attachment.

## Neonatal period

❑ Studies have proven that breast milk provides preterm neonates with better protection from infection, such as necrotizing enterocolitis, because of the antibodies contained in the milk.

❑ Commercial formula doesn't provide any better nutrition than breast milk.

❑ Breast milk feedings can be started as soon as the neonate is stable.

❑ Surfactant works by reducing surface tension in the lung and allows the lung to remain slightly expanded, decreasing the amount of work required for inspiration.

- Acrocyanosis, a normal finding also called peripheral cyanosis, is a bluish discoloration of the hands and feet in the neonate and shouldn't last more than 24 hours after birth.

- The supine position is recommended for the neonate to reduce the risk of sudden infant death syndrome in infancy (put the baby *"back"* to sleep).

- Neonates of mothers with diabetes are at risk for hypoglycemia due to increased insulin levels because the neonate's liver can't initially adjust to the changing glucose levels after birth.

- Bronchopulmonary dysplasia is a complication common in neonates who receive prolonged mechanical ventilation at birth.

- Esophageal atresia is a structural defect in which the esophagus and trachea communicate with each other.

- Soft, smooth skin in a neonate is a sign of adequate hydration.

- A sunken fontanel and no urine output in the first 24 hours of life are signs of poor hydration.

- A positive Babinski's sign is present in infants until approximately age 1.

- The appearance of "sunset" eyes, in which the sclera is visible above the iris, results from cranial nerve palsies and may indicate increased intracranial pressure.

- A neonate's pupils normally react to light in the same way as an adult's.

- Hepatitis B immune globulin should be given within 12 hours to a neonate born to a woman infected with hepatitis B.

- Eye prophylaxis is administered to the neonate immediately or soon after birth to prevent ophthalmia neonatorum.

- The neonate with an ABO blood incompatibility with its mother would have a positive Coombs' test result and will have jaundice within the first 24 hours of life.

- Jaundice after the first 24 hours of life is called physiologic jaundice.

- Preterm birth is the single most important risk factor for developing respiratory distress syndrome.

- A yellow-white exudate around the head of the neonate's penis 2 days after circumcision is a normal finding. It is part of the granulation process for a healing penis after circumcision; it shouldn't be removed.

- Postdate fetuses lose the vernix caseosa, and the epidermis may become desquamated.

- The small-for-gestational age neonate is at risk for developing polycythemia due to chronic hypoxia during intrauterine life.

- The small-for-gestational age neonate is at risk for hypoglycemia and hypothermia due to decreased glycogen stores.

❑ Temperature instability, especially when it results in a low temperature in the neonate, may be a sign of infection.

❑ The neonate's color commonly changes with an infectious process and generally becomes ashen or mottled.

❑ The neonate with an infection will usually show a decrease in activity level or lethargy.

❑ A respiratory rate of 40 to 60 breaths/minute is normal for a neonate during the transitional period.

❑ Nasal flaring and audible grunting are signs of respiratory distress in a neonate.

❑ An Apgar score of 5 or less indicates a need for resuscitative efforts.

❑ A neonate experiencing drug withdrawal should be swaddled to prevent him from flailing and stimulating himself; he should be moved to a quiet area of the nursery to minimize environmental stimuli.

❑ Medications, such as phenobarbital, should be given as needed to neonates experiencing drug withdrawal.

❑ Neonates of mothers with diabetes are at increased risk for macrosomia (excessive fetal growth) as a result of the combination of the increased supply of maternal glucose and an increase in fetal insulin.

❑ Along with macrosomia, neonates of diabetic mothers are at risk for respiratory distress syndrome, hypoglycemia, hypocalcemia, hyperbilirubinemia, and congenital anomalies.

❑ Microcephaly is usually the result of congenital cytomegalovirus or congenital rubella virus infection.

❑ Neonates have coagulation deficiencies because of a lack of organisms that help produce vitamin K in the intestines, which helps the liver synthesize clotting factors II, VII, IX, and X.

❑ Convection heat loss is the flow of heat from the body surface to cooler air.

❑ Conduction is the loss of heat from the body surface to cooler surfaces in direct contact.

❑ Evaporation is the loss of heat that occurs when a liquid is converted to a vapor.

❑ Radiation is the loss of heat from the body surface to cooler solid surfaces not in direct contact but in relative proximity.

❑ Hyperbilirubinemia is caused almost exclusively by unconjugated bilirubin.

❑ Jaundice usually appears in a cephalocaudal progression from head to feet.

❑ Caput succedaneum is a boggy edematous swelling present at birth that crosses the suture line; it most commonly occurs in the occipital area and usually resolves within 3 to 4 days.

❑ A cephalhematoma is a collection of blood between the skull and periosteum that doesn't cross cranial suture lines and resolves in 3 to 6 weeks.

❑ The neonate's eyes and genitalia must be covered with eye patches to prevent damage from phototherapy for hyperbilirubinemia.

❑ The temperature of a neonate receiving phototherapy should be monitored at least every 2 to 4 hours because of the risk of hyperthermia with phototherapy.

❑ Neonates of Rh-negative mothers tend to have hyperbilirubinemia.

❑ Low Apgar scores may indicate a risk for hyperbilirubinemia.

❑ *Escherichia coli, Klebsiella,* and *Pseudomonas aeruginosa* species are gram-negative rods that produce 78% to 85% of bacterial infections in neonates.

❑ Transmission of group B beta-hemolytic streptococci to the fetus results in respiratory distress that can rapidly lead to septic shock.

❑ *Escherichia coli* is the second most common cause of neonatal sepsis.

❑ Candidiasis may be acquired from the birth canal and causes infection that may manifest in the neonate more than 24 hours after birth.

❑ *Chlamydia trachomatis* infection causes neonatal conjunctivitis and pneumonia.

❑ Both chlamydia and gonorrhea are common causes of neonatal *conjunctival infections*.

❑ Hypoglycemia in a neonate is expressed as jitteriness, lethargy, diaphoresis, and a serum glucose level below 40 mg/dL.

❑ A hyperalert state in a neonate is more suggestive of neurologic irritability and has no correlation to blood glucose levels.

❑ Vernix caseosa, which protects the fetus in utero, is a white, cheesy material that may be present on the neonate's skin at birth.

❑ Lecithin and sphingomyelin are phospholipids that help compose surfactant in the lungs; lecithin peaks at 36 weeks' gestation, and sphingomyelin concentrations remain stable.

❑ The presence of phosphatidylglycerol indicates lung maturity.

❑ Chronic fetal stress tends to increase lung maturity.

❑ Conjunctival hemorrhages are commonly seen in neonates secondary to the cranial pressure applied during the birth process.

❑ Simian creases are present in 40% of neonates with trisomy 21.

❑ Bulging fontanels are a sign of intracranial pressure.

❑ Erythema toxicum is small, white or yellow papules or vesicles with erythematous dermatitis; they resemble flea bites that come and go on the neonate's face, trunk, and limbs.

❑ If a neonate's environment is too cold, his metabolism must increase to warm his body cells, resulting in increased oxygen demand with resultant hypoxia.

❑ If a neonate's environment is too warm, his metabolism must decrease to cool his body.

❑ Neonates use nonshivering thermogenesis to increase body temperature.

❑ Immediately drying the neonate after birth decreases evaporative heat loss from his moist body.

❑ Placing the neonate on a warm, dry towel decreases conductive heat losses.

❑ Preterm neonates are not able to thermoregulate due to the lack of brown fat; the more preterm the infant, the more immature the thermoregulation system.

❑ Infants born to diabetic mothers and those with jaundice are not more at risk for problems with thermoregulation than a preterm infant.

❑ Increased bilirubin levels result from the impaired conjugation and excretion of bilirubin and difficulty clearing bilirubin from plasma.

❑ Clinical jaundice arising before age 36 hours or lasting beyond 14 days, or serum bilirubin level increasing by more than 5 mg/dL/day, suggests pathologic jaundice.

❑ An absent Moro reflex, lethargy, and seizures are symptoms of bilirubin encephalopathy, which can be life-threatening.

❑ A maculopapular rash, greenish stools, and bronze-colored skin are minor side effects of phototherapy that should be monitored but don't require immediate intervention.

❑ Transient tachypnea of a newborn is caused by a delay in removing excessive amounts of lung fluid.

❑ Choanal atresia is caused by a protrusion of bone or membrane into nasal passages, causing blockage or narrowing.

❑ Meconium aspiration is meconium aspirated into the lungs during birth.

❑ Mask ventilation should be avoided in the neonate born with diaphragmatic hernia to prevent air from being introduced into the GI tract by this technique.

❑ An orogastric tube is needed to decompress the bowel and stomach within the chest in the neonate born with diaphragmatic hernia.

❑ Distinctive facial dysmorphology of children with fetal alcohol syndrome most commonly involves the eyes (microphthalmia).

❑ Microcephaly is generally seen with fetal alcohol syndrome, as are short palpebral fissures and a poorly developed philtrum.

❑ Meconium ileus is a luminal obstruction of the distal small intestine by abnormal meconium seen in neonates with cystic fibrosis.

❑ VACTERL or VATER association is an acronym used to describe a series of characteristics that have been found to occur together (V = vertebrae; A = imperforate anus or anal atresia, or an anus that does not open to the outside of the body; C = cardiac anomalies; TE = tracheoesophageal fistula; R = renal or kidney anomalies; and L = limb anomalies [radial agenesis]).

❑ Auscultation of the precordium should be the primary means to assess heart rate in a neonate.

❑ Heart rate assessment should be the primary vital sign by which to assess the need for resuscitation in a neonate.

❑ For an uncomplicated birth at term there is benefit in delaying umbilical cord clamping for a minimum time ranging from 1 minute until the cord stops pulsating after birth.

❑ A telangiectatic hemangioma is a salmon pink coloration found at the nape of the neck, eyelids, or forehead.

❑ Molding refers to the overlapping of cranial sutures that occurs as the fetus passes through the birth canal, which causes the neonate's head to appear cone-shaped.

❑ Hydrocephalus is an increase in the size of the entire head as a result of increased cerebrospinal fluid volume.

❑ A neonate's lacrimal glands are immature, resulting in tearless crying for up to 2 months.

❑ Erythema toxicum neonatorum causes a transient maculopapular rash—a normal finding in all neonates.

❑ Greenish brown stools at 48 hours are normal and indicate that the neonate is eliminating formula instead of meconium.

❑ To elicit a plantar grasp reflex, which usually disappears around age 9 months, the nurse would touch the sole of the foot near the base of the digits, causing flexion or grasping.

❑ The neonate experiences prolonged coagulation time after birth because maternal stores of vitamin K become depleted and the neonate's immature liver can't produce enough to maintain adequate levels.

❑ The full-term neonate's neurologic system should produce equal strength and symmetry in responses and reflexes.

❑ Diminished or absent reflexes in a neonate may indicate a serious neurologic problem, and asymmetrical responses may indicate trauma during birth, including nerve damage, paralysis, or fracture.

❑ Normal neonatal apical heart rate is 120 to 160 beats/minute.

❑ Normal neonatal respirations are 30 to 60 breaths/minute.

❑ Normal neonatal blood pressure reading ranges from 60/40 mm Hg to 90/45 mm Hg.

❑ The Apgar scoring system provides a way to evaluate the neonate's cardiopulmonary and neurologic status using assessments performed at 1 and 5 minutes after birth and repeated every 5 minutes until the infant stabilizes.

❑ An Apgar score of 8 to 10 indicates that the neonate is in no apparent distress; a score below 8 indicates that resuscitative measures may be needed.

❑ The neonatal skull has two fontanels: a diamond-shaped anterior fontanel and a triangular-shaped posterior fontanel.

❑ Epispadias means the urinary meatus is located on the dorsal surface of the penis.

❑ The anterior fontanel is formed by the junction of the sagittal, frontal, and coronal sutures.

❑ The anterior fontanel is shaped like a diamond and normally measures 4 to 5 cm at its widest point.

❑ Hypospadias means the urinary meatus is located on the ventral surface of the penis.

❑ Neonates may have polydactyly (more than five digits on an extremity) or syndactyly (two or more digits fused together).

❑ A port-wine stain (nevus flammeus) is a capillary angioma located below the dermis and is commonly found on the face.

❑ A strawberry hemangioma (nevus vasculosus) is a capillary angioma located in the dermal and subdermal skin layers, indicated by a rough, raised, sharply demarcated birthmark.

❑ The sucking reflex is elicited when a nipple is placed in the neonate's mouth.

❑ The Moro reflex is elicited when the neonate is lifted above the crib and suddenly lowered; the arms and legs symmetrically extend and then abduct while the fingers spread to form a "C."

❑ The rooting reflex is elicited when the neonate's cheek is stroked; the neonate turns his head in the direction of the stroke.

❑ The tonic neck (fencing position) reflex is elicited when the neonate's head is turned while the neonate is lying supine; the extremities on the same side straighten while those on the opposite side flex.

❑ The palmar grasp reflex is elicited when a finger is placed in each of the neonate's hands; fingers grasp tightly enough to be pulled to a sitting position.

❑ The dancing or stepping reflex is elicited when the neonate is held upright with the feet touching a flat surface; the neonate exhibits dancing or stepping movements.

❑ The startle reflex is elicited when a loud noise, such as a hand clap, elicits neonatal arm abduction and elbow flexion; the neonate's hands stay clenched.

❑ The trunk incurvature reflex is elicited when a finger is run laterally down the neonate's spine; the trunk flexes and the pelvis swings toward the stimulated side.

# Pediatric care

## Growth and development

❑ An infant holds on to furniture while walking (cruising) at 10 months, walks with support at 11 months, and takes his first steps at 12 months.

❑ By 12 months, a child can say a few words, with more words and short phrases being added each month.

❑ At 16 months, a child engages in solitary play and has little interaction with other children.

❑ At age 3 months, the most primitive reflexes begin to disappear, except for the protective and postural reflexes (blink, parachute, cough, swallow, and gag reflexes), which remain for life.

❑ At age 3 months, the infant reaches out voluntarily but is uncoordinated.

❑ At 2 to 3 months of age, the infant begins to hold up his head, begins to put hand to mouth, develops binocular vision, and cries to express needs.

❑ The instinctual smile appears at 2 months and the social smile at 3 months.

❑ At age 5 to 6 months, the infant rolls over from stomach to back, cries when the parent leaves, attempts to crawl when prone, and voluntarily grasps and releases objects.

❑ At age 7 to 9 months, the infant can self-feed crackers and a bottle.

❑ Fear of strangers appears to peak during the 8th month of age.

❑ At age 10 to 12 months, birth weight triples and birth length increases about 50%.

❑ The infant says "mama" and "dada" and responds to his own name at age 10 months. He can say about five words but understands many more.

❑ The toddler period includes ages 1 to 3 and is a slow growth period with a weight gain of 4 to 9 lb (2 to 4 kg) over 2 years.

❑ The toddler's normal pulse rate is 100 beats/minute, normal respiratory rate is 26 breaths/minute, and normal blood pressure is 99/64 mm Hg.

❑ The toddler uses at least 400 words as well as two- to three-word phrases and comprehends many more by age 2; the toddler uses about 11,000 words by age 3.

❑ In the preschool child, ages 3 to 5 years, the normal pulse rate is from 90 to 100 beats/minute, normal respiratory rate is 25 breaths/minute, and normal blood pressure ranges from 85/60 to 90/70 mm Hg.

❑ In the school-age child, ages 5 to 12 years, the normal pulse rate is from 75 to 115 beats/minute, normal blood pressure ranges from 106/69 to 117/76 mm Hg, and normal respiratory rate ranges from 20 to 25 breaths/minute.

❑ Accidents are a major cause of death and disability in children ages 5 to 12.

❑ A child may regress in his behaviors when hospitalized.

❑ Preschoolers see death as temporary, a type of sleep or separation.

❑ Thinking about the future is typical of an adolescent facing death.

❑ Ages 12 to 18 years encompass the adolescent period, which is a period of rapid growth characterized by puberty-related changes in body structure and psychosocial adjustment.

❑ According to Piaget's theory of cognitive development, an 8-month-old child will look for an object after it disappears from sight to develop the cognitive skill of object permanence.

❑ A strong hand grasp is demonstrated within the first month of life.

❑ Holding one object while looking for another is accomplished by the 20th week.

❑ During the school-age years, the most important social interactions typically are those with peers, and children socialize more frequently with friends than with parents.

❑ Peer-to-peer interactions lead to the formation of intimate friendships between same-sex children.

❑ Friendships with opposite-sex children are uncommon during the school-age years.

❑ Interest in peers of the opposite sex generally doesn't begin until ages 10 to 12.

❑ Magical thinking and fantasy play are more characteristic during the preschool years.

❑ At age 3, gross motor development and refinement in hand-eye coordination enable a child to ride a tricycle.

❑ A preschooler typically asks for a bandage after having blood drawn because he has poorly defined body boundaries and believes he will lose all of his blood from the hole the needle has made.

❑ An adolescent might be upset about a surgical scar because he's concerned about body image.

❑ A school-age child might ask why his friends don't visit because peers become important by that age.

❑ Object permanence is exhibited by the infant looking for objects that have been hidden from sight.

❑ Returning blocks to the same spot on the table is imitative behavior.

❑ Recognizing that a ball of clay is the same object even when flattened out is an example of the theory of conservation, which occurs during Piaget's concrete operational stage in early school-age children (ages 7 to 11).

❑ Gross motor skills of the 6-month-old infant include rolling from front to back and back to front.

❑ Teething usually begins around age 6 months; therefore, offering a teething ring is appropriate at this age.

❑ Visual coordination is usually resolved by age 6 months.

❑ At age 6 months, fine motor skills include purposeful grasps.

❑ The 6-month-old infant should have good head control and should no longer display head lag when pulled up to a sitting position.

❑ Chest circumference is most accurately measured by placing the measuring tape around the infant's chest with the tape covering the nipples.

❑ If chest circumference is measured above or below the nipples, a false measurement is obtained.

❑ Sexual maturity in males and females is classified according to Tanner's stages, named after the original researcher on sexual maturity.

❑ The diamond-shaped anterior fontanel normally closes between ages 9 and 18 months.

❑ The triangular posterior fontanel normally closes between ages 2 and 3 months.

❑ The palmar grasp reflex disappears around age 3 to 4 months.

❑ The plantar grasp reflex disappears at age 6 to 8 months.

❑ The Moro reflex disappears around age 4 months.

## Cardiovascular system

❑ Hypotension is considered a late sign of shock in children.

❑ Infants and children with heart defects tend to have poor nutritional intake and weight loss, indicating poor cardiac output, heart failure, or hypoxemia.

❑ The child can appear lethargic or tired because of the heart failure or hypoxia.

❑ Premature atrial contractions are common in fetuses, neonates, and children.

❑ Atrial fibrillation is an uncommon arrhythmia in children that arises from a disorganized state of electrical activity in the atria.

❑ Bradyarrhythmias are congenital, surgically acquired, or caused by infection.

❑ Premature ventricular contractions are more common in adolescents.

❑ In the immediate postcatheterization phase, the child should avoid raising the head, sitting, straining the abdomen, or coughing.

❑ Aldosterone and antidiuretic hormone increase sodium levels, decrease potassium levels, increase water retention, and decrease urine output.

❑ When the heart stretches beyond efficiency, an extra heart sound, or $S_3$ gallop, may be audible.

❑ Respiratory symptoms, such as tachypnea and dyspnea, are seen as a result of pulmonary congestion in heart failure.

❑ Energy expenditures need to be limited to reduce metabolic and oxygen needs in the child with heart failure.

❑ In older children with heart failure, fluids may be restricted but fluid restriction is contraindicated in infants because their nutritional requirements depend on fluid needs.

❑ In a child with heart failure, an upright position facilitates lung expansion, provides less restrictive movement of the diaphragm, relieves pressure from abdominal organs, and decreases pulmonary congestion.

❑ For an infant in heart failure, formulas with increased caloric content are given to meet the greater caloric requirements from the overworked heart and labored breathing.

❑ A neonate's vascular system changes with birth; certain factors help to reverse the flow of blood through the ductus arteriosus and ultimately favor its closure.

❑ Ductus arteriosus closure typically begins within the first 24 hours after birth and ends within a few days after birth.

❑ At birth, oxygenated blood normally causes the ductus arteriosus to constrict, and the vessel closes completely by age 6 weeks.

❑ Patent ductus arteriosus is considered an acyanotic defect with increased pulmonary blood flow. It can cause excessive blood flow to the lungs because of the high pressure in the aorta.

❑ Heart failure is common in premature infants with a patent ductus arteriosus.

❑ Preterm neonates having patent ductus arteriosus with good renal function may receive oral indomethacin, a prostaglandin inhibitor, to encourage ductal closure.

❑ If indomethacin isn't effective in closing a patent ductus arteriosus, surgery is suggested.

❑ The continuous, turbulent flow of blood from the aorta through the patent ductus arteriosus to the pulmonary artery produces a machinelike murmur.

❑ With an acyanotic heart defect, the increase in blood flow to the lungs may cause tachycardia and increased respiratory rates to compensate.

❑ Poor growth and development may be seen in a child with an acyanotic heart defect because of the increased energy required for breathing.

❏ Failure of a septum to develop between the ventricles results in a left-to-right shunt, which is noted as a ventricular septal defect.

❏ When the septum fails to develop between the atria, it's considered an atrial septal defect.

❏ For small ventricular septal defects, a stitch closure is performed; larger ventricular septal defects may be repaired by sewing a patch over the defect.

❏ Surgery with pulmonary artery banding may be a palliative procedure for a child with a ventricular septal defect in heart failure who is too small or too ill for surgical repair of the defect.

❏ The pulse below the catheterization site should be strong and equal to the pulse in the unaffected extremity.

❏ A weakened pulse below the cardiac catheterization site may indicate vessel obstruction or perfusion problems.

❏ Atrial septal defects shunt from left to right because pressures are greater on the left side of the heart.

❏ Pulmonic stenosis, tetralogy of Fallot, and total anomalous pulmonary venous return will show a right-to-left shunting of blood.

❏ With coarctation of the aorta, as blood is pumped from the left ventricle to the aorta, some blood flows to the head and upper extremities while the rest meets obstruction and jets through the constricted area.

❏ A child with tetralogy of Fallot will be mildly cyanotic at rest and have increasing cyanosis with crying, activity, or straining, as with a bowel movement.

❏ Higher pressures in the upper extremities are characteristic of coarctation of the aorta.

❏ Chronic hypoxia of longer than 6 months' duration causes clubbing of the fingers and toes when untreated, such as with a child with tetralogy of Fallot.

❏ Hypoxia varies with the degree of pulmonic stenosis in a child with tetralogy of Fallot.

❏ Growth and development may appear normal in a child with tetralogy of Fallot.

❏ A child with tetralogy of Fallot may squat or assume a knee-chest position in order to breathe more easily.

❏ The arterial oxygen saturation of infants with tetralogy of Fallot can suddenly drop markedly; called a "tetralogy spell," this usually results from a sudden increased constriction of the outflow tract to the lungs, which further restricts the pulmonary blood flow.

❏ The lips and skin of infants who have a sudden decrease in arterial oxygen level from a "tetralogy spell" will appear acutely more blue.

❑ Decreased or absent pulses in the lower extremities is a sign of coarctation of the aorta.

❑ In tetralogy of Fallot, chest X-rays will show right ventricular hypertrophy pushing the heart apex upward, resulting in a boot-shaped cardiac silhouette.

❑ Echocardiogram scans define such defects as large ventricular septal defects, pulmonic stenosis, and malposition of the aorta.

❑ Tricuspid atresia is failure of the tricuspid valve to develop, leaving no communication between the right atrium and right ventricle.

❑ Narrowing at the aortic outflow tract is called aortic stenosis.

❑ Total anomalous pulmonary venous return is a defect in which the pulmonary veins don't return to the left atrium, but instead return to the right side of the heart.

❑ Narrowing at the entrance of the pulmonary artery represents pulmonic stenosis.

❑ Cyanosis is the most consistent clinical sign of tricuspid atresia.

❑ Tachypnea and dyspnea are commonly present in tricuspid atresia because of the decreased pulmonary blood flow and right-to-left shunting.

❑ A child who has pulmonary venous obstruction will exhibit signs of increasing respiratory distress, such as increased respiratory rate, dyspnea, and shortness of breath.

❑ Children with total anomalous pulmonary venous return defects are prone to repeated respiratory infections due to increased pulmonary blood flow.

❑ The child with tricuspid atresia will be dusky, particularly around mucous membranes and nail beds, for the rest of his life as a result of chronic hypoxemia.

❑ Increasing pulmonary blood flow causes bounding pulses and a widened pulse pressure in a child with truncus arteriosus.

❑ Systemic and pulmonary blood mixing leads to mild or moderate cyanosis, so mucous membranes may appear dull or gray in a child with truncus arteriosus.

❑ Patent foramen ovale, patent ductus arteriosus, and ventricular septal defect are associated defects related to transposition of the great arteries.

❑ An atrial septal defect is common in association with total anomalous pulmonary venous return.

❑ Hypoplasia of the left ventricle and mitral atresia are two defects associated with hypoplastic left heart syndrome.

❑ In treating transposition of the great arteries, prostaglandin $E_1$ is necessary to maintain the patency of the ductus arteriosus and improve systemic arterial flow in children with inadequate intracardiac mixing.

❑ Balloon atrial septostomy is a palliative procedure used during cardiac catheterization for septal defects for those children without a coexisting lesion.

❑ The Blalock-Taussig operation is used to palliate tricuspid atresia and pulmonic atresia.

❑ In pulmonic stenosis, right-to-left shunting develops through a patent foramen ovale, an atrial septal defect, or a ventricular septal defect due to right ventricular failure and an increase in pressure in the right side of the heart.

❑ Children with aortic stenosis may develop chest pain similar to angina when they're active.

❑ The most common causes of heart failure in children are congenital heart defects.

❑ Some congenital heart defects result from the blood being pumped from the left side of the heart to the right side of the heart.

❑ Infective endocarditis is usually caused by the bacteria *Streptococcus viridans* and commonly affects children with acquired or congenital anomalies of the heart or great vessels.

❑ Bacteria in endocarditis may grow into adjacent tissues and may break off and embolize elsewhere, such as the spleen, kidney, lung, skin, and central nervous system.

❑ Endocardial cushion defects represent inappropriate fusion of the endocardial cushions in fetal life.

❑ Symptoms of bacterial endocarditis may include a low-grade intermittent fever, decrease in hemoglobin level, tachycardia, anorexia, weight loss, and decreased activity level.

❑ In bacterial endocarditis, bacterial organisms can enter the bloodstream from any site of infection, such as a urinary tract infection.

❑ Gram-negative bacilli are common causative agents of bacterial endocarditis.

❑ Dental work is a common portal of entry in bacterial endocarditis if the client is not pretreated with antibiotics.

❑ In a child with suspected Kawasaki disease, inflammation of the pharynx and oral mucosa develops, causing red, cracked lips and a "strawberry" tongue in which the normal coating of the tongue sloughs off.

❑ The subacute phase of Kawasaki disease shows characteristic desquamation of the hands and feet.

❑ The most serious complication of Kawasaki disease is cardiac involvement.

❑ Abdominal pain, vomiting, and restlessness are the main symptoms of an acute myocardial infarction in children with Kawasaki disease.

❑ Pain in the joints is an expected sign of arthritis that usually occurs in the subacute phase of Kawasaki disease.

❏ An increased erythrocyte sedimentation rate is a reflection of the inflammatory process and may be seen for 2 to 4 weeks after the onset of symptoms in Kawasaki disease.

❏ In Kawasaki disease, black, tarry stools are abnormal and are signs of bleeding that should be reported to the physician immediately.

❏ Because of the risk of coronary artery involvement and possible aneurysm development in Kawasaki disease, repeat echocardiography and electrocardiography will be required for the first few weeks and at 6 months.

❏ In acute rheumatic fever, leukocytosis can be seen as an immune response triggered by colonization of the pharynx with group A streptococci.

❏ In acute rheumatic fever, the electrocardiogram will show a prolonged PR interval as a result of carditis.

❏ The inflammatory response in acute rheumatic fever will cause an elevated erythrocyte sedimentation rate.

❏ Blood cultures would be positive for *Streptococcus* organisms in acute rheumatic fever.

❏ Carditis is a major diagnostic criteria of acute rheumatic fever; it's the only manifestation that can lead to death or long-term sequelae.

❏ In acute rheumatic fever, prolonged PR interval, low-grade fever, and previous heart disease are considered minor diagnostic components of Jones criteria.

❏ A regurgitant murmur, cardiomegaly, and a pericardial friction rub are clinical signs of rheumatic carditis.

❏ Sinus tachycardia is commonly seen in children with a fever.

❏ Sinus arrhythmia is a common occurrence in childhood and adolescence.

❏ Sinus block, sinus bradycardia, and sinus tachycardia are respiration-independent arrhythmias.

❏ Sinus arrest may occur in children when vagal tone is increased, such as during Valsalva's maneuver elicited when vomiting, gagging, or straining during a bowel movement.

❏ A heart rate of 100 beats/minute is a normal finding for a 1-year-old child.

❏ A heart rate of around 180 beats/minute in a 1-year-old child may represent sinus tachycardia.

❏ A heart rate of less than 80 beats/minute in a 1-year-old child can be characterized as sinus bradycardia.

❏ Vagal maneuvers, such as immersion of the hands in cold water, are commonly tried first as a mechanism to decrease the heart rate in a 2-year-old child experiencing supraventricular tachycardia.

❏ Synchronized cardioversion may be required if vagal maneuvers and drugs are ineffective for supraventricular tachycardia.

❏ If a child has low cardiac output, cardioversion may be used instead of drugs for supraventricular tachycardia.

❏ A heart rate of 180 beats/minute is normal in an infant with a fever.

❏ In patent ductus arteriosus, an accessory fetal structure that connects the pulmonary artery to the aorta fails to close at birth, allowing blood to shunt from the aorta to the pulmonary artery.

## Hematologic and immune systems

❏ In naturally acquired active immunity, the immune system makes anti-bodies after exposure to disease. This requires contact with the disease.

❏ In naturally acquired passive immunity, no active immune process is involved; antibodies are passively received through placental transfer by immunoglobu-lin G (the smallest immunoglobulin) and breast-feeding (colostrum).

❏ Because of passive antibody transmission, all infants born to human immunodeficiency virus (HIV)-infected mothers test positive for antibod-ies to HIV up to about age 18 months; confirmation of diagnosis during this time requires detection of the HIV antigen.

❏ The human immunodeficiency virus (HIV) has a much shorter incuba-tion period in children than in adults; children who receive the virus by placental transmission are usually HIV-positive by age 6 months and develop clinical signs by age 3.

❏ There are two types of hemophilia: hemophilia A and hemophilia B.

❏ Hemophilia A is called factor VIII deficiency or classic hemophilia and is the most common type (75% of all cases).

❏ Hemophilia B is also called factor IX deficiency or Christmas disease.

❏ Hemophilia is an X-linked recessive disorder.

❏ The most common nutritional anemia during childhood is iron deficiency anemia, which is characterized by poor red blood cell production.

❏ In iron deficiency anemia, insufficient body stores of iron lead to depleted red blood cell mass, decreased hemoglobin concentration (hypochromia), and decreased oxygen-carrying capacity of the blood.

❏ Most commonly, iron deficiency anemia occurs when the child experiences rapid physical growth, low iron intake, inadequate iron absorption, or loss of blood.

❏ Peak incidence of iron deficiency anemia occurrence is at age 12 to 18 months.

❏ In children, the most common type of leukemia is acute lymphocytic leukemia.

❏ Acute lymphocytic leukemia is marked by extreme proliferation of immature lymphocytes (blast cells).

❏ In adolescents, acute myelogenous leukemia is more common and is believed to result from a malignant transformation of a single stem cell.

❏ In a child with acute lymphocytic leukemia, blast cells appear in the peripheral blood (where they don't normally appear).

❏ Children between ages 3 and 7 have the best prognosis for acute lymphocytic leukemia.

❏ In sickle cell anemia, a defect in the hemoglobin molecule changes the shape of red blood cells, altering their oxygen-carrying capacity.

❏ The altered hemoglobin molecule in sickle cell anemia is referred to as hemoglobin S.

❏ In sickle cell anemia, red blood cells acquire a sickle shape.

❏ The child with sickle cell anemia may experience periodic, painful attacks called sickle cell crises, which may be triggered or intensified by dehydration, deoxygenation, or acidosis.

❏ Sickle cell anemia is an autosomal recessive trait; the child inherits the gene that produces hemoglobin S from two healthy parents who carry the defective gene.

## Respiratory system

❏ Preterm infants, especially those with low birth weight, have an increased risk for sudden infant death syndrome.

❏ Infants with apnea, central nervous system disorders, or respiratory disorders have a higher risk of sudden infant death syndrome.

❏ Peak age for sudden infant death syndrome is 2 to 4 months.

❏ There is an increased risk of sudden infant death syndrome (SIDS) with prematurity, low birth weight, maternal smoking, and multiple births and in subsequent siblings of two or more SIDS victims.

❏ Lungs aren't fully developed at birth and alveoli continue to grow and increase in size through age 8.

❏ A child's respiratory tract has a narrower lumen than an adult's until age 5; the narrow airway makes the young child prone to airway obstruction and respiratory distress from inflammation, mucus secretion, or a foreign body.

❏ The American Academy of Pediatrics endorses placing infants face-up in their cribs (or "back to sleep") as a way to reduce sudden infant death syndrome.

❏ A warm, running shower provides a mist that may be helpful to moisten and decrease the viscosity of airway secretions and may also decrease laryngeal spasm, but cool liquids would be best for the child with acute spasmodic laryngitis.

❑ If the child with acute spasmodic laryngitis is unable to take liquid, the child needs to be in the emergency department.

❑ A resonant cough described as "barking" is the most characteristic sign of croup.

❑ With worsening croup, intercostal retractions occur as the child's breathing becomes more labored and the use of other muscles is necessary to draw air into the lungs.

❑ The client with epiglottitis shouldn't be allowed anything by mouth during the initial phases of the infection to prevent aspiration.

❑ Respiratory isolation isn't required with epiglottitis.

❑ The assessment sequence of airway, breathing, and compressions needs to be followed when a child is found unresponsive.

❑ A compression-ventilation ratio of 30:2 is recommended for the lone rescuer performing cardiopulmonary resuscitation (CPR) on infants and children.

❑ For health care providers performing 2-rescuer CPR on infants and children, a compression-ventilation ratio of 15:2 is recommended.

❑ If a tracheal tube is in place when performing CPR on an infant or child, compressions should not be interrupted for ventilations.

❑ When performing chest compressions, the depth of compressions corresponds to about 1½" (4 cm) in an infant and 2" (5 cm) in most children.

❑ After the airway is open in an unconscious choking 10-month-old infant, the nurse should check for a foreign object and remove it with a finger sweep if it can be seen.

❑ If ventilation is unsuccessful in the unconscious choking 10-month-old infant, the nurse should then give five back blows and five chest thrusts in an attempt to dislodge the object.

❑ Blind finger sweeps should never be performed in an infant or child because this may push the object further back into the airway.

❑ A child between ages 1 and 8 years should receive abdominal thrusts to help dislodge the object.

❑ Infants younger than age 1 year should receive back blows before chest thrusts and should never receive abdominal thrusts.

❑ After a 4-year old child has a tonsillectomy, laying the child on his stomach with the head turned to the side allows blood and other secretions to drain from the mouth and pharynx, reducing the risk of aspiration.

❑ Children with chronic otitis media commonly require surgery for a myringotomy and ear tube placement.

❑ Ear tubes allow normal fluid to drain from the middle ear, improve ventilation, and permit pressure to equalize in the middle ear.

❑ For infants receiving eardrops, the parent should be told to gently pull the earlobe down and back to visualize the external auditory canal.

❑ For children receiving eardrops over age 3 and for adults, the earlobe is gently pulled slightly up and back.

❑ The child with chronic otitis media should be positioned on the affected side to facilitate drainage after returning from surgery for myringotomy and placement of ear tubes.

❑ After myringotomy and placement of ear tubes, warm compresses may help to facilitate drainage when used on the affected ear.

❑ With acute otitis media, the tympanic membrane may present as bright red or yellow, bulging or retracted.

❑ A pearl-gray tympanic membrane is a normal finding.

❑ Dull gray membrane fluid is consistent with subacute or chronic otitis media.

❑ In an infant or child, the eustachian tubes are short, wide, and straight and lie in a horizontal plane, allowing them to be more easily blocked by conditions such as large adenoids and infections.

❑ Until the eustachian tubes change in size and angle, children are more susceptible to otitis media.

❑ Cartilage lining is underdeveloped in the 1-year-old child, making the eustachian tubes more distensible and more likely to open inappropriately.

❑ The usual lying-down position of infants favors the pooling of fluid such as formula in the pharyngeal cavity.

❑ Immature humoral defense mechanisms in a 1-year-old child increase the risk of otitis media infection.

❑ Eardrum perforation is the most common complication of acute otitis media as the exudate accumulates and pressure increases.

❑ Antibiotics should be given for the full prescribed course of therapy regardless of whether the child has symptoms with otitis media.

❑ Oral antibiotics are used to treat otitis media.

❑ Tongue blades are contraindicated with acute epiglottitis and may cause the epiglottis to spasm.

❑ The classic signs of epiglottitis are drooling, sitting upright, and leaning forward with chin thrust out, mouth open, and tongue protruding.

❑ The child with epiglottitis should be kept in an upright position to ease the work of breathing and to avoid aspiration of secretions and obstruction of the airway by the swollen epiglottis.

❑ The gag reflex of a child with epiglottitis should never be checked unless emergency personnel and equipment are immediately available to perform a tracheotomy if the airway should become obstructed by the swollen epiglottis.

❑ The child with right lower lobe pneumonia should be placed on the left side.

❑ Placing the lobe with pneumonia upward places the unaffected lung in a position in which gravity will promote blood flow to the healthy lung tissue, improving gas exchange.

❑ Preterm neonates with low birth weight on high-pressure ventilators are at highest risk for developing bronchopulmonary dysplasia.

❑ The infant with bronchopulmonary dysplasia will have impaired gas exchange related to retention of carbon dioxide and borderline oxygenation secondary to fibrosis of the lungs.

❑ Thermoregulation is important for the infant with bronchopulmonary dysplasia because both hypothermia and hyperthermia will increase oxygen consumption and may increase oxygen requirements.

❑ Tachypnea, dyspnea, and wheezing are intermittently or chronically present secondary to airway obstruction and increased airway resistance in bronchopulmonary dysplasia.

❑ Infants with bronchopulmonary dysplasia usually show increased work of breathing and increased use of accessory muscles.

❑ Pulmonary hypertension is a common finding resulting from fibrosis and chronic hypoxia occurring with bronchopulmonary dysplasia.

❑ Infants with bronchopulmonary dysplasia require frequent, prolonged rest periods.

❑ Patient teaching for the parents of an infant with bronchopulmonary dysplasia should include the causes of the dysplasia, and care of their infant at the time of discharge.

❑ Before and after suctioning a tracheostomy tube, provide hyperventilation to the child to prevent hypoxia.

❑ When suctioning a tracheostomy tube, insert the catheter 0.5 cm beyond the tracheostomy tube.

❑ Allergies elicit consistent bouts of sneezing, are seldom accompanied by fever, and tend to cause itching of the eyes and nose.

❑ Excessively cold air, wet or humid changes in weather and seasons, and air pollution are some of the most common asthma triggers.

❑ Asthma frequently presents with wheezing and coughing.

❑ Airway inflammation and edema in asthma increase mucus production.

❑ A history of prior admission to an intensive care unit for asthma indicates that a child has an increased risk of asthma severity and of asthma-related death and needs immediate therapy.

❑ Hyperexpansion, atelectasis, and a flattened diaphragm are typical X-ray findings for a child with asthma.

❑ In asthma, air becomes trapped behind the narrowed airways and the residual capacity rises, leading to hyperinflation.

❑ Hypoxemia in asthma results from areas of the lung not being well-perfused.

❑ Overhydration to correct dehydration in a 2-year-old client with asthma may increase interstitial pulmonary fluid and exacerbate small-airway obstruction.

❑ Basements or cellars should be avoided by the child with asthma to lessen the child's exposure to molds and mildew.

❑ Ineffective oxygen supply and demand may lead to activity intolerance in the child with asthma.

❑ The nurse should promote rest for the child with asthma and encourage developmentally appropriate activities.

❑ Nutrition may be decreased in the child with asthma due to respiratory distress and GI upset.

❑ Dehydration is common in the child with asthma due to diaphoresis, insensible water loss, and hyperventilation.

❑ In bronchiolitis, the bronchioles become narrowed and edematous, which can cause wheezing.

❑ Infants with bronchiolitis typically have a 2- to 3-day history of an upper respiratory infection and feeding difficulties with loss of appetite due to nasal congestion and increased work of breathing.

❑ In most cases, bronchiolitis is caused by a viral agent, most commonly respiratory syncytial virus.

❑ Respiratory syncytial virus is most prevalent in the winter and early spring months.

❑ Most children develop the respiratory syncytial virus (RSV) infection between ages 2 and 6 months, and RSV infection generally occurs during the first 3 years of life.

❑ Respiratory syncytial virus is highly contagious and is spread through direct contact with infectious secretions via hands, droplets, and fomites.

❑ When caring for a client with respiratory syncytial virus, gowns, gloves, and masks should be worn to prevent the spread of infection.

❑ Infants with cardiac or pulmonary conditions are at highest risk for developing respiratory syncytial virus.

❑ Measurement of urine specific gravity is recommended when monitoring an infant with bronchiolitis to assess for dehydration. This can be obtained with diaper changes.

❑ Weighing diapers is a way of measuring output only.

❑ Infants with bronchiolitis will have impaired gas exchange related to bronchiolar obstruction, atelectasis, and hyperinflation.

❑ It's essential for parents of infants with bronchiolitis to be able to recognize signs of increasing respiratory distress and know how to count the respiratory rate.

❑ The child with bronchiolitis should be positioned with the head of the bed elevated for comfort and to facilitate removal of secretions.

❑ Use of cool mist for the child with bronchiolitis may help to replace insensible fluid loss.

❑ Bronchiolitis is a severe infection of the bronchioles.

❑ *Mycoplasma* pneumonia is a primary atypical pneumonia seen in children between ages 5 and 12.

❑ Infections with enteric bacilli, staphylococcal pneumonia, and streptococcal pneumonia are mostly seen in children from age 3 months to 5 years.

❑ Pertussis is characterized by consistent short, rapid coughs followed by a sudden inspiration with a high-pitched whooping sound.

❑ A barking cough and inspiratory stridor are noted with croup.

❑ Pertussis is usually accompanied by a low-grade fever.

❑ A sputum culture is the definitive test for tuberculosis.

❑ For a child with a possible foreign body aspiration, a cough with stridor and changes in phonation would occur if the foreign body were in the larynx.

❑ For a child with a possible foreign body aspiration, asymmetrical breath sounds indicate that the object may be located in the bronchi.

❑ Bronchoscopy can give a definitive diagnosis of the presence of foreign bodies and is also the best choice for removal of the object with direct visualization.

❑ Chest X-ray and lateral neck X-ray may also be used to detect foreign bodies, but findings vary.

❑ Some X-ray films may appear normal or show changes such as inflammation related to the presence of the foreign body.

❑ Fluoroscopy is valuable in detecting and localizing foreign bodies in the bronchi.

❑ Meconium ileus is commonly a presenting sign of cystic fibrosis.

❑ Thick, mucilaginous meconium blocks the lumen of the small intestine, causing intestinal obstruction, abdominal distention, and vomiting in cystic fibrosis.

❑ A chloride concentration greater than 60 mEq/L is diagnostic of cystic fibrosis.

❑ Normal sweat chloride content is less than 40 mEq/L, with the average being 18 mEq/L.

❑ Chloride levels between 40 and 60 mEq/L are highly suggestive of cystic fibrosis.

❑ Fat restriction isn't required for a child with cystic fibrosis because digestion and absorption of fat in the intestine is impaired.

❑ Low-sodium foods can lead to hyponatremia for a child with cystic fibrosis; therefore, high-sodium foods are recommended, especially during hot weather or when the child has a fever.

❑ For a child with cystic fibrosis, pancreatic enzymes are administered with each feeding, meal, and snack to optimize absorption of the nutrients consumed.

❑ To promote growth and development in a child with cystic fibrosis, the child should eat a high-calorie, high-protein diet, and consume higher than usual amounts of fluids and sodium.

❑ The child with cystic fibrosis should be given water-soluble forms of fat-soluble vitamins (A, D, E, and K).

❑ Chest physiotherapy is recommended for the child with cystic fibrosis two to four times per day to help loosen and move secretions to facilitate expectoration.

❑ Cystic fibrosis is an autosomal recessive disease.

❑ When both parents carry the gene for cystic fibrosis, with each pregnancy there's a 25% chance of the child having cystic fibrosis, a 25% chance of the child being normal, and a 50% chance of the child being a carrier.

❑ In recessive disorders such as cystic fibrosis, both parents must pass the defective gene or set of genes to the child.

❑ Sex-linked genetic disorders are carried on the X chromosome.

❑ Dominant disorders are characterized by only one defective gene or set of genes passed by one parent.

❑ A child with an XXY karyotype would have Klinefelter's syndrome.

❑ Pulmonary obstruction related to thickened mucus secretions can lead to a progressive pulmonary disturbance. Secondary infections can lead to death in the child with cystic fibrosis.

❑ In the child with cystic fibrosis, gastroesophageal reflux can be managed with medications and proper reflux precautions.

❑ Clients with cystic fibrosis are at risk for developing diabetes mellitus because the pancreatic duct becomes obstructed as pancreatic tissues are destroyed.

❑ Clients with cystis fibrosis can expect to have normal sexual relationships, but fertility becomes difficult because thick secretions obstruct the cervix and block sperm entry.

## Neurosensory system

❑ During the first 12 hours of life, the most life-threatening event for a child with a myelomeningocele would be an infection.

❑ Hydrocephalus is caused by an alteration in circulation of the cerebrospinal fluid (CSF), causing an increase in CSF, resulting in bulging of the fontanel.

❑ The increase in intracranial pressure that occurs with hydrocephalus causes the neonate's eyes to deviate downward (the "setting sun sign"), and the neonate's cry becomes high-pitched.

❑ After shunt insertion on the right side of the head to relieve hydrocephalus, the child should be placed flat in bed to avoid rapid decompression of cerebrospinal fluid (CSF), and on the left side or on his back to avoid occlusion of the shunt and blockage of the drainage of CSF.

❑ After shunt insertion, placing the child in a semi-Fowler's or upright position may promote too-rapid decompression of cerebrospinal fluid.

❑ Tactile stimulation may increase seizure activity; therefore, it must be limited as much as possible.

❑ Normal serum sodium level for an infant is 135 to 145 mmol/L.

❑ Hyponatremia is one of the causes of seizures in infants.

❑ Neonates can be either hypothermic or hyperthermic with meningitis.

❑ The irritation to the meninges causes the neonates to be irritable and to have a decreased appetite.

❑ The infant with meningitis may be pale and mottled with a bulging, full fontanel.

❑ Older children and adults with meningitis have headaches, nuchal rigidity, and hyperthermia as clinical manifestations.

❑ Two of the most common characteristics of children with attention deficit hyperactivity disorder are inattention and impulsiveness.

❑ Children who reverse letters and words while reading have dyslexia.

❑ The child with cerebral palsy needs continual treatment and therapy to maintain or improve functioning.

❑ Without therapy, muscles with cerebral palsy will get progressively weaker and more spastic.

❑ Although some children with cerebral palsy are mentally retarded, many have normal intelligence.

- ❏ Absence seizures are commonly misinterpreted as daydreaming.

- ❏ The child loses awareness but no alteration in motor activity is exhibited with absence seizures.

- ❏ A bulging fontanel and high-pitched cry are typical signs of a brain tumor in an infant due to increased intracranial pressure.

- ❏ A change in vital signs is a late sign of increased intracranial pressure.

- ❏ Noise and bright lights stimulate the child with meningitis and can be irritating, causing the child to cry. This, in turn, increases intracranial pressure.

- ❏ After ventriculoperitoneal shunt placement for hydrocephalus, the child should be placed on the side opposite the surgical site to prevent pressure on the shunt valve.

- ❏ Febrile seizures usually occur after age 6 months and are unusual after age 5 years.

- ❏ For febrile seizures, the treatment is to decrease the temperature because seizures occur as the temperature rises.

- ❏ By definition, cerebral palsy is a nonprogressive neuromuscular disorder that can be mild or quite severe; it is believed to be the result of a hypoxic event during the pregnancy or birth process.

- ❏ A finding of dilated and nonreactive pupils in a client who has sustained trauma may indicate that anoxia or ischemia of the brain has occurred.

- ❏ After a trauma, if the pupils are fixed (don't move) in addition to being dilated and nonreactive, herniation of the brain stem has occurred.

- ❏ For a lumbar puncture, the nurse should position the client on his side with his back curved. Curving the back maximizes the space between the lumbar vertebrae, facilitating needle insertion.

- ❏ The mechanism producing the headache that accompanies increased intracranial pressure may be the stretching of the meninges and pain fibers associated with blood vessels.

- ❏ Cervical flexion is painful in meningitis due to the stretching of the inflamed meninges. The pain triggers a reflex spasm of the neck extensors to splint the area against further cervical flexion, producing nuchal rigidity.

- ❏ Cerebral ischemia occurs in meningitis because of vascular obstruction and decreased perfusion of the brain tissue.

- ❏ A positive Kernig's sign indicates nuchal rigidity, caused by an irritative lesion of the subarachnoid space.

- ❏ Fever, change in feeding pattern, vomiting, and diarrhea are commonly observed in children with bacterial meningitis.

- ❏ Hemorrhagic rashes, petechiae, photophobia, fever, lethargy, and purpura are common manifestations in older children with meningitis.

❏ The glucose level in the cerebrospinal fluid is reduced in acute bacterial meningitis.

❏ Atonic seizures are frequently accompanied by falling.

❏ Focal seizures are partial seizures.

❏ Absence seizures are generalized seizures.

❏ Anticonvulsant drugs, such as phenytoin (Dilantin), suppress the influx of sodium, thereby decreasing the ability of the neurons to fire.

❏ Some anticonvulsant drugs, such as valproate sodium (Depakene), used for absence seizures, suppress the influx of calcium.

❏ Until seizure control is certain, clients shouldn't participate in activities (such as riding a bicycle) that could be hazardous if a seizure were to occur.

❏ Meningeal irritation may cause seizures and heightens a child's sensitivity to all stimuli, including noise, lights, movement, and touch.

❏ Because the child with meningitis is already at increased risk of cerebral edema and increased intracranial pressure due to inflammation of the meningeal membranes, the nurse should monitor fluid intake and output to avoid fluid volume overload.

❏ Unilateral or bilateral posturing of one or more extremities during the onset of seizure activity can occur.

❏ Striped wallpaper, ceiling fans, and blinking lights on a Christmas tree can all be triggers to seizure activity if the child is photosensitive.

❏ Position the child with his head midline, not hyperextended, to promote a good airway and adequate ventilation during a seizure.

❏ During a seizure, don't attempt to prop the child up into a sitting position. Ease him to the floor to prevent falling and unnecessary injury.

❏ Don't put anything in the child's mouth during a seizure because it could cause infection or obstruct the airway.

❏ When a spinal cord lesion exists at birth, it commonly leads to altered development or function of other areas of the central nervous system.

❏ Sound discrimination is present at birth.

❏ By ages 5 to 6 months, the infant can localize sounds presented on a horizontal plane and begins to imitate selected sounds.

❏ By ages 7 to 12 months, the infant can localize sounds in any plane.

❏ By age 18 months, the child can hear and follow a simple command without visual cues.

❏ Children who have difficulty with language development by age 18 months should have their hearing evaluated.

❑ Key signs and symptoms of Down syndrome include mild to moderate retardation, short stature with pudgy hands, simian crease, small head with slow brain growth, and upward slanting eyes.

❑ Sixty percent of patients with Down syndrome have congenital heart defects, respiratory infections, chronic myelogenous leukemia, and a weak immune response to infection.

❑ In noncommunicating hydrocephalus, an obstruction occurs in the free circulation of cerebrospinal fluid, causing increased pressure on the brain or spinal cord.

❑ In most cases, congenital hydrocephalus is noncommunicating.

❑ Communicating hydrocephalus involves the free flow of cerebrospinal fluid (CSF) between the ventricles and the spinal cord; increased pressure on the spinal cord is caused by defective absorption of CSF.

❑ Spina bifida is a complex neurologic defect that heavily impacts the physical, cognitive, and psychosocial development of the child.

❑ Spina bifida requires collaborative, life-long management due to the chronicity and multiplicity of the problems involved.

❑ Chiari II malformation may lead to a possibility of respiratory function problems, such as respiratory stridor associated with paralysis of the vocal cords, apneic episodes of unknown cause, difficulty swallowing, and an abnormal gag reflex.

❑ Damage to the white matter (association area) caused by ventricular enlargement has been linked to impairment of intellectual and perceptual abilities often seen in children with spina bifida.

❑ The child with a myelomeningocele will undergo sac closure within the first 24 to 48 hours after birth to replace the nerve tissue into the vertebral canal, cover the spinal defect, and achieve a watertight sac closure.

❑ There's complete loss of nervous function below the level of the spinal cord lesion with myelomeningocele.

❑ Prone position is used preoperatively for myelomeningocele because it minimizes tension on the sac and the risk of trauma.

❑ The head is turned to one side for feeding in the client with myelomeningocele.

❑ A side-lying or partial side-lying position is best used after myelomeningocele repair, unless the position permits undesirable hip flexion.

❑ For a child with myelomeningocele, areas of sensory and motor impairment require meticulous care, including gentle range-of-motion exercises to prevent contractures as well as stretching of contractures when indicated.

❑ Frequent turning is indicated for the child with myelomeningocele in order to maintain skin integrity, but the supine position shouldn't be used to avoid pressure on the surgical site.

❑ Children with spina bifida are at high risk for developing a latex allergy because of repeated exposure to latex products during multiple surgeries and from numerous bladder catheterizations related to lack of bladder function.

❑ Classic signs of increased intracranial pressure are a decrease in respirations, an increase in blood pressure, and a decrease in pulse rate.

❑ A widened, bulging fontanel is a sign of increased intracranial pressure.

❑ Common signs and symptoms of viral meningitis include fever, nuchal rigidity, irritability, and photophobia.

❑ A bulging anterior fontanel is a sign of hydrocephalus.

❑ A petechial, purpuric rash may be seen with bacterial meningitis.

❑ Hypothermia is a common sign of bacterial meningitis in an infant younger than age 3 months.

❑ Persistence of the tonic neck reflex beyond 2 months suggests asymmetrical central nervous system development.

## Musculoskeletal system

❑ In Bryant's traction, the child's hips should be slightly elevated off the bed at a 15-degree angle.

❑ Duchenne muscular dystrophy is a progressive muscular degenerative disorder in which children lose their ability to walk independently by age 12.

❑ Surgery may be done to correct contractures in Duchenne muscular dystrophy, but it doesn't change the course of the disease.

❑ Death occurs by early adulthood in the client with Duchenne muscular dystrophy, usually from respiratory failure.

❑ After hip-spica cast application, a client is at risk for peripheral neurovascular dysfunction due to swelling within the confined space of the cast.

❑ The Milwaukee brace is commonly used in the treatment of scoliosis.

❑ Strengthening of the evertor muscle group of the foot is important in a client diagnosed with talipes equinovarus.

❑ Clinical manifestations of fat emboli include dyspnea, hypoxia, tachypnea, tachycardia, and chest pain.

❑ Scoliosis of greater than 60 degrees can cause shifting of organs and decreased ability for the ribs to expand, thus decreasing vital capacity.

❑ Residual volume will increase secondary to decreased ability of the lungs to expel air with scoliosis greater than 60 degrees.

❑ Cerebral palsy is usually associated with some degree of hypotonia or hypertonia.

❑ To walk down the stairs with crutches, the crutches are first placed on the lower step, and then the affected leg is lowered, followed by the unaffected leg.

❏ A raised iliac crest may be indicative of a leg length discrepancy or a curvature in the lumbar spine.

❏ Scoliosis is eight times more prominent in adolescent girls than boys; the peak incidence is between ages 8 and 15.

❏ Bone lengthening occurs in the epiphyseal plates at the ends of bones; when the epiphyses close, growth stops.

❏ Bone healing occurs much faster in a child than in an adult because the child's bones are still growing.

❏ The younger the child, the faster the bone heals.

❏ Bone healing takes approximately 1 week for every year of life up to age 10.

❏ The most common fractures in the child are clavicular fractures and greenstick fractures.

❏ Greenstick fractures of the long bones are related to the increased flexibility of the young child's bones; the compressed side of the bone bends while the side under tension fractures.

❏ Clubfoot occurs in these five forms: equinovarus, talipes calcaneus, talipes equinus, talipes valgus, and talipes varus.

❏ Talipes calcaneus clubfoot involves dorsiflexion of the foot, as if walking on one's heels.

❏ Talipes equinus clubfoot involves plantar flexion, as if pointing one's toes.

❏ Talipes valgus clubfoot involves eversion of the ankles, with the feet turning out.

❏ Talipes varus clubfoot involves inversion of the ankles, with the soles of the feet facing each other.

❏ Developmental dysplasia of the hip results from an abnormal development of the hip socket and occurs when the head of the femur is still cartilaginous and the acetabulum (socket) is shallow; as a result, the head of the femur comes out of the hip socket.

❏ Developmental dysplasia of the hip can affect one or both hips and occurs in varying degrees of dislocation, from partial (subluxation) to complete.

❏ In developmental dysplasia of the hip, Barlow's sign is present; a click is felt when the infant is placed supine with hips flexed 90 degrees, knees fully flexed, and the hip brought into midabduction.

❏ Barlow's sign, Ortolani's sign, and Trendelenburg's test are all used to diagnose developmental dysplasia of the hip.

❏ Duchenne muscular dystrophy is an X-linked genetic disorder (defect on the X chromosome) that occurs only in males.

- ❏ Duchenne muscular dystrophy (also called pseudohypertrophic dystrophy) is marked by muscular deterioration due to a lack of production of dystrophin that progresses throughout childhood.

- ❏ In Duchenne muscular dystrophy, the absence of dystrophin results in breakdown of muscle fibers; muscle fibers are replaced with fatty deposits and collagen in muscles.

- ❏ Neonates with developmental dysplasia of the hip are treated with Bryant's traction (if the acetabulum doesn't deepen) or a Pavlik harness or casting to keep the neonate's hips and knees flexed and the hips abducted for at least 3 months

- ❏ Treatment for developmental dysplasia of the hip in older children is a hip-spica cast or corrective surgery.

- ❏ Juvenile rheumatoid arthritis is an autoimmune disease of the connective tissue and is characterized by chronic inflammation of the synovia and possible joint destruction.

- ❏ Pauciarticular juvenile rheumatoid arthritis is asymmetrical involvement of fewer than five joints, usually affecting large joints such as the knees, ankles, and elbows.

- ❏ Polyarticular juvenile rheumatoid arthritis is symmetrical involvement of five or more joints, especially the hands and weight-bearing joints, such as the hips, knees, and feet.

- ❏ In polyarticular juvenile rheumatoid arthritis, involvement of the temporomandibular joint may cause earache; involvement of the sternoclavicular joint may cause chest pain.

- ❏ The third type of juvenile rheumatoid arthritis is systemic disease with polyarthritis, which involves the lining of the heart and lungs, blood cells, and abdominal organs.

- ❏ Legg-Calve-Perthes disease is ischemic necrosis that leads to eventual flattening of the head of the femur caused by vascular interruption.

- ❏ Osgood-Schlatter disease is a common cause of knee pain in adolescents and is most common in active adolescent boys; however, it may also be seen in girls ages 10 to 11.

- ❏ Scoliosis is a lateral curvature of the spine that is commonly identified at puberty and throughout adolescence.

- ❏ The causes of scoliosis are congenital, neuromuscular, and idiopathic.

- ❏ In congenital scoliosis, abnormal formation of the vertebrae or fused ribs occurs during prenatal development.

- ❏ Neuromuscular scoliosis occurs as a result of poor muscle control or weakness secondary to another condition, such as cerebral palsy or muscular dystrophy.

❑ In idiopathic scoliosis, there is an unknown reason for the curvature in a previously straight spine.

❑ A paralytic ileus is common with Harrington instrumentation rod placement, and the client may have a nasogastric tube in place for the first 48 hours after surgery.

❑ Spinous processes are the best bony landmark to identify when attempting to screen for scoliosis because this will show lateral deviation of the column.

❑ Serial casting is a treatment choice for talipes equinovarus in attempts to change the length of soft tissue.

❑ Corrective shoes are used for talipes equinovarus instead of short leg braces.

❑ Eversion exercise will help in talipes equinovarus.

❑ Placing several diapers on the infant with developmental dysplasia of the hip will keep the hips and knees flexed and the hips abducted.

❑ In the infant with developmental dysplasia of the hip, swaddling him tightly straightens the legs and doesn't allow abduction of the hips.

❑ X-rays show the location of the femur head and a shallow acetabulum, confirming the diagnosis of developmental dysplasia of the hip.

❑ Myelography is an invasive procedure used to evaluate abnormalities of the spinal canal and cord.

❑ Internal rotation of the hip is an unstable position and should be avoided in infants with hip instability.

❑ Typically, the child with developmental dysplasia of the hip is placed in slight abduction while in a hip-spica cast.

❑ A positive Galeazzi sign (one knee being higher than the other) is used to help diagnose hip dislocation.

❑ Avascular necrosis is common with fractures to the subcapital region, secondary to possible compromise of blood supply to the femoral head.

❑ Positional muscles of the hip and shoulder are affected first in muscular dystrophy, followed by the muscles of the foot and hand.

❑ Involuntary muscles, such as the muscles of respiration, are affected last in muscular dystrophy.

❑ A muscle biopsy, used to confirm the diagnosis of muscular dystrophy, shows the degeneration of muscle fibers and infiltration of fatty tissue.

❑ Creatine kinase values aid in the diagnosis of muscular dystrophy, as these enzymes rise due to muscle damage or deterioration and may reveal some forms of this disease.

❑ Duchenne muscular dystrophy, also known as pseudohypertrophic muscular dystrophy, accounts for 50% of all cases of muscular dystrophy and affects cardiac and respiratory muscles, as well as all voluntary muscles.

❏ An increased lumbar lordosis would be seen in a child suffering from muscular dystrophy secondary to paralysis of lower lumbar postural muscles; it also occurs to increase lower extremity support.

❏ Upper extremity spasticity isn't seen with muscular dystrophy because this disease isn't due to upper motor neuron lesions.

❏ Muscular dystrophy is hereditary and acquired through a recessive sex-linked trait.

❏ Respiratory infection can be fatal for clients with muscular dystrophy due to poor chest expansion and decreased ability to mobilize secretions.

❏ A shortened Achilles tendon may cause a child to walk on his toes.

❏ A hamstring release is done only when there's a knee flexion contracture.

❏ Muscular dystrophy is a result of a gene mutation.

❏ Studies have shown that children diagnosed with muscular dystrophy usually show some form of weakness by around age 3 years.

❏ In the child with muscular dystrophy, muscles will commonly be firm on palpation secondary to the infiltration of fatty tissue and connective tissue into the muscle.

❏ Gowers sign is a description of a transfer technique present during some phases of muscular dystrophy, in which the child turns on his side or abdomen, extends his knees, and pushes his torso to an upright position by walking his hands up the legs.

❏ For the infant with a hip-spica cast, the infant's body and cast should be at a 180-degree angle.

❏ Studies have shown that Duchenne muscular dystrophy is the most severe form of muscular dystrophy.

❏ After casting for a fracture of the radius, pain over a bony prominence, such as in the wrist or elbow, signals an impending pressure ulcer and requires prompt attention.

❏ Studies show that subluxation accounts for the greatest number of cases of developmental dysplasia of the hip.

❏ In developmental dysplasia of the hip, the femoral head loses contact with the acetabulum and is displaced posteriorly.

❏ The ligamentum teres is lengthened in developmental dysplasia of the hip.

❏ Buck's traction is a form of skeletal traction that pulls directly on the skeleton using a pin placed into the bone.

❏ Pin site care involves cleaning the insertion sites to reduce the risk of infection and observing the site for signs and symptoms of infection.

❏ The child's position should be changed every 2 hours to prevent skin breakdown when using Buck's traction.

❑ In Trendelenburg gait, the pelvis tilts downward on weight bearing secondary to a weakness of the abductors on the affected side.

❑ In developmental dysplasia of the hip, the internal rotation with subsequent dislocation will cause the leg to be shorter.

❑ There's usually decreased abduction as well as muscle and leg length changes in developmental dysplasia of the hip.

❑ In developmental dysplasia of the hip, internal rotation increases the risk of hip dislocation.

❑ After a spinal fusion, the child is usually placed on bed rest and ordered to lie flat.

❑ The child is allowed to sit up and get out of bed 2 to 4 days after spinal fusion.

❑ To prevent venous stasis after skeletal traction application, antiembolism stockings or an intermittent compression device is used on the unaffected leg.

❑ In scoliosis, the scapula on one side becomes more prominent, and the opposite side hollows; as the child bends over, the curvature of the spine is more apparent.

❑ In Bryant's traction, both legs are suspended 90 degrees off the bed, even though only one is fractured, with the child's body weight providing the countertraction.

❑ For the child in traction, all joints, except those immediately proximal and distal to the fracture, should be placed through range of motion every shift.

❑ For itching under the cast, cool air from a hair dryer may soothe the itchiness.

❑ Elevating the cast above the heart helps reduce swelling.

❑ To prevent foot drop in a casted leg, the foot should be supported with 90 degrees of flexion.

❑ Touch-down weight bearing prevents the client from putting weight on the extremity, but the client may touch the floor with the affected extremity.

❑ Full weight bearing allows for full weight bearing on the affected extremity.

❑ Partial weight bearing allows for only 30% to 50% weight bearing on the affected extremity.

❑ Nonweight bearing is no weight on the extremity, and the extremity must remain elevated.

❑ After repair of clubfoot, walking will stimulate all of the involved muscles and help with strengthening.

❑ Because an infant grows quickly, a series of casts will be needed for clubfoot as often as every 2 weeks to correct the deformity as the child grows.

❑ Casting for clubfoot should be complete by the time the child is crawling and walking.

❑ A greenstick fracture occurs when the bone is bent beyond its limits, causing an incomplete fracture.

❑ A plastic deformation or bend occurs when there is a microscopic fracture line where the bone bends.

❑ A buckle fracture occurs due to compression of the porous bone, causing a raised area or bulge at the fracture site.

❑ A complete fracture is one in which the bone is broken into separate pieces.

❑ Foul odors from the cast may be a sign of infection and should be reported to the physician immediately.

❑ Capillary refill of less than 3 seconds is a normal finding in a casted extremity.

❑ During the first 24 hours, the client may feel warmth under the cast as it dries.

❑ Breech presentation is a factor commonly associated with developmental dysplasia of the hip.

❑ After placement of Harrington rods, the client must remain flat in bed.

❑ After placement of Harrington rods, the gatch on a manual bed should be taped, and electric beds should be unplugged to prevent the client from raising the head or foot of the bed.

❑ A Frejka splint maintains abduction through padding of the diaper area.

❑ Soft abduction devices, such as the Frejka splint, must be worn continually except for diaper changes and skin care.

❑ The abduction position must be maintained in a child with developmental dysplasia of the hip to establish a deep hip socket.

❑ Bryant's traction is the usual method for treating a simple fracture of the femur in a child younger than age 3 and weighing less than 35 lb (15.9 kg).

❑ For a femur fracture to heal properly, it usually requires traction before casting.

❑ Assessing sensation, circulation, and motion is necessary in all children with a cast.

❑ Deep pain unrelieved by analgesics is an important sign of compartment syndrome, which may occur with a crush injury or when a fracture is reduced.

❑ Compartment syndrome occurs when swelling associated with inflammation reduces blood flow to the affected areas; casting causes additional constriction of blood flow.

❑ Volkmann's contracture is a contraction of the fingers, and sometimes the wrist, that occurs after severe injury or improper use of a tourniquet or cast.

❑ A brace for scoliosis must be worn at all times except for bathing.

❑ Most scoliosis braces must be worn for several months to 1 year.

❑ The client with a full body cast may exhibit signs and symptoms of anxiety most likely caused by the feeling of being claustrophobic.

❑ A client with compartment syndrome would exhibit signs of intense pain unrelieved by analgesics.

❑ Compression of the mesenteric blood supply can cause constipation.

## Gastrointestinal system

❑ The mother of a child diagnosed with celiac disease should be taught to read the packages of all foods carefully to ensure that they're gluten-free.

❑ Steatorrhea (fatty, foul-smelling, frothy, bulky stools) is common with celiac disease because of the inability to absorb fat.

❑ Clay-colored stools are characteristic of a decrease or absence of conjugated bilirubin.

❑ Red currant jelly stool is an indication of intussusception.

❑ Within a day or two of starting a gluten-free diet, most children with celiac disease show improved appetite, disappearance of diarrhea, and weight gain.

❑ To prevent trauma to the suture line of an infant who underwent cleft lip repair, arm restraints are used to prevent the infant from rubbing the sutures.

❑ After surgery for cleft lip repair (staphylorraphy), the suture line must be cleaned after each feeding to reduce the risk of infection, which could adversely affect the healing and cosmetic results.

❑ In the infant with cleft lip or palate, feedings are usually given in the upright position to prevent formula or breast milk from coming through the nose.

❑ Various special nipples have been devised for infants with cleft lip or palate; a normal nursery nipple isn't effective.

❑ Sometimes, especially if the cleft isn't severe, breast-feeding may be easier because the human nipple conforms to the shape of the infant's mouth.

❑ On return from surgery after repair of a cleft palate, the infant should be positioned on his side to allow oral secretions to drain from the mouth and avoid suctioning.

❑ Pacifiers shouldn't be used after repair of a cleft palate because they can damage the suture line.

❑ A soft diet is recommended for a small child who has just had surgical repair of a cleft palate; no food harder than mashed potatoes can be eaten.

❑ After surgical repair of a cleft palate, the nurse should irrigate the infant's mouth with the infant in an upright position and head tilted forward to prevent aspiration.

❑ The prone position isn't appropriate after surgical cleft lip repair because this may put pressure on the suture line.

❑ A sunken anterior fontanel is a sign of dehydration in the neonate whose fontanel hasn't yet closed.

❑ Because the GI system is so crucial to other body systems, a problem in this system can quickly affect the overall health, growth, and development of the child.

❑ Celiac disease is intolerance to gliadin—a gluten protein found in grains, such as wheat, rye, oats, and barley—that causes poor food absorption.

❑ In celiac disease, a decrease in the amount and activity of enzymes in the intestinal mucosal cells causes the villi of the proximal small intestine to atrophy, decreasing intestinal absorption.

❑ Celiac disease usually becomes apparent between ages 6 and 18 months.

❑ Esophageal atresia with tracheoesophageal fistula occurs when either the distal end of the esophagus ends in a blind pouch and the proximal end of the esophagus is linked to the trachea via a fistula, or the proximal end of the esophagus ends in a blind pouch and the distal portion of the esophagus is connected to the trachea via a fistula.

❑ Other birth defects may coexist with esophageal atresia with tracheoesophageal fistula and should be assessed at birth.

❑ In neonates, peristalsis occurs within 2½ to 3 hours of eating. It occurs within 3 to 6 hours in older infants and children.

❑ Gastric stomach capacity of the neonate is 30 to 60 mL, which gradually increases to 200 to 350 mL by age 12 months, and to 1,500 mL as an adolescent.

❑ The neonatal abdomen is larger than the chest up to ages 4 to 8 weeks, and the musculature is poorly developed.

❑ The extrusion reflex (or tongue-thrust reflex), which protects the infant from food substances that his system is too immature to digest, persists to ages 3 to 4 months.

❑ At age 4 months, saliva production begins and aids in the process of digestion.

❑ The sucking reflex begins to diminish at age 6 months.

❑ The neonate has immature muscle tone of the lower esophageal sphincter and low volume capacity of the stomach, which cause the neonate to "spit up" frequently.

❑ Increased myelination of nerves to the anal sphincter allows for physiologic control of bowel function, usually around age 2.

❑ The liver's slow development of glycogen storage capacity makes the infant prone to hypoglycemia.

❑ From ages 1 to 3, composition of intestinal flora becomes more adultlike and stomach acidity increases, reducing the number of GI infections.

❑ Cheiloplasty is performed between birth and age 3 months in an infant with cleft lip. It unites the lip and gum edges in anticipation of teeth eruption, providing a route for adequate nutrition and sucking.

❑ Cleft palate repair surgery (staphylorrhaphy) is usually scheduled at about age 18 months to allow for growth of the palate and to be done before the infant develops speech patterns.

❑ Before cleft palate repair surgery (staphylorrhaphy), the infant must be free from ear and respiratory infections.

❑ A sonorous seal bark cough may be heard in the birthing room after the birth of a neonate with esophageal atresia and tracheoesophageal fistula.

❑ The nurse caring for an infant suspected of having esophageal atresia and tracheoesophageal fistula would initially observe for abdominal distention when the infant cries. Crying may force air into the stomach, causing distention.

❑ Secretions in a client with esophageal atresia and tracheoesophageal fistula may be more visible, although normal in quantity, because of the client's inability to swallow effectively.

❑ Dietary management in a child diagnosed with ulcerative colitis should include a high-calorie diet.

❑ After surgical repair of a tracheoesophageal fistula and esophageal atresia, the neonate should be kept in an upright position after feeding to reduce the risk of refluxed stomach contents and aspiration pneumonia.

❑ Because the chest cavity is entered during repair of a tracheoesophageal fistula and esophageal atresia, the neonate may have a chest tube in place during recovery that's removed before discharge.

❑ Gastroschisis is a herniation of the bowel through an abnormal opening in the abdominal wall.

❑ Tracheoesophageal fistula is a malformation of the trachea and esophagus.

❑ The spleen has commonly been seen in the thorax of infants with a diaphragmatic hernia on the left side.

❑ The presence of abdominal organs in the chest cavity due to a diaphragmatic hernia causes the mediastinum to shift to the unaffected side, which causes a partial collapse of that lung.

❑ Positioning the infant with a diaphragmatic hernia on his affected side lets the lung on the unaffected side expand, making breathing easier.

❑ The stomach and intestine in the chest cavity may also become distended with swallowed air from crying with a diaphragmatic hernia.

❑ Careful positioning and handling prevent infection and rupture of the omphalocele.

❑ The infant with pyloric stenosis should be weighed daily.

❑ Because the obstruction in pyloric stenosis doesn't allow food to pass through to the duodenum, the infant vomits for relief when the stomach becomes full.

❏ When assessing a neonate, visible peristaltic waves across the epigastrium are indicative of hypertrophic pyloric stenosis.

❏ Positioning the infant with pyloric stenosis slightly on the right side in high semi-Fowler's position will help facilitate gastric emptying.

❏ Infants with pyloric stenosis usually swallow a lot of air from sucking on their hands and fingers because of their intense hunger.

❏ Burping frequently during feeding will lessen gastric distention in infants with pyloric stenosis and increase the likelihood that the infant will retain the feeding.

❏ In infants with pyloric stenosis, record the type, amount, and character of the vomit as well as its relation to the feeding.

❏ Even with successful surgery, most infants with pyloric stenosis have some vomiting during the first 24 to 48 hours after the surgical repair.

❏ Minimal handling of the infant with pyloric stenosis, especially after a feeding, will help prevent vomiting.

❏ Infants with pyloric stenosis are constantly hungry because of their inability to retain feedings.

❏ Bowel sounds decrease with pyloric stenosis because food can't pass into the intestines.

❏ Normal respiratory effort is affected by the abdominal distention that pushes the diaphragm up into the pleural cavity with pyloric stenosis.

❏ In the recovery phase following ingestion of drain cleaner by a child, scar tissue develops as the burn from ingestion heals, leading to esophageal strictures.

❏ Chemical pneumonitis is the most common complication of ingestion of a hydrocarbon, such as kerosene.

❏ The first step parents should take if their child has ingested a poisonous substance is to call the poison control center for instructions.

❏ Home administration of syrup of ipecac is no longer recommended by the American Academy of Pediatrics for poisoning.

❏ If a child ingests poisonous hydrocarbons, keeping the child calm and relaxed will help prevent vomiting, which can damage the esophagus from regurgitation of the gastric poison.

❏ The risk of chemical pneumonitis exists if vomiting occurs in a child who has ingested poisonous hydrocarbons.

❏ The most common pain medications accidentally ingested are acetaminophen-containing (Tylenol-containing) drugs, nonsteroidal anti-inflammatory drugs, and opioids.

❏ Recurrent or persistent diarrhea is a common feature of ulcerative colitis.

❑ After ingestion of poisonous amounts of salicylates, there's usually a delay of 6 hours before evidence of toxicity is noted.

❑ Gastric lavage is used in the immediate treatment for salicylate poisoning because the stomach contents and salicylates will move from the stomach to the remainder of the GI tract, where vomiting will no longer result in the removal of the poison.

❑ Acetaminophen poisoning damages the liver, leading to elevated serum alanine aminotransferase and aspartate aminotransferase levels.

❑ After therapy with acetylcysteine is started for acetaminophen poisoning, liver enzymes should begin to fall.

❑ During the first 12 to 24 hours after ingestion, profuse sweating is a significant sign of acetaminophen poisoning.

❑ Weak pulse, hypothermia, and decreased urine output are common findings with acetaminophen poisoning.

❑ If the client is seen within 4 hours of ingestion, activated charcoal should be given to prevent absorption of acetaminophen.

❑ Gastric lavage is recommended only if the client is seen within 1 hour of ingestion in acetaminophen poisoning.

❑ In older homes that contain lead-based paint, paint chips may be eaten directly by the child or they may cling to toys or hands that are then put into the child's mouth.

❑ Ingested lead is initially absorbed by bone; X-rays reveal a characteristic "lead line" at the epiphyseal line.

❑ Chronic ingestion of lead produces effects on the central nervous, renal, and hematologic systems.

❑ Lead is dangerously toxic to the biosynthesis of heme, and the reduced amounts of heme molecule in red blood cells cause anemia.

❑ Paralysis may occur in lead toxicity as toxic damage to the brain progresses.

❑ Lead intoxification produces damage to the central nervous system that is difficult to repair.

❑ One diagnostic characteristic of lead poisoning is a gingival or Burton line, which refers to black lines along the gums.

❑ Chelation therapy is the main treatment for lead poisoning and involves the removal of metal by combining it with another substance.

❑ Sometimes exchange transfusions may be needed to rid the blood of lead quickly.

❑ A calcium-chelating agent is used for the treatment of lead poisoning, resulting in hypocalcemia.

❏ The sudden cessation of abdominal pain in the client with appendicitis may indicate perforation or infarction of the appendix, requiring emergency surgery.

❏ The client with abdominal pain, fever, and vomiting (the cardinal signs of appendicitis) should seek immediate emergency care to reduce the risk of complications if the appendix should rupture.

❏ Pain can be generalized or periumbilical in appendicitis; it usually descends to the lower right quadrant.

❏ Enemas may aggravate appendicitis.

❏ Only a single dose of medication, such as mebendazole, is needed to treat pinworms.

❏ Right lower quadrant pain, a low-grade fever, nausea, rebound tenderness, and a positive psoas sign are all consistent with appendicitis.

❏ Gastroenteritis is characterized by generalized abdominal tenderness.

❏ Pancreatitis is characterized by pain in the left abdominal quadrant.

❏ Cholecystitis is characterized by pain in the right upper abdominal quadrant.

❏ Neonates with a cleft lip and a cleft palate may have an excessive amount of saliva and usually have a difficult time with feedings.

❏ Special feeding techniques, such as using a flanged nipple, may be necessary to prevent aspiration in neonates with a cleft lip and a cleft palate.

❏ In type III/C tracheoesophageal fistula, the proximal end of the esophagus ends in a blind pouch and a fistula connects the distal end of the esophagus to the trachea.

❏ In type III/C tracheoesophageal fistula, because the distal end of the esophagus is connected to the trachea, the neonate can't vomit, but he can aspirate. Stomach acid may go into the lungs through this fistula, causing pneumonitis.

❏ Pyloric stenosis involves hypertrophy of the circular (or olive-shaped) muscle fibers of the pylorus.

❏ The hypertrophy with pyloric stenosis is palpable in the right upper quadrant of the abdomen.

❏ A "sausage" mass is palpable in the right upper quadrant in children with intussusception.

❏ Infants with pyloric stenosis vomit hydrochloric acid, causing them to become alkalotic and hypochloremic.

❏ Projectile vomiting in an infant is a sign of pyloric stenosis, a condition that requires surgical intervention to correct.

❏ After surgery for pyloric stenosis, the infant is at risk for infection because the incision is near the diaper area.

❑ Necrotizing enterocolitis is an ischemic disorder of the gut.

❑ The cause of necrotizing enterocolitis is unknown, but it's more common in premature neonates who had a hypoxic episode.

❑ In necrotizing enterocolitis, the neonate's intestines become dilated and necrotic, and the abdomen becomes distended.

❑ Young children with gastroenteritis are at high risk for developing a fluid volume deficit because their intestinal mucosa allows for more fluid and electrolytes to be lost when they have gastroenteritis.

❑ The main goal of the health care team in young children with gastroenteritis should be to rehydrate the infant; deficient fluid volume is life-threatening.

❑ Diarrhea in infants can rapidly lead to dehydration and electrolyte imbalances, especially hyponatremia and hypokalemia.

❑ It's important to continue the gluten-free diet in celiac disease to avoid symptoms and the associated risk of colon cancer.

❑ Cellophane tape placed near the anal edge will capture the eggs and assist in diagnosing pinworms.

❑ An intussusception begins suddenly and leads to bloody stools and vomiting.

❑ A meconium ileus is nonpassage of meconium by 24 hours of age.

❑ Signs of pyloric stenosis include projectile vomiting and weight loss.

❑ Celiac disease presents with steatorrhea, weight loss, and inability to digest gluten foods.

❑ Allowing only clear liquids while recovering from gastroenteritis gives the intestine time to heal, but the fluids should be reintroduced slowly to determine the child's ability to tolerate and retain them.

❑ Adverse effects of corticosteroids include acne, hirsutism, mood swings, osteoporosis, and adrenal suppression.

❑ Steroid use in children and adolescents may cause delayed growth.

❑ Children with school phobia commonly complain of vague symptoms, such as stomachaches, nausea, headaches, and dizziness, to avoid going to school.

## Genitourinary system

❑ The goal of acute glomerulonephritis involves interventions, such as decreased fluid and salt intake, designed to minimize or prevent fluid retention and edema.

❑ The child with acute glomerulonephritis should be monitored for fluid imbalance, which is done through daily weights.

❑ Urinalysis findings consistent with acute glomerulonephritis include a specific gravity less than 1.030, proteinuria, hematuria, and the presence of red blood cell casts.

❏ One of the first signs of improvement during the acute phase of glomerulonephritis is an increase in urine output.

❏ Antihypertensive drugs may be needed to stabilize the blood pressure in a client with glomerulonephritis.

❏ Acute glomerulonephritis is an immunocomplex disease that occurs as a by-product of a streptococcal infection.

❏ Moderate sodium restriction with a diet that has no added salt after cooking is usually effective in acute glomerulonephritis.

❏ A latent period of 10 to 14 days occurs between streptococcal infection of the throat or skin and the onset of clinical manifestations of acute glomerulonephritis.

❏ A sign of periorbital edema would lead the nurse to investigate the possibility of glomerulonephritis, especially if reported to be worse in the morning.

❏ Acute glomerulonephritis can occur at any age, but it primarily affects early school-age children, with a peak age of onset of 6 to 7.

❏ Acute glomerulonephritis is uncommon in children younger than age 2.

❏ Enuresis is involuntary urination after age 5 years that generally occurs while the child is sleeping.

❏ The major complications during the acute phase of glomerulonephritis are hypertensive encephalopathy, acute cardiac decompensation, and acute renal failure.

❏ When collecting a clean-catch urine specimen, the first-voided specimen of the day should never be used because of urinary stasis; this also applies after a nap.

❏ The clean-catch urine specimen should be collected midstream, not at the beginning or end of urination.

❏ Because hypertension is a complication of acute glomerulonephritis, the nurse should check the child's blood pressure every 4 hours.

❏ Foods that are high in sodium content, such as hot dogs, should be eliminated from the diet of a child who has acute glomerulonephritis.

❏ Chordee, or ventral curvature of the penis, results from the replacement of normal skin with a fibrous band of tissue and usually accompanies more severe forms of hypospadias.

❏ Because undescended testes may also be present with hypospadias, the small penis may appear to be an enlarged clitoris.

❏ Hypospadias shouldn't be mistaken for ambiguous genitalia; if there's any doubt, more tests should be performed.

❏ The principal objectives of surgical corrections for hypospadias are to enhance the child's ability to void in the standing position with a straight stream, to improve the physical appearance of the genitalia for psychological reasons, and to preserve a sexually adequate organ.

❏ After hypospadias repair, a pressure dressing is applied to the penis to reduce bleeding and tissue swelling.

❏ After hypospadias repair, the penile tip should be assessed frequently for signs of circulatory impairment.

❏ The preferred time for surgical repair of hypospadias is age 6 to 18 months, before the child has developed body image and castration anxiety.

❏ Parents are taught to care for the indwelling catheter or stent and irrigation techniques after surgical repair of hypospadias, if indicated.

❏ Long-term complications of pelvic inflammatory disease include abscess formation in the fallopian tubes and adhesion formation, leading to increased risk of ectopic pregnancy or infertility.

❏ Clinical manifestations of chlamydia include meatal erythema, tenderness, itching, dysuria, and urethral discharge in the male and mucopurulent cervical exudate with erythema, edema, and congestion in the female.

❏ The treatment of choice for chlamydia is doxycycline or azithromycin.

❏ Human papilloma virus doesn't increase the risk of gonorrhea, chlamydia, or urinary tract infections.

❏ Gonorrhea is caused by *Neisseria gonorrhoeae*.

❏ Teenagers find sexually transmitted diseases a very difficult topic to discuss with their parents and will usually seek out a peer or another adult to obtain information.

❏ Gonorrhea can occur with or without symptoms.

❏ The younger the client when sexual activity begins, the higher the incidence of human immunodeficiency virus and AIDS.

❏ Pelvic inflammatory disease is an infection of the upper female genital tract most commonly caused by sexually transmitted diseases.

❏ Presenting symptoms of pelvic inflammatory disease in the adolescent may be generalized with fever, abdominal pain, urinary tract symptoms, and vague, influenza-like symptoms.

❏ A hard, painless, red defined lesion indicates syphilis.

❏ Small, painful vesicles on the genital area indicate herpes genitalis.

❏ Cervical discharge with redness and edema indicates chlamydia.

❏ Human immunodeficiency virus can be spread through many routes, including sexual contact and contact with infected blood or other body fluids.

❏ Only about 25% of all new human immunodeficiency virus infections in the United States occur in people under age 22.

❑ In a urinary tract infection, infected urine usually contains more than 100,000 colonies/mL, usually of a single organism.

❑ The urine of a client with a urinary tract infection is usually cloudy, hazy, and may have strands of mucus; it has a foul, fishy odor even when fresh.

❑ Drinking highly acidic juices, such as cranberry juice, may help maintain urinary health.

❑ Reflux of urine into the ureters and then back into the bladder after voiding sets up the client for a urinary tract infection; this can lead to renal damage due to scarring of the parenchyma.

❑ Glomerulonephritis is an autoimmune reaction to a beta-hemolytic streptococcal infection.

❑ Cotton is a more breathable fabric and allows for dampness to be absorbed from the perineum in young girls to help prevent urinary tract infections.

❑ The perineum should always be cleaned from front to back in young girls to help prevent urinary tract infection.

❑ Under normal conditions, the act of completely and repeatedly emptying the bladder flushes away any organisms before they have an opportunity to multiply and invade surrounding tissue.

❑ There's an increased incidence of urinary tract infection in uncircumcised infants under 1 year, but not after that age.

❑ In infants and children less than 2 years old, the signs of a urinary tract infection are characteristically nonspecific; feeding problems are usually the first indication.

❑ The most accurate tests of bacterial content in urine are suprapubic aspiration (for children less than 2 years old) and properly performed bladder catheterization.

❑ Bagged urine specimen, clean-catch urine specimen, and first-voided urine specimen have a high incidence of contamination not related to infection.

❑ Caffeinated or carbonated beverages are avoided in the child with a urinary tract infection because of their potentially irritating effect on the bladder mucosa.

❑ Wilms tumor is the most frequent intra-abdominal tumor of childhood and the most common type of renal cancer.

❑ The peak incidence of Wilms tumor is age 3 years.

❑ There's an increased incidence of Wilms tumor among siblings and identical twins.

❑ The most common presenting sign of Wilms tumor is a swelling or mass within the abdomen.

❏ The mass associated with Wilms tumor is characteristically firm, nontender, confined to one side, and deep within the flank.

❏ Blood pressure is characteristically increased with Wilms tumor.

❏ Wilms tumor usually involves only one kidney and is usually staged during surgery so that an effective course of treatment can be established.

❏ Wilms tumor has a slightly higher occurrence in the left kidney, and it stays encapsulated for an extended period of time.

❏ Children with Wilms tumor who have stage I or II localized tumor have a 90% chance of cure with multimodal therapy.

❏ If both kidneys are involved with Wilms tumor, the child may be treated with radiation therapy or chemotherapy preoperatively to shrink the tumor, allowing more conservative therapy.

❏ Surgery is the preferred treatment for Wilms tumor and is scheduled as soon as possible after confirmation of a renal mass, usually within 24 to 48 hours of admission, to be sure the encapsulated tumor remains intact.

❏ An infant has a much greater percentage of total body water in extracellular fluid (42% to 45%) than an adult does (20%).

❏ Because of the increased percentage of water in a child's extracellular fluid, a child's water turnover rate is two to three times greater than that of an adult.

❏ Every day, 50% of an infant's extracellular fluid is exchanged, compared with only 20% of an adult's; therefore, a child is more susceptible to dehydration than an adult.

❏ A neonate has a greater ratio of body surface area to body weight than an adult; this ratio results in greater fluid loss through the skin.

❏ A child's kidneys attain the adult number of nephrons (about a million in each kidney) shortly after birth.

❏ The nephrons, which form urine, continue to mature throughout early childhood.

❏ An infant's renal system can maintain a healthy fluid and electrolyte status; however, it doesn't function as efficiently as an adult's during periods of stress.

❏ An infant's kidneys don't concentrate urine at an adult level (average specific gravity is less than 1.010 for an infant, compared with 1.010 to 1.030 for an adult).

❏ Children have short urethras; therefore, organisms can be easily transmitted into the bladder, increasing the risk of bladder infection.

❏ In infants, the infecting organism that causes a chlamydia infection is passed from the infected mother to the fetus during passage through the birth canal.

❑ Chlamydia is the most common cause of ophthalmia neonatorum (eye infection at birth or during the first month of life) and a major cause of pneumonia in infants in the first 3 months of life.

❑ Hypospadias is a congenital anomaly of the penis in which the urethral opening may be anywhere along the ventral side of the penis.

❑ Hypospadias shortens the distance to the bladder, offering easier access for bacteria.

❑ Treatment for hypospadias includes a tubularized incised plate procedure (for distal and midshaft hypospadias), the most commonly used repair for primary tubularization of the ureteral plate.

❑ Urethroplasty is a procedure in which the urethra is extended into a normal position with a meatus at the tip of the penis and may initially be performed to restore normal urinary function.

❑ Orthoplasty is performed to treat hypospadias when the child is 12 to 18 months old. It releases the adherent chordee (fibrous band that causes the penis to curve downward); if extensive repair is needed, delay until age 4.

❑ Nephritis is a sudden inflammation that primarily affects the interstitial area and the renal pelvis or, less commonly, the renal tubules.

❑ Types of nephritis include acute tubulointerstitial nephritis, pyelonephritis, and glomerulonephritis.

❑ One of the most common renal diseases, nephritis is more common in females, probably because of a shorter urethra and the proximity of the urinary meatus to the vagina and the rectum.

❑ In the client with nephritis, encourage fluid intake to achieve urine output of more than 2 L/day; however, discourage intake greater than 3 L/day because excessive fluid intake may decrease the effectiveness of antibiotics.

❑ Nephroblastoma, also known as Wilms tumor, is an embryonal cancer of the kidney.

❑ The prognosis for Wilms tumor is excellent if metastasis hasn't occurred.

❑ Don't palpate the abdomen in a client with nephroblastoma and prevent others from doing so; palpating the abdomen may cause tumor rupture.

❑ The risk of urinary tract infections varies depending on the child's age and the presence of obstructive uropathy or voiding dysfunction.

❑ In the neonatal period, urinary tract infections occur most commonly in males, possibly because of the higher incidence of congenital abnormalities in male neonates.

❑ By age 4 months, urinary tract infections are much more common in girls than in boys.

❑ The increased incidence of urinary tract infections in girls continues throughout childhood.

❑ Assess the child's toileting habits for proper front-to-back wiping and proper hand washing to prevent recurrent infection.

❑ Because the child is left with only one kidney after removal of the other for a Wilms tumor, certain precautions, such as avoiding contact sports, are recommended to prevent injury to the remaining kidney.

❑ Fluid intake is essential for renal function of the remaining kidney.

❑ After surgery for Wilms tumor the child is at risk for intestinal obstruction; GI abnormalities, such as absent bowel sounds, require notification of the physician.

❑ A stage IV tumor has a poor prognosis because other organs are involved.

❑ Wilms tumor can be genetically inherited and is associated with other congenital anomalies.

## Endocrine system

❑ Clinical manifestations of thyroid hormone overdose in an infant include tachycardia, irritability, and diaphoresis.

❑ Preterm neonates are usually affected by hypothyroidism due to hypothalamic and pituitary immaturity.

❑ The most serious consequence of congenital hypothyroidism is delayed development of the central nervous system, which leads to severe mental retardation.

❑ The severity of the intellectual deficit is related to the degree of hypothyroidism and the duration of the condition before treatment.

❑ Heelstick blood tests for congenital hypothyroidism are mandatory in all states and are usually performed on neonates between 2 and 6 days of life.

❑ Treatment of congenital hypothyroidism involves lifelong thyroid hormone replacement therapy that begins as soon as possible after diagnosis. Treatment abolishes all signs of hypothyroidism and reestablishes normal physical and mental development.

❑ If a neonate begins to look yellow, hyperbilirubinemia may be the cause.

❑ The importance of compliance with the levothyroxine (Synthroid) regimen for the neonate to achieve normal growth and development must be stressed.

❑ Children with congenital hypothyroidism will have dry skin.

❑ Education about congenital hypothyroidism should occur as soon as the parents are ready so they'll understand the genetic implications for future children.

❑ Food intake should be increased in children with diabetes when they are more physically active.

❏ The child with diabetes has an increased risk of insulin shock and a decreased risk of hyperglycemia when he's more physically active.

❏ Adolescents appear to have the most difficulty in adjusting to diabetes.

❏ Teenagers may believe that alcohol will increase blood glucose levels, when in fact the opposite occurs.

❏ Teens with diabetes mellitus who drink alcohol may become hypoglycemic, but their symptoms of hypoglycemia may be misinterpreted as being intoxicated.

❏ When a child exhibits signs of hypoglycemia, the majority of cases can be treated with a simple concentrated sugar, such as honey, that can be held in the mouth for a short time.

❏ Diabetic ketoacidosis, the most complete state of insulin deficiency, is a life-threatening situation.

❏ Children with diabetes can learn to collect their own blood for glucose testing at a relatively young age (4 to 5 years), and most are able to check their blood glucose level and administer insulin at about age 9; some children may be able to do it earlier.

❏ Diabetic ketoacidosis is determined by the presence of hyperglycemia (blood glucose level of 300 mg/dl or higher), accompanied by acetone breath, dehydration, weak and rapid pulse, and a decreased level of consciousness.

❏ A child who complains of feeling shaky, is sweating, and appears pale may be having symptoms of hypoglycemia.

❏ During an illness involving vomiting or loss of appetite in a client with diabetes, the NPH insulin dose may be lowered by 25% to 30% to avoid hyperglycemia; regular insulin is given according to home glucose monitoring results.

❏ A glycosylated hemoglobin level provides an overview of a person's blood glucose level over the previous 2 to 3 months.

❏ Glycosylated hemoglobin values are reported as a percentage of the total hemoglobin within a red blood cell.

❏ Rapid heart rate, headache, and hunger are signs and symptoms of hypoglycemia.

❏ The simplest test used to diagnose diabetes insipidus is restriction of oral fluids and observation of consequent changes in urine volume and concentration.

❏ Unresponsiveness to exogenous vasopressin usually indicates nephrogenic diabetes insipidus.

❏ The usual treatment for diabetes insipidus is hormone replacement with vasopressin or desmopressin acetate.

❏ Idiopathic growth hormone deficiency is commonly associated with other pituitary hormone deficiencies, such as deficiencies of thyroid-stimulating hormone and corticotropin, and may be secondary to hypothalamic deficiency.

❑ During the school-age years, growth slows and doesn't accelerate again until adolescence.

❑ Familial short stature refers to otherwise healthy children who have ancestors with adult height in the lower percentiles and whose height during childhood is appropriate for genetic background.

❑ Children with delayed linear growth and skeletal and sexual maturation that is behind that of their peers are considered to have constitutional growth delay.

❑ Clinical features of hypopituitarism develop slowly and vary with the severity of the disorder and the number of deficient hormones.

❑ Epiphyseal maturation is retarded in hypopituitarism consistent with retardation in height.

❑ Definitive diagnosis of hypopituitarism is based on absent or subnormal reserves of pituitary growth hormone.

❑ The definitive treatment of growth hormone deficiency is replacement of the growth hormone; it is successful in 80% of affected children.

❑ The thyroid gland, many times larger in children than in adults, is functional at age 2 weeks and is thought to play a role in immune function.

❑ The ovaries, present at birth, remain inactive until puberty.

❑ Male secondary sexual development consists of genital growth and the appearance of pubic and body hair.

❑ Congenital hypothyroidism is present at birth.

❑ Acquired hypothyroidism is commonly due to thyroiditis, an inflammation of the thyroid gland that results in injury or damage to thyroid tissue.

❑ Infants with hypothyroidism treated before age 3 months usually grow and develop normally.

❑ Children with hypothyroidism who remain untreated beyond age 3 months, and children with acquired hypothyroidism who remain untreated beyond age 2, suffer irreversible cognitive impairment.

❑ Type 1 diabetes mellitus (formerly referred to as juvenile diabetes or insulin-dependent diabetes) is a chronic metabolic disease characterized by absolute insulin insufficiency.

❑ Assessment findings for a neonate with congenital hypothyroidism include depressed nasal bridge, short forehead, puffy eyelids, and large tongue; thick, dry, mottled skin that feels cold to the touch; coarse, dry, lusterless hair; abdominal distention; umbilical hernia; hyporeflexia; bradycardia; hypothermia; hypotension; anemia; and wide cranial sutures.

❑ Weight loss, lack of energy, acetone odor to breath, and a blood glucose level of 325 mg/dL indicate diabetic ketoacidosis.

❑ Common findings of Cushing syndrome include obesity, moon-shaped face, and emotional instability.

❑ Hypopituitarism presents with a retarded growth pattern, appearance younger than chronological age, and normal skeletal proportions and intelligence.

❑ Symptoms of pheochromocytoma include hypertension, headaches, hyperglycemia with weight loss, diaphoresis, and hyperventilation.

❑ Generally, children with hypopituitarism are of average birth weight and grow at a normal pace for the first 2 or 3 years, then fall behind their peers in height, usually below the third percentile.

❑ Polydipsia and polyuria with normal serum glucose may be indicative of diabetes insipidus.

## Integumentary system

❑ Caloric intake with a burn injury should be 1½ to 2 times the basal metabolic rate, with a minimum of 1.5 to 2 g/kg of body weight of protein daily.

❑ Full-thickness burns usually need surgical closure and grafting for complete healing.

❑ Healing in 10 to 12 days with little or no scarring is associated with superficial partial-thickness burns.

❑ With superficial partial-thickness burns, pigment is expected to return to the injured area after healing.

❑ Deep partial-thickness burns heal in 6 weeks with scarring.

❑ A client with a deep partial-thickness burn will have tissue necrosis to the epidermis and dermis layers.

❑ Erythema and pain are characteristic of superficial burn injury.

❑ With deep burns, the nerve fibers are destroyed and the client won't feel pain in the affected area.

❑ Necrosis through all skin layers is seen with full-thickness injuries.

❑ Circumferential burns can compromise blood flow to an extremity, causing numbness.

❑ Absence of pain and full range of motion implies good tissue oxygenation from intact circulation in a burn injury.

❑ The cutaneous eruption of fifth disease can reappear for up to 4 months.

❑ The child with fifth disease should be isolated from pregnant women, immunocompromised clients, and clients with chronic anemia for up to 2 weeks.

❑ A child with fifth disease is contagious during the first stage, when symptoms of headache, body aches, fever, and chills are present, not after the rash appears.

❑ The classic symptoms of fifth disease begin with intense redness of both cheeks.

❑ An erythematous rash with a sandpaper-like texture is associated with scarlet fever, which is a bacterial infection.

❑ Children with varicella typically have vesicular lesions of the trunk, face, and scalp after a low-grade fever.

❑ An erythematous rash after a fever is characteristic of roseola.

❑ A bull's eye rash is a classic symptom of Lyme disease and is located primarily at the site of the bite.

❑ Necrotic, painful rashes are associated with the bite of a brown recluse spider.

❑ A linear, papular, vesicular rash indicates exposure to the leaves of poison ivy.

❑ Once every varicella lesion is crusted over, the child is no longer considered contagious.

❑ The rash with varicella is typically a maculopapular vesicular rash.

❑ The incubation period of varicella is 10 to 20 days.

❑ Teardrop vesicles of varicella-zoster virus on an erythematous base generally begin on the trunk, face, and scalp, with minimal involvement of the extremities.

❑ Koplik's spots are diagnostic of rubeola.

❑ A descending maculopapular rash is characteristic of rubeola.

❑ Yellow ulcers of the hands and feet are associated with hand, foot, and mouth disease caused by the coxsackievirus.

❑ Signs and symptoms of frostbite include tingling, numbness, burning sensation, and white skin.

❑ A paronychia is a localized infection of the nail bed caused by either staphylococci or streptococci.

❑ *Borrelia burgdorferi* is responsible for Lyme disease.

❑ Pruritic papules, vesicles, and linear burrows are diagnostic for scabies.

❑ Nits, seen as white oval dots, are characteristic of head lice and are empty eggshells in the child's hair.

❑ Stings from honeybees are associated with a stinger, pain, and erythema.

❑ In cases of suspected child abuse, an accurate precise examination of all lesions must be properly and legally documented.

❑ Contusions that result from falls are typically confined to a single body area and are considered a reasonable finding in a child still learning to walk.

❑ Injuries from normal falls are usually not linear in nature.

❑ The bleeding from contusions can cause variations, but the color change is consistent.

❑ The clinical sign of pinworms is perianal itching that increases at night.

❏ Anal fissures are associated with rectal bleeding and pain with bowel movements.

❏ Scabies are associated with a pruritic rash, characterized as linear burrows of the webs of the fingers and toes.

❏ Detection of pinworms by the clear cellophane tape test is virtually 100% accurate with five tests.

❏ The most common intestinal parasitic infection in the United States is giardiasis, prevalent among children attending group day care or nursery school.

❏ Papules are elevated up to 0.5 cm; nodules and tumors are elevated more than 0.5 cm.

❏ Erosions are characterized as loss of the epidermis layer.

❏ Fluid-filled lesions are vesicles and pustules.

❏ Macules and patches are described as nonpalpable flat changes in skin color.

❏ Pustules are pus-filled lesions, such as acne and impetigo.

❏ A wheal is a superficial area of localized edema.

❏ Vesicles are serous-filled lesions up to 0.5 cm in diameter.

❏ Bullae are serous-filled lesions greater than 0.5 cm in diameter.

❏ Tinea versicolor is a superficial fungus infection.

❏ Depigmented areas are signs of vitiligo.

❏ After 7 to 10 days, the bruise from an injury becomes greenish yellow.

❏ Contusions of the back and buttocks are highly suspicious of abuse related to punishment.

❏ Contusions at various stages of healing are red flags to potential abuse.

❏ Contusions of the shins and forehead are usually related to an active toddler falling and bumping into objects.

❏ Like most body systems, the integumentary system isn't mature at birth; therefore, it provides a less effective barrier to physical elements or microorganisms during birth and infancy than during childhood. This helps to explain why infants and young children are more prone to infection.

❏ The skin of infants and young children appears smoother than that of adults.

❏ A child's skin has less terminal hair and hasn't been subjected to long-term exposure to environmental elements.

❏ Infants have poorly developed subcutaneous fat, predisposing them to hypothermia.

❏ Children have thinner and more sensitive skin than adults.

❏ Irritation in the neonate's skin can result from sensitivity or clogged pores.

❑ In diascopy, a lesion is covered with a glass slide or piece of clear plastic and pressure is applied; the area is observed to identify purpura (the lesion remains red) or erythema (the lesion blanches).

❑ Side lighting shows minor elevations or depressions in lesions; it also helps determine the configuration and degree of eruption.

❑ Subdued lighting, another test, highlights the difference between normal skin and circumscribed lesions that are hypopigmented or hyperpigmented.

❑ Acne vulgaris primarily affects adolescents, although lesions can appear as early as age 8.

❑ Although acne is more common and more severe in boys, it usually occurs in girls at an earlier age and tends to last longer, sometimes into adulthood.

❑ Most pediatric burns occur to children younger than age 5.

❑ Overall, burns are the third leading cause of accidental death in children after motor vehicle accidents and drowning.

❑ The Lund and Browder chart, a body surface area chart that's corrected for age to determine the extent of injury, estimates extent of the burn.

❑ The Rule of Nines is inaccurate for children because the head can account for 13% to 19% of body surface area; the legs account for 10% to 16%, depending on the child's age and size.

❑ Impetigo is a highly contagious superficial infection of the skin, marked by patches of tiny blisters that erupt.

❑ Impetigo is common in children ages 2 to 5 and is caused by infection with staphylococci.

❑ Impetigo is spread by direct contact; incubation period is 2 to 10 days after contact.

❑ Port-wine stains are associated with syndromes of the neonate, such as Sturge-Weber syndrome.

❑ Port-wine stains found on the face or extremities may be associated with soft tissue and bone hypertrophy.

❑ Harlequin color change is a benign disorder related to the immaturity of hypothalamic centers that control the tone of peripheral blood vessels.

❑ A newborn that has been lying on its side may appear reddened on the dependent side; the color fades on position change.

❑ Koplik's spots are consistent with measles.

❑ Tonsillar exudate is consistent with pharyngitis caused by group A beta-hemolytic streptococci.

❑ Vesicular lesions are associated with coxsackie virus.

❑ Strawberry hemangiomas are rapidly growing vascular lesions that reach maximum growth by age 1 year, followed by an involution period of 6 to 12 months, and complete involution by age 2 or 3 years.

❑ Herpes zoster is caused by the varicella zoster virus and presents as papulovesicular lesions that erupt along a dermatome, usually with hyperesthesia, pain, and tenderness.

❑ When salmon patches appear on the nape of the neck, they're commonly called "stork bites."

❑ The rash in measles occurs on the face, trunk, and extremities.

❑ Seborrheic dermatitis is cradle cap and occurs in infants.

❑ Filiform warts are long spiny projections from the skin surface.

❑ Flat warts are flat-topped, smooth-surfaced lesions.

❑ Plantar warts are rough papules, commonly found on the soles of the feet.

❑ Tinea pedis is a superficial fungal infection on the feet, commonly called athlete's foot.

❑ Tinea corporis, or ringworm, is a flat scaling papular lesion with raised borders.

❑ Erosion is a depressed vesicular lesion.

❑ A fissure is a cleavage in the surface of skin.

❑ Striae are linear depressions of the skin.

❑ Cherry-red skin changes are seen when a child has been exposed to high levels of carbon monoxide.

❑ First-degree or superficial burns involve only the epidermis.

❑ Second degree or partial-thickness burns affect the epidermis and dermis.

❑ A third-degree or full-thickness burn involves all of the skin layers and the nerve endings.

❑ Fourth-degree burns involve all skin layers, nerve endings, muscles, tendons, and bone.

❑ I.V. fluids must be started immediately in all children who sustain a major burn injury to prevent the child from going into hypovolemic shock.

❑ Fluid resuscitation should be started on all clients with burns over more than 20% of their body surface area.

❑ Hand, foot, and mouth disease is caused by coxsackie virus and usually occurs in preschool children.

❑ Vesicular lesions accompanied by a low-grade fever are typical signs of varicella.

❑ Burns that are bilateral as well as symmetrical are typical of child abuse.

❑ The shape of the burn may resemble the item used to create it, such as a cigarette.

# Psychiatric care

## Essentials of psychiatric care

❑ Electroconvulsive therapy is most commonly used to treat major depression in clients who haven't responded to antidepressants or who have medical problems that contraindicate the use of antidepressants.

❑ Transference is the unconscious assignment of negative or positive feelings evoked by a significant person in the client's past to another person.

❑ Intellectualization is a defense mechanism in which the client avoids dealing with emotions by focusing on facts.

❑ Triangulation refers to conflicts involving three family members.

❑ Splitting is a defense mechanism commonly seen in clients with personality disorders in which the world is perceived as all good or all bad.

❑ "Unconditional positive regard" is a phrase from Carl Rogers's client-centered therapy that describes a supportive, nonjudgmental, neutral approach by a therapist.

❑ Analysis of free association is characteristic of Freudian psychoanalysis.

❑ Classical conditioning is characteristic of a pure behavioral intervention.

❑ Examination of negative thought patterns is an intervention typical of a nurse using a cognitive-behavioral approach to a client experiencing low self-esteem.

❑ Yalom's curative, or therapeutic, factors of group therapy include instillation of hope, universality, imparting of information, group cohesiveness, altruism, catharsis, and existential factors.

❑ Universality assists group participants in recognizing common experiences and responses, helps reduce anxiety, and allows group members to provide support and understanding to each other.

❑ Altruism refers to finding meaning through helping others.

❑ Catharsis is an open expression of previously suppressed feelings.

❑ Nonverbal clues to suicidal ideation include giving away personal possessions, a sudden calmness, and risk-taking behaviors.

❑ Clients with major depression generally don't exhibit suicidal behavior until their outlook on their problems begins to improve.

❑ Setting limits and removing the client from the situation is the best way to handle aggression.

❑ Neuroleptic malignant syndrome is a life-threatening adverse effect of antipsychotic medications such as haloperidol and is associated with a rapid increase in temperature.

❑ In the technique called focusing, the nurse assists the client in redirecting his attention toward something specific.

❑ During milieu therapy, the nurse utilizes all aspects of the hospital environment in a therapeutic manner to encourage communication and decision-making and provides opportunities for enhancing self-esteem and learning new skills and behaviors.

❑ Therapeutic communication is the foundation for developing a nurse-client relationship.

❑ Biological therapy includes psychoactive drugs, electroconvulsive therapy, and nonconvulsive electrical stimulation.

❑ Cognitive therapy uses strategies such as role-playing and thought substitution to modify the beliefs and attitudes that influence a client's feelings and behaviors.

❑ The Mini-Mental Status Examination measures orientation, registration, recall, calculation, language, and motor skills.

❑ The Cognitive Capacity Screening Examination measures orientation, memory, calculation, and language.

❑ The Global Deterioration Scale assesses and stages primary degenerative dementia based on orientation, memory, and neurologic function.

❑ The Functional Dementia Scale measures orientation, affect, and the ability to perform activities of daily living.

❑ The Beck Depression Inventory helps diagnose depression, determine its severity, and monitor the client's response during treatment.

❑ The Eating Attitudes Test detects patterns that suggest an eating disorder.

❑ The Minnesota Multiphasic Personality Inventory helps assess personality traits and ego function in adults and adolescents.

❑ The CAGE Questionnaire includes four questions in which two or three positive responses indicate alcoholism.

❑ Reality therapy focuses on assisting the client to love and be loved and to feel worthwhile and feel that others are worthwhile.

❑ Family therapy involves the entire family to improve family function.

❑ Group therapy aims to increase self-awareness, change maladaptive behaviors, and improve interpersonal relationships.

❑ In the technique called sharing impressions, the nurse attempts to describe the client's feelings and then seeks corrective feedback from the client.

❑ In a physical examination of the psychiatric client, the nurse should assess the client's general appearance, behavior, mood, thought processes and cognitive function, coping mechanisms, and potential for self-destructive behavior.

❑ The *Diagnostic and Statistical Manual of Mental Disorders* (*DSM*) includes a complete description of psychiatric disorders and other conditions and describes diagnostic criteria that must be met to support each diagnosis.

❑ To add diagnostic detail, the *DSM-IV-TR* uses a multiaxial approach and specifies that every client be evaluated on each of the five axes.

❑ The *DSM-IV-TR* Axis I describes a clinical disorder, the diagnosis that best describes the presenting complaint.

❑ The *DSM-IV-TR* Axis II describes personality disorders and mental retardation.

❑ The *DSM-IV-TR* Axis III is used to describe any concurrent medical conditions or disorders.

❑ The *DSM-IV-TR* Axis IV describes psychosocial and environmental problems.

❑ The *DSM-IV-TR* Axis V is a global assessment of functioning based on a scale of 1 to 100.

❑ The global assessment of functioning scale allows evaluation of the client's overall psychological, social, and occupational functioning.

❑ Shifting of an emotion from its original object to a substitute is a coping mechanism called displacement.

❑ Avoiding the awareness of truth or reality is a coping mechanism called denial.

❑ Creation of unrealistic or improbable images to escape from daily pressures and responsibilities is a coping mechanism called fantasy.

❑ Unconscious adoption of the personality characteristics, attitudes, values, and behavior of another person is a coping mechanism called identification.

❑ Displacement of negative feelings onto another person is a coping mechanism called projection.

❑ Substitution of acceptable reasons for the real or actual reasons motivating behavior is a coping mechanism called rationalization.

❑ Conduct in a manner opposite from the way the person feels is a coping mechanism called reaction formation.

❑ Returning to the behavior of an earlier, less worrisome time in life is a coping mechanism called regression.

❑ Exclusion of acceptable thoughts and feelings from the conscious mind, leaving the client to operate in the subconscious, is a coping mechanism called repression.

## Anxiety and mood disorders

❑ People who fear loss of control during a panic attack commonly make statements about feeling trapped, getting hurt, or having little or no personal control over their situations.

❑ During a panic attack, the nurse should remain with the client and direct what's said toward changing the physiologic response, such as having the client take deep breaths.

❑ The client with agoraphobia typically restricts himself to home and can't carry out normal socializing and life-sustaining activities.

❑ A group therapy intervention that is of primary importance to a client with panic disorder is discussing new ways of thinking and feeling about panic attacks.

❑ Restructuring an anxiety-producing event allows the client with panic disorder to gain control over the situation during therapy.

❑ People who have a social phobia fear social gatherings and dislike being the center of attention; they are very critical of themselves and believe that others will also be critical.

❑ Systematic desensitization is a common behavior modification technique successfully used to help treat phobias.

❑ Clients who experience posttraumatic stress disorder are at high risk for suicide and other forms of violent behaviors.

❑ Sundowner syndrome is an increase in agitation that occurs in the evening accompanied by confusion and is commonly seen in clients with dementia.

❑ After experiencing a trauma, the client with posttraumatic stress disorder may have strong reactions to stimuli similar to those that occurred during the traumatic event.

❑ Denial can act as a protective response.

❑ Perfectionism is more commonly seen in clients with eating disorders.

❑ Clients who have had a severe trauma commonly experience an inability to trust others.

❑ The use of substances is a way for the client to deny problems and self-medicate distress.

❑ An effective communication strategy for a nurse to use with a client with posttraumatic stress disorder is listening attentively and staying with the client.

❑ Symptoms of posttraumatic stress disorder usually appear 6 or more months after the event has occurred; symptoms persist or recur for at least one month.

❑ Hypnosis is one of the main therapies for clients who dissociate.

❑ Approximately 75% of clients with generalized anxiety disorder also may have a diagnosis of phobia, panic disorder, or substance abuse.

❑ A client with generalized anxiety disorder may refuse to take medication because he believes that requiring medication is a sign of personal weakness and of an inability to solve problems by himself. Intrusive dreams and nightmares are associated with posttraumatic stress disorder.

❑ Clients with anxiety disorders commonly experience somatic symptoms, such as a headache or upset stomach.

❑ To decrease stimulation in the client with mania, the nurse should attempt to redirect and focus the client's communication and not allow the client to talk about different topics.

❑ For a manic client, it's best to ask closed questions because open-ended questions may enable the client to talk endlessly, again possibly contributing to the client feeling out of control.

❑ The nurse must check the client's gag reflex before allowing the client to have a drink after an electroconvulsive therapy procedure.

❑ During episodes of hypomania, the client may demonstrate an elevated and irritable mood, along with mild or beginning symptoms of mania.

❑ Indecision and vacillation with a diminished ability to think are symptoms likely seen in a major depressive episode.

❑ A client with hypomania tends to be creative and more productive than usual.

❑ Headache, agitation, and indigestion are symptoms suggestive of mania in a client with a history of bipolar disorder.

❑ Thoughtless or reckless spending is a common symptom of a manic episode.

❑ During episodes of mania, a client may in fact interact with many people and participate in unsafe sexual behavior.

❑ Cognitive impairment is typically associated with delirium or dementia.

❑ Establishing a suicide contract with the client demonstrates that the nurse's concern for his safety is a priority and that his life is of value.

❑ Agoraphobia is characterized by fear of public places.

❑ Dissociative disorder is characterized by lost periods of time.

❑ Posttraumatic stress disorder is characterized by hypervigilance and sleep disturbance.

❑ Flight of ideas is a speech pattern characterized by rapid transition from topic to topic, typically without finishing one idea, and is common in mania.

❑ Echolalia is the repetition of words heard.

❑ Clang associations are the use of rhyming.

❑ Neologism is invented words.

❑ Dysthymic disorder is a mood disorder similar to major depression, but it remains mild to moderate in severity.

❑ Cyclothymic disorder is a mood disorder characterized by a mood range from moderate depression to hypomania.

❑ Bipolar I disorder is characterized by a single manic episode with no past major depressive episodes.

❑ Seasonal affective disorder is a form of depression occurring in the fall and winter.

❑ Clients with blood injection-injury phobia may avoid all medical care, which is dangerous to their health.

❑ Improving stress management skills, verbalizing feelings, and anticipating and planning for stressful situations are adaptive responses to stress.

❑ Verbalizing the relationship between stress and behaviors indicates that the client understands the disease process.

❑ Avoiding, rationalizing, and hiding behaviors demonstrate maladaptive methods for managing stress and anxiety.

❑ Impulsive behavior, overwhelming guilt, chronic illness, and anger repression are factors that contribute to suicide potential.

❑ Anxiety disorders are characterized by anxiety and avoidant behavior.

❑ Clients with anxiety cling to maladaptive behaviors in an attempt to alleviate their own distress, but these behaviors only increase their symptoms.

❑ Mood disorders are characterized by depressed or elevated moods that alter the client's ability to cope with reality and to function normally.

❑ Major mood disorders include bipolar disorder and major depression.

❑ Major anxiety disorders include generalized anxiety, obsessive-compulsive disorder, panic disorder, phobias, and posttraumatic stress disorder.

## Cognitive disorders

❑ Cognitive disorders result from any condition that alters or destroys brain tissue and, in turn, impairs cerebral functioning.

❑ Symptoms of cognitive disorders include cognitive impairment, behavioral dysfunction, and personality changes.

❑ The most common cognitive disorders described in the *DSM-IV-TR* are delirium, dementia, and amnestic disorders.

❑ Cognitive disorders are characterized by the disruption of cognitive functioning.

❑ Cognitive disorders may result from a primary brain disease, the brain's response to a systemic disturbance such as a medical condition, or the brain tissue's reaction to a toxic substance, as in substance abuse.

❑ Delirium is commonly caused by the disruption of brain homeostasis; when the source of the disturbance is eliminated, cognitive deficits generally resolve.

❑ Common causes of delirium include postoperative conditions or metabolic disorders, withdrawal from alcohol and drugs, and exposure to toxic substances.

❑ Unlike delirium, dementia is caused by primary brain pathology; therefore, reversal of cognitive defects is less likely.

❑ Dementia can easily be mistaken for delirium, so the cause needs to be thoroughly investigated.

❑ A client with Alzheimer-type dementia suffers from a global impairment of cognitive functioning, memory, and personality.

❑ The dementia with Alzheimer-type dementia occurs gradually but with continuous decline.

❑ Damage from Alzheimer-type dementia is irreversible.

❑ Because of the difficulty in obtaining direct pathologic evidence of Alzheimer disease, the diagnosis can be made only when other etiologies for the dementia have been eliminated.

❑ The Clinical Dementia Rating scale delineates five stages in Alzheimer-type dementia; the Global Deterioration Scale delineates seven stages.

❑ Most health care providers categorize three stages of Alzheimer-type dementia: mild, moderate, and severe.

❑ Causes of Alzheimer-type dementia include alterations in acetylcholine levels (a neurotransmitter), altered immune function, with autoantibody production in the brain; familial history, increased brain atrophy with wider sulci and cerebral ventricles than seen in normal aging; and presence of neurofibrillary tangles and beta-amyloid neuritic plaques, mainly in the cerebral cortex and hippocampus (early) and later in the frontal, parietal, and temporal lobes.

❑ A client with stage 1 (mild) Alzheimer-type dementia demonstrates confusion and memory loss, disorientation to time and place, difficulty performing routine tasks, changes in personality and judgment, and sleep disturbances.

❑ A client with stage 2 (moderate) Alzheimer-type dementia demonstrates difficulty performing activities of daily living, such as feeding and bathing; anxiety; suspiciousness; agitation; wandering; pacing; repetitive behaviors; sleep disturbances; and difficulty recognizing family members.

❑ A client with stage 3 (severe) Alzheimer-type dementia demonstrates loss of speech, loss of appetite, weight loss, loss of bowel and bladder control, and total dependence on caregiver.

❑ In amnestic disorder, the client experiences a loss of both short-term and long-term memory; he can't recall some or many past events.

❑ Delirium is characterized by an acute onset and may last from several hours to several days; it's potentially reversible but can be life-threatening if not treated.

❑ Also called multi-infarct dementia, vascular dementia impairs the client's cognitive functioning, memory, and personality but doesn't affect the client's level of consciousness.

❑ Vascular dementia is caused by an irreversible alteration in brain function that damages or destroys brain tissue.

## Dissociative disorders

❏ A client with a dissociative disorder experiences a disruption in the usual relationship among memory, identity, consciousness, and perceptions; the disturbance may occur suddenly or appear gradually.

❏ Dissociative disorder is more common in women than in men.

❏ Typically, dissociation is a mechanism used to protect the self and gain relief from overwhelming anxiety.

❏ Common dissociative disorders include depersonalization disorder, dissociative amnesia, dissociative fugue, and dissociative identity disorder.

❏ In depersonalization disorder, the client may feel like a detached observer, passively watching his mental or physical activity as if in a dream, but reality testing remains intact.

❏ Reality testing is the ability to distinguish fact from fantasy.

❏ In dissociative amnesia, the client may not recall important life events in an attempt to avoid traumatic memories.

❏ Recovery from dissociative amnesia is common; recurrences are rare.

❏ In dissociative fugue, the client may travel from home or work and become suddenly confused about his personal identity; the client may take on a new identity and can't recall the past.

❏ Contributing factors to dissociative amnesia are emotional abuse, low self-esteem, past traumatic event, physical abuse, or sexual abuse.

❏ In dissociative identity disorder, formerly known as multiple personality disorder, the client has at least two unique identities; each identity can have unique behavior patterns and unique memories, although usually one primary identity is associated with the client's name.

❏ In dissociative identity disorder, the client may also have traumatic memories that intrude into his awareness.

❏ Dissociative identity disorder tends to be chronic and recurrent.

❏ Contributing factors in dissociative identity disorder include emotional, physical, or sexual abuse; genetic predisposition; lack of nurturing experiences to assist in recovery from abuse; low self-esteem; and a traumatic experience before age 15.

## Eating disorders

❏ Eating disorders are characterized by severe disturbances in eating behaviors.

❏ The two most common eating disorders, anorexia nervosa and bulimia nervosa, put the client at risk for severe cardiovascular and GI complications and can ultimately result in death. In anorexia nervosa, the client deliberately starves herself or engages in binge eating and purging.

❏ A client with anorexia nervosa wants to become as thin as possible and refuses to maintain an appropriate weight.

❏ A key clinical finding in anorexia nervosa is a refusal to sustain weight at or above minimum requirements for the client's age and height and an intense fear of gaining weight or becoming fat.

❏ If left untreated, anorexia nervosa can be fatal.

❏ Bulimia nervosa is characterized by episodic binge eating, followed by purging in the form of vomiting; the client may also use laxatives, enemas, diuretics, or syrup of ipecac.

❏ Contributing factors to bulimia nervosa are thought to include a distorted body image, history of sexual abuse, low self-esteem, neurochemical changes, and poor family relations.

❏ Russell's sign (bruised knuckles due to repeated self-induced vomiting) may be observed in bulimia nervosa. In bulimia nervosa, metabolic acidosis may occur from diarrhea caused by enemas and excessive laxative use.

❏ In bulimia nervosa, metabolic alkalosis (the most common metabolic complication) may occur from frequent vomiting.

❏ Prevent the client with bulimia nervosa from using the bathroom for 90 minutes after eating to help the client avoid purging behavior.

❏ Clients with eating disorders commonly use manipulative ploys and countertransference to resist weight gain (if they restrict food intake) or to maintain purging practices (if they're bulimic).

❏ Constant binging and purging behaviors can result in severe electrolyte imbalances, erosion of tooth enamel from constant exposure to gastric acids, menstrual irregularities, esophageal tears and, in severe cases, gastric rupture.

## Personality disorders

❏ Personality traits are patterns of behavior that reflect how people perceive and relate to others and themselves. Personality disorders occur when these traits become rigid and maladaptive.

❏ According to the *DSM-IV-TR*, a personality disorder is a problematic pattern occurring in two of the following four areas: cognition, affectivity, interpersonal functioning, and impulse control.

❏ A client with a personality disorder uses maladaptive behavior to relate to others and fulfill basic emotional needs.

❏ Major personality disorders include antisocial personality disorder, borderline personality disorder, dependent personality disorder, and paranoid personality disorder.

❑ Antisocial personality disorder leads the client to have a total disregard for the rights of others.

❑ Borderline personality disorder results in a pattern of instability in a person's mood, interpersonal relationships, self-esteem, self-identity, behavior, and cognition.

❑ Impulsiveness is the most prominent characteristic of borderline personality disorder.

❑ Borderline personality disorder appears to originate in early childhood.

❑ Aggressive behavior makes caring for the client with antisocial personality disorder a challenge because these clients are typically impulsive and tend to lash out at those who interfere with their need for immediate gratification.

❑ The client with dependent personality disorder experiences an extreme need to be taken care of that leads to submissive, clinging behavior and fear of separation.

❑ The need to be taken care of that leads to the submissive, clinging behavior and fear of separation that occurs with dependent personality disorder begins by early adulthood, when behaviors designed to elicit caring from others become predominant and arise from the client's perception that he's unable to function adequately without others.

❑ Paranoid personality disorder is characterized by extreme distrust of others.

❑ Paranoid people avoid relationships in which they aren't in control or have the potential of losing control.

## Schizophrenic and delusional disorders

❑ Schizophrenic and delusional disorders fall under the diagnostic umbrella of psychosis.

❑ A psychotic illness is a brain disorder characterized by an impaired perception of reality, commonly coupled with mood disturbances.

❑ Psychosis can be either progressive or episodic.

❑ Schizophrenia is characterized by disturbances (for at least 6 months) in thought content and form, perception, affect, sense of self, volition, interpersonal relationships, work and self-care, and psychomotor behavior.

❑ Schizophrenia is usually a chronic disorder, equally prevalent in men and women, that begins in young adulthood, and is more common in African and Asian Americans.

❑ Positive schizophrenia symptoms focus on a *distortion* of normal functions; negative symptoms focus on a *loss* of normal functions.

❑ Examples of positive symptoms of schizophrenia are delusions, hallucinations, disorganized speech, and grossly disorganized or catatonic behavior.

❑ Examples of negative symptoms of schizophrenia include flat affect, alogia (poverty of speech), avolition (lack of self-initiated behaviors), and anhedonia (minimal enjoyment of activities).

❑ Delusions are false, fixed beliefs that aren't shared by other members of the client's social, cultural, or religious background.

❑ Delusions may occur in the form of thought broadcasting, in which the client believes that his personal thoughts are broadcast to the external world.

❑ Many times, the client with delusions believes that his feelings, thoughts, or actions aren't his own.

❑ Delusional themes are described as persecutory, somatic, erotomanic, jealous, or grandiose.

❑ An example of a persecutory delusion is the idea that one is being followed, tricked, tormented, or made the subject of ridicule.

❑ The client with erotomanic delusions falsely believes he shares an idealized relationship with another person, usually someone of higher status such as a celebrity.

❑ An example of a somatic delusion is a client who believes his body is deteriorating from within.

❑ An example of a jealous delusion is a client who feels that his spouse or partner is unfaithful with no evidence of unfaithfulness.

❑ The client with grandiose delusions has an exaggerated sense of self-importance.

❑ In disorganized thinking, or looseness of associations, the client's speech shifts randomly from one topic to another, with only a vague connection between topics.

❑ The client with disorganized thinking or looseness of associations may digress to unrelated topics, make up new words (neologisms), repeat words involuntarily (perseveration), or repeat words or phrases similar in sound only (clang association).

❑ The client with schizophrenia may demonstrate a blunted, flat, or inappropriate affect manifested by poor eye contact; a distant, unresponsive facial expression; and very limited body language.

❑ Most commonly, schizophrenics experience auditory hallucinations.

❑ When the client with schizophrenia hears voices, he perceives these voices as being separate from his own thoughts.

❑ The content of the voices a client with schizophrenia hears is usually threatening and derogatory; many times, the voices tell the client to commit an act of violence against himself or others.

❑ Major psychotic disorders include catatonic schizophrenia, disorganized schizophrenia, paranoid schizophrenia, and delusional disorder.

❑ Clients with catatonic schizophrenia show little reaction to their environment.

❑ The client with catatonic schizophrenia may exhibit bizarre postures, waxy flexibility (posture held in odd or unusual fixed positions for extended periods), and resistance to being moved.

❑ Disorganized schizophrenics have a flat or inappropriate affect and incoherent thoughts.

❑ Clients with disorganized schizophrenia exhibit loose associations and disorganized speech and behaviors.

❑ If a client experiences hallucinations, don't attempt to reason with him or challenge his perception of the hallucinations; instead, ensure the client's safety and provide comfort and support.

❑ Attempts to reason with the client experiencing hallucinations will increase his anxiety and possibly make his hallucinations worse.

❑ Encourage the client with auditory hallucinations to reveal what the voices are telling him to help prevent harm to the client and others.

❑ Clients with paranoid schizophrenia have delusions or frequent auditory hallucinations unrelated to reality.

❑ The client with paranoid schizophrenia commonly displays bizarre behavior, is easily angered, and is at high risk for violence.

❑ The prognosis for independent functioning in clients with paranoid schizophrenia is usually better than for other types of schizophrenia.

❑ Clients with delusional disorder hold firmly to false belief despite contradictory information; they tend to be intelligent and can have a high level of competence but impaired social and personal relationships.

❑ One indication of delusional disorder is an absence of hallucinations.

❑ Explore events that trigger delusions with the client with delusional disorder; also discuss anxiety associated with triggering events, which can help you understand the dynamics of the client's delusional system.

❑ Don't directly attack the client's delusion; doing so will increase the client's anxiety.

❑ When the dynamics of the delusions are understood, discourage repetitious talk about delusions and refocus the conversation on the client's underlying feelings.

## Sexual and gender identity disorders

❑ Sexual disorders described in the *DSM-IV-TR* include gender identity disorder, paraphilias, and sexual dysfunctions.

❑ Gender identity disorder is characterized by intense and ongoing cross-gender identification.

❑ Paraphilias are characterized by an intense, recurring sexual urge centered on inanimate objects or on human suffering and humiliation.

❑ Sexual dysfunctions are characterized by a deficiency or loss of desire for sexual activity or by a disturbance in the sexual response cycle.

❑ Clients with gender identity disorders want to become or be like the opposite sex and are extremely uncomfortable with their assigned gender roles.

❑ A paraphilia is defined as a recurrent, intense sexual urge or fantasy, generally involving nonhuman subjects, children, nonconsenting partners, or the degradation, suffering, and humiliation of the client or partners.

❑ The client with a paraphilia may report that the fantasy is always present but that the frequency of the fantasy and intensity of the urge may vary.

❑ Paraphilia tends to be chronic and lifelong, but in adults both the fantasy and behavior commonly diminish with advancing age.

❑ Inappropriate sexual behavior may increase in response to psychological stressors, in relation to other mental disorders, or when opportunity to engage in the paraphilia becomes more available.

❑ Common paraphilias include exhibitionism, fetishism, and frotteurism.

❑ Exhibitionism is exposing one's genitals and occasionally masturbating in public.

❑ Fetishism is use of an object to become sexually aroused.

❑ Frotteurism is rubbing one's genitals on another nonconsenting person to become aroused.

❑ The most common sexual dysfunctions are orgasmic disorders, sexual arousal disorders, sexual desire disorders, sexual pain disorders, and substance-induced sexual dysfunction.

❑ The *DSM-IV-TR* lists orgasmic disorders as female orgasmic disorder, male orgasmic disorder, and premature ejaculation.

❑ Male and female orgasmic disorders are characterized by a persistent or recurrent delay in or absence of orgasm following a normal sexual excitement phase.

❑ Premature ejaculation is marked by persistent and recurrent onset of orgasm and ejaculation with minimal sexual stimulation.

❑ Sexual arousal disorders include female sexual arousal disorder and male erectile disorder.

❑ With female sexual arousal disorder, the client has a persistent or recurrent inability to attain or maintain adequate lubrication, swelling, and response of sexual excitement until the completion of sexual activity.

❑ In male erectile disorder, the client has a persistent or recurrent inability to attain or maintain an adequate erection until completion of sexual activity.

❏ Sexual desire disorders include hypoactive sexual desire disorder and sexual aversion disorder.

❏ The key feature of hypoactive sexual desire disorder is a deficiency or absence of sexual fantasies and the desire for sexual activity; the client usually doesn't initiate sexual activity and may only engage in it reluctantly when it's initiated by the partner.

❏ With sexual aversion disorder, the client has an aversion to and active avoidance of genital sexual contact with a sexual partner.

❏ Sexual pain disorders include dyspareunia and vaginismus.

❏ In sexual dysfunction due to a medical condition, the sexual dysfunction may occur as a result of a physiologic problem.

❏ The essential feature of dyspareunia is genital pain associated with sexual intercourse.

❏ Most commonly experienced during intercourse, dyspareunia may also occur before or after intercourse.

❏ Vaginismus is recurrent or persistent involuntary contraction of the perineal muscles surrounding the outer third of the vagina when vaginal penetration is attempted.

❏ In some clients with vaginismus, even the anticipation of vaginal insertion may result in muscle spasm; the contractions may be mild to severe.

❏ Substance-induced sexual dysfunction refers to sexual dysfunction resulting from direct physiologic effects of a substance, such as from drug abuse, medication use, or toxin exposure.

## Somatoform and sleep disorders

❏ The client with a sleep disorder commonly suffers from excessive daytime sleepiness and impaired ability to perform daily tasks safely or properly.

❏ The client with a somatoform disorder commonly suffers physical symptoms related to an inability to handle stress; the physical symptoms have no physiologic cause but are overwhelming to the client.

❏ Because the client with a somatoform disorder doesn't produce the symptoms intentionally or feel a sense of control over them, he's usually unable to accept that his illness has a psychological cause.

❏ Psychosomatic is a term used to describe conditions in which a psychological state contributes to the development of a physical illness.

❏ Somatization is the manifestation of physical symptoms that result from psychological distress.

❏ A somatic symptom (such as the pain of a sore throat or the ache of flu) isn't considered somatization unless the physical symptoms are an expression of emotional stress.

❑ Internalization refers to the condition in which a client's anxiety, stress, and frustration are expressed through physical symptoms rather than confronted directly.

❑ The client with a primary sleep disorder is unable to initiate or maintain sleep.

❑ Primary sleep disorders may be categorized as dyssomnias or parasomnias.

❑ Dyssomnias involve excessive sleep or difficulty initiating and maintaining sleep.

❑ Examples of dyssomnias include primary insomnia, circadian rhythm sleep disorder, obstructive sleep apnea syndrome, primary hypersomnia, and narcolepsy.

❑ Parasomnias are physiologic or behavioral reactions during sleep.

❑ Examples of parasomnias include nightmare disorder, sleep terror disorder, and sleepwalking disorder.

❑ Sleep can be broken down into two major phases, rapid-eye-movement (REM) sleep and non–REM sleep, which alternate throughout the sleep period.

❑ Stage 1 non–rapid-eye-movement sleep is a transition from wakefulness to sleep characterized by low-voltage mixed-frequency EEG and slow eye movement; it occupies about 5% of time spent asleep in healthy adults.

❑ Stage 2 non–rapid-eye-movement sleep is characterized by specific EEG waveforms (sleep spindles and K complexes); it occupies about 50% of time spent asleep.

❑ Stages 3 and 4 non–rapid-eye-movement sleep (also known collectively as slow-wave sleep or delta sleep) are the deepest levels of sleep; they occupy about 10% to 20% of sleep time, declining to 0% in the elderly.

❑ Rapid-eye-movement sleep, during which the majority of typical storylike dreams occur, occupies about 20% to 25% of total sleep.

❑ Rapid-eye-movement sleep periods increase in duration during the last half of the night, toward the morning.

❑ Polysomnography generally includes measurement of EEG activity, electro-oculographic activity (electrographic tracings made by movement of the eye), and electromyographic activity (electrographic tracings made by skeletal muscles at rest).

❑ Additional polysomnographic measures may include measurement of oral or nasal airflow, respiratory effort, chest and abdominal wall movement, oxyhemoglobin saturation, and exhaled carbon dioxide concentration.

❑ The onset of symptoms in a client with conversion disorder is preceded by psychological trauma or conflict.

❑ The physical symptoms associated with conversion disorder are a manifestation of the conflict, and resolution of the symptoms usually occurs spontaneously.

❑ In hypochondriasis, the client is preoccupied by fear of a serious illness, despite medical assurance of good health.

❑ The client with hypochondriasis interprets all physical sensations as indications of illness, impairing his ability to function normally.

❑ In pain disorder, the client experiences pain in which psychological factors play a significant role in the onset, severity, exacerbation, or maintenance of the pain.

❑ The pain with hypochondriasis isn't intentionally produced or feigned by the client; the pain becomes a major focus of life, and the client is often unable to function socially or at work.

❑ The client with hypochondriasis may have a physical ailment but shouldn't be experiencing such intense pain.

❑ Primary insomnia is characterized by subjective complaint of difficulty initiating or maintaining sleep that lasts for at least 1 month; alternatively, the client may report that sleep isn't refreshing.

❑ A key symptom of primary insomnia is the client's intense focus and anxiety about not getting sleep, resulting in significant distress or impairment; commonly, the client reports being a "light sleeper."

❑ In circadian rhythm sleep disorder, there's a mismatch between the internal sleep-wake circadian rhythm and the timing and duration of sleep.

❑ In circadian rhythm sleep disorder, the client may report insomnia at particular times during the day and excessive sleepiness at other times.

❑ Causes of circadian rhythm sleep disorder can be intrinsic, such as delays in the sleep phases, or extrinsic, as in jet lag or shift work.

❑ In primary hypersomnia, the client experiences excessive sleepiness lasting at least 1 month.

❑ People with primary hypersomnia have great difficulty with morning obligations.

❑ In circadian rhythm sleep disorder, polysomnography shows short sleep latency (length of time it takes to fall asleep), reduced sleep duration, and sleep continuity disturbances.

❑ Parasomnias are characterized by abnormal, unpleasant motor or verbal arousals and behaviors that occur during sleep.

❑ Nightmare disorder is characterized by the recurrence of frightening dreams that cause the client to awaken from sleep.

❑ When the client with nightmare disorder awakens, he's fully alert and experiences persistent anxiety or fear; typically, the client can recall details of the dream involving physical danger.

❏ Sleep terror disorder is characterized by episodes of sleep terrors that cause distress or impairment of social or occupational functioning.

❏ In sleep terror disorder, the client may sit up in bed screaming or crying with a frightened expression and signs of intense anxiety.

❏ During sleep terror disorder episodes, the client is difficult to awaken and, if he does awaken, he's generally confused or disoriented and has no recollection of the dream content.

❏ In sleepwalking disorder, the client arises from bed and walks about; the client has limited recall of the event upon awakening.

❏ Sleepwalkers may also sit up, talk, or engage in inappropriate behavior with little or no recall of the incident.

## Substance abuse disorders

❏ Substance intoxication is the development of a reversible substance-specific syndrome due to ingestion of or exposure to a substance.

❏ The clinically significant maladaptive behavior or psychological changes in substance abuse disorders vary depending on the substance.

❏ The essential feature of substance abuse is a maladaptive pattern of substance use coupled with recurrent and significant adverse consequences.

❏ Substance dependence is characterized by physical, behavioral, and cognitive changes resulting from persistent substance use.

❏ Persistent drug use can result in tolerance and withdrawal.

❏ Tolerance is defined as an increased need for a substance or a need for an increased amount of the substance to achieve an effect.

❏ Withdrawal occurs when the tissue and blood levels of a substance decrease in a person who has engaged in prolonged, heavy use of the substance.

❏ When uncomfortable withdrawal symptoms persist, the person usually takes the drug to relieve the symptoms.

❏ Withdrawal symptoms vary depending on the substance.

❏ Although alcohol abuse and dependence are considered substance-related abuse disorders, assessment findings and treatment differ somewhat from that for other substances.

❏ Alcohol is a sedative but it creates a feeling of euphoria; sedation increases with the amount ingested, and respiratory depression and coma can occur with excessive intake.

❏ Individuals exposed to cocaine develop dependence after a very short period followed by maladaptive behavior resulting in social dysfunction.

❏ Cocaine use can cause serious physical complications, such as cardiac arrhythmias, myocardial infarction, seizures, and stroke.

# Pharmacology

## Interactions

❑ A drug interaction occurs when a drug given with or shortly after another drug increases or decreases the effect of either or both drugs.

❑ Combination drug therapy is based on drug interaction; one drug may be given to complement the effects of another.

❑ An example of combination drug therapy is administering probenecid, which blocks the excretion of penicillin, with penicillin to maintain an adequate blood level of penicillin for a longer time.

❑ Aspirin and codeine are commonly given in combination because together they provide greater pain relief than if either is given alone.

❑ Drug interactions are sometimes used to prevent or antagonize certain adverse reactions.

❑ The diuretics hydrochlorothiazide and spironolactone are often given together because hydrochlorothiazide is potassium-depleting and spironolactone is potassium-sparing.

❑ Many drugs interact and decrease efficacy or increase toxicity, such as occurs when a tetracycline is given with drugs or foods that contain calcium or magnesium (such as antacids or milk); these bind with tetracycline in the GI tract and cause inadequate drug absorption.

❑ When mixed with alcohol, metronidazole causes a disulfiram-like effect involving nausea, vomiting, and other unpleasant symptoms.

❑ Antacids may decrease digoxin absorption.

❑ The client taking spironolactone should avoid potassium-rich foods and potassium supplements.

❑ Carbamazepine decreases blood levels of phenytoin and hormonal contraceptives.

❑ Antihypertensives should be used cautiously in clients already taking thioridazine.

❑ Because spironolactone is a potassium-sparing diuretic, the client should avoid salt substitutes because of their high potassium content.

❑ Alcohol decreases phenytoin activity, diminishing its effectiveness.

❑ Phenytoin is compatible only with saline solutions; dextrose causes an insoluble precipitate to form.

❑ Nutritional supplements and milk interfere with the absorption of phenytoin, decreasing its effectiveness.

❑ Anabolic steroids, salicylates, alcohol, and monoamine oxidase inhibitors may increase the hypoglycemic effects of insulin.

❑ Beta-adrenergic blockers may prolong the hypoglycemic effects of insulin and may mask signs and symptoms of hypoglycemia.

❑ Acetylcysteine is used to treat acetaminophen toxicity but should never be given with activated charcoal.

❑ Don't give activated charcoal in or with ice cream, milk, or sherbet because these foods reduce the adsorption capacities of charcoal.

❑ Use Alzheimer disease drugs cautiously with nonsteroidal anti-inflammatory drugs because the drug increases gastric acid secretion; there is increased risk of developing ulcers and active or occult GI bleeding.

❑ Use of gemfibrozil with lovastatin may cause myopathy.

❑ Ferrous gluconate shouldn't be taken with antacids, milk, or whole-grain cereals because these foods reduce iron absorption.

## Adverse drug effects and adverse reactions

❑ Drugs cause adverse effects; clients have adverse reactions.

❑ An adverse reaction may be tolerated to obtain a therapeutic effect, or it may be hazardous and unacceptable.

❑ Some adverse reactions subside with continued use.

❑ A common side effect of oxybutynin is dry mouth.

❑ Rifampin and its metabolites turn urine, feces, sputum, tears, and sweat orange.

❑ Rifampin may cause GI upset, headache, drowsiness, dizziness, visual disturbances, and fever.

❑ Common adverse effects of albuterol include tachycardia, nervousness, tremors, insomnia, irritability, and headache.

❑ Atropine dries up secretions and lessens the response of ciliary and iris sphincter muscles in the eye, causing mydriasis as an adverse effect.

❑ Atropine usually causes paradoxical excitement in children.

❑ Common adverse effects of erythromycin include nausea, vomiting, diarrhea, abdominal pain, and anorexia.

❑ The rubella vaccine is made from duck eggs, so an allergic reaction may occur in clients with egg allergies.

❑ Antiparkinsonian medications cause vivid dreams and nightmares.

❑ Beta-adrenergic blockers decrease rapid-eye-movement sleep and can cause the client to have nightmares.

❑ Oxytocin has an antidiuretic effect and can cause fluid overload.

❏ Oxytocin may cause maternal tachycardia.

❏ Oxytocin, given to induce or augment labor, may cause uterine tachysystole, which increases the risk of uterine rupture.

❏ Amphetamines, tricyclic antidepressants, monoamine oxidase inhibitors, barbiturates, and benzodiazepines decrease rapid-eye-movement sleep.

❏ Selective serotonin reuptake inhibitors decrease rapid-eye-movement sleep and cause vivid dreams.

❏ Benzodiazepines and barbiturates cause decreased waking after sleep onset.

❏ A client with schizophrenia would be at risk for secondary Parkinson disease caused by taking chlorpromazine.

❏ Atropine allows more light onto the retina and may cause photophobia and blurred vision.

❏ Phenytoin levels are checked before giving the drug; the drug is withheld if levels are elevated to avoid compounding toxicity.

❏ Levodopa-carbidopa may require that the client take a drug holiday.

❏ Steroids, opioids, beta-adrenergic blockers, alcohol, and selective serotonin reuptake inhibitors cause increased waking after sleep onset.

❏ Because propranolol can cause light-headedness, the client should be told to rise slowly when standing.

❏ Serum aspartate aminotransferase and serum alanine aminotransferase levels become elevated soon after ingestion of acetaminophen.

❏ Steroid use tends to increase blood glucose levels, particularly in clients with diabetes and prediabetes.

❏ Magnesium sulfate crosses the placenta and can produce adverse neonatal effects, including respiratory depression, hypotonia, and bradycardia.

❏ Furosemide is a potassium-depleting diuretic that can cause hypokalemia.

❏ If a client reports difficulty swallowing and excessive respiratory secretions 1 hour after receiving pyridostigmine bromide, it suggests cholinergic crisis or excessive acetylcholinesterase medication.

❏ Immunosuppression with repeated use is an adverse effect of steroid administration, a medication used to treat myasthenia gravis.

❏ Trihexyphenidyl is an anticholinergic agent that causes blurred vision, dry mouth, constipation, and urine retention.

❏ Phenothiazines such as chlorpromazine deplete dopamine, which may lead to tremor and rigidity (extrapyramidal effects).

❏ Long-term therapy with levodopa-carbidopa can result in drug tolerance or toxicity.

❑ Flushing, chest pain, palpitations, anxiety, shortness of breath, and itching occur in some clients after administration of glatiramer.

❑ Levels of aminophylline below 10 mcg/mL are considered to be less than therapeutic.

❑ Symptoms of aminophylline toxicity, such as nausea, tachycardia, and irritability, can appear when levels exceed 20 mcg/mL.

❑ Levels of aminophylline greater than 30 mcg/mL can cause seizures and arrhythmias.

❑ Changing phenytoin brands may alter the therapeutic effect.

❑ When given through an I.V. catheter in the hand, phenytoin may cause purple glove syndrome.

❑ Abrupt phenytoin withdrawal may trigger status epilepticus; therefore, a client should be warned not to stop taking the drug unless the physician instructs them to do so.

❑ Rapid administration of phenytoin can depress the myocardium, causing arrhythmias.

❑ Adverse effects of phenytoin include sedation, somnolence, gingival hyperplasia, blood dyscrasia, and toxicity.

❑ A phenytoin level of 32 mg/dL indicates phenytoin toxicity.

❑ Symptoms of phenytoin toxicity include confusion and ataxia.

❑ Carbamazepine causes agranulocytosis because of the reduction in white blood cells.

❑ Complications of carbamazepine administration include diplopia, dizziness, ataxia, and rash.

❑ Hypersensitivity reactions to cephalosporins are more common in clients with penicillin allergy.

❑ Symptoms of cholinergic crisis or excessive acetylcholinesterase medication typically appear 45 to 60 minutes after the last dose of acetylcholinesterase inhibitor.

❑ Many adverse reactions are dosage related and lessen or disappear only if the dosage is reduced.

❑ Most adverse reactions aren't therapeutically desirable, but a few can be put to clinical use.

❑ Drug hypersensitivity, or drug allergy, is the result of an antigen–antibody immune reaction that occurs in the body when a drug is given to a susceptible client.

❑ Idiosyncratic reactions are highly unpredictable and unusual reactions, such as aplastic anemia caused by the antibiotic chloramphenicol.

❏ A common idiosyncratic drug reaction is extreme sensitivity to very low doses of a drug or insensitivity to higher-than-normal doses.

❏ To deal with adverse reactions correctly, the nurse needs to be alert to even minor changes in the client's clinical status, which may be an early warning of his reactions to a drug.

❏ The client needs to be told which adverse effects to expect so that he won't become worried or even stop taking the drug on his own if these effects occur.

❏ Always advise the client to report adverse reactions to the physician immediately.

❏ If you suspect a severe adverse reaction, withhold the drug until you can check with the pharmacist and the physician.

❏ Chronic drug toxicities are usually caused by the cumulative effect and resulting buildup of the drug in the body; these effects may be extensions of the desired therapeutic effect.

❏ Normal doses of glyburide normalize the glucose level, but higher doses can produce hypoglycemia.

❏ Alpha blockers may cause severe orthostatic hypotension and syncope, especially with the first few doses, an effect commonly called the "first-dose effect."

❏ The most common adverse effects of alpha$_1$ blockade are dizziness, headache, drowsiness, somnolence, and malaise.

❏ Alpha blockers may cause tachycardia, palpitations, fluid retention (from excess renin secretion), nasal and ocular congestion, and aggravation of respiratory tract infection.

❏ Drugs used to treat Alzheimer disease may cause weight loss, diarrhea, anorexia, nausea, vomiting, dizziness, headache, bradyarrhythmias, hypertension, and diarrhea.

❏ Ototoxicity and nephrotoxicity are the most serious complications of aminoglycosides.

❏ Neuromuscular blockade may also occur with aminoglycosides.

❏ Oral forms of aminoglycosides most commonly cause diarrhea, nausea, and vomiting.

❏ Parenteral forms of aminoglycosides may cause vein irritation, phlebitis, and sterile abscess.

❏ The most common adverse effects of therapeutic doses of angiotensin-converting enzyme inhibitors are angioedema of the face and limbs, dry cough, dysgeusia, fatigue, headache, hyperkalemia, hypotension, proteinuria, rash, and tachycardia.

❏ Severe hypotension may occur at toxic drug levels of angiotensin-converting enzyme inhibitors.

❑ Ranolazine may cause dizziness and nausea.

❑ Beta blockers may cause bradycardia, cough, diarrhea, disturbing dreams, dizziness, dyspnea, fatigue, fever, heart failure, hypotension, lethargy, nausea, peripheral edema, and wheezing.

❑ Calcium channel blockers may cause bradycardia, confusion, constipation, depression, diarrhea, dizziness, dyspepsia, edema, transient elevations in liver enzyme levels, fatigue, flushing, headache, hypotension, insomnia, nervousness, and rash.

❑ Nitrates may cause flushing, headache, orthostatic hypotension, reflex tachycardia, rash, syncope, and vomiting.

❑ Most antiarrhythmics can aggravate existing arrhythmias or cause new ones.

❑ Antiarrhythmics may produce central nervous system disturbances, such as dizziness or fatigue; GI problems, such as nausea, vomiting, or altered bowel elimination; hypersensitivity reactions; and hypotension.

❑ Some antiarrhythmics may worsen heart failure.

❑ Class II antiarrhythmic drugs may cause bronchoconstriction.

❑ Anticoagulants commonly cause bleeding and may cause hypersensitivity reactions.

❑ Warfarin may cause agranulocytosis, alopecia (with long-term use), anorexia, dermatitis, fever, nausea, tissue necrosis or gangrene, urticaria, and vomiting.

❑ Heparin derivatives may cause thrombocytopenia and may increase liver enzyme levels.

❑ Nonhemorrhagic adverse reactions associated with thrombin inhibitors may include back pain, bradycardia, and hypotension.

❑ Anticonvulsants can cause adverse central nervous system effects, such as ataxia, confusion, somnolence, and tremor.

❑ Many anticonvulsants cause cardiovascular disorders, such as arrhythmias and hypotension; GI effects, such as vomiting; and hematologic disorders, such as agranulocytosis, bone marrow depression, leukopenia, and thrombocytopenia.

❑ Stevens-Johnson syndrome, severe skin rashes, and abnormal liver function test results may occur with certain anticonvulsants.

❑ Sulfonylureas cause dose-related reactions that usually respond to decreased dosage: anorexia, headache, heartburn, nausea, paresthesia, vomiting, and weakness.

❑ The most serious adverse reaction linked to metformin is lactic acidosis; although rare, it's most likely to occur in clients with renal dysfunction.

❑ Other reactions to metformin include dermatitis, GI upset, megaloblastic anemia, rash, and unpleasant or metallic taste.

❏ Thiazolidinediones may cause fluid retention leading to or exacerbating heart failure.

❏ Alpha-glucosidase inhibitors can cause abdominal pain, diarrhea, and flatulence.

❏ Antiemetics may cause asthenia, fatigue, dizziness, headache, insomnia, abdominal pain, anorexia, constipation, diarrhea, epigastric discomfort, gastritis, heartburn, nausea, vomiting, neutropenia, hiccups, tinnitus, dehydration, and fever.

❏ Fluconazole may cause transient elevations of liver enzymes, alkaline phosphatase, and bilirubin levels, as well as dizziness, nausea, vomiting, abdominal pain, diarrhea, rash, headache, hypokalemia, and elevated blood urea nitrogen and creatinine levels.

❏ Adverse reactions to itraconazole include headache and nausea.

❏ The most common adverse reactions to ketoconazole are nausea and vomiting.

❏ Adverse reactions to voriconazole are uncommon; however, the drug may alter renal function and cause vision changes.

❏ Common adverse reactions to caspofungin include paresthesia, tachycardia, anorexia, anemia, pain, myalgia, tachypnea, chills, and sweating.

❏ Reactions to nystatin seldom occur, but may include diarrhea, nausea, vomiting, and abdominal pain.

❏ Terbinafine may cause abdominal pain, jaundice, diarrhea, flatulence, nausea, anaphylaxis, headache, rash, and vision disturbances.

❏ Administer I.V. amphotericin under close clinical observation; acute infusion reactions can occur, including fever, shaking chills, hypotension, anorexia, nausea, vomiting, and tachypnea.

❏ Antilipemics commonly cause GI upset.

❏ Bile-sequestering drugs may cause bloating, cholelithiasis, constipation, and steatorrhea.

❏ Fibric acid derivatives may cause cholelithiasis and have other GI or central nervous system effects.

❏ HMG-CoA reductase inhibitors may affect liver function or cause rash, pruritus, increased creatine kinase levels, rhabdomyolysis, and myopathy.

❏ The most serious adverse reactions associated with the antirheumatic drugs abatacept and adalimumab include serious infections and malignancies.

❏ Serious adverse reactions to gold therapy include anaphylactic shock, bradycardia, and angioneurotic edema.

❏ The most common adverse reactions to gold therapy include dermatitis, pruritus, and stomatitis.

❏ Isoniazid may precipitate seizures in clients with a seizure disorder and produce optic or peripheral neuritis, as well as elevated liver enzymes.

❑ Optic neuritis is the only significant reaction to ethambutol.

❑ The most common adverse reactions to rifampin include epigastric pain, nausea, vomiting, flatulence, abdominal cramps, anorexia, and diarrhea.

❑ Cycloserine can cause seizures, confusion, dizziness, headache, and somnolence.

❑ Prolonged or frequent use of a benzodiazepine can cause physical dependency and withdrawal syndrome when the drug is stopped.

❑ In pregnant clients, benzodiazepines increase the risk of congenital malformation if taken in the first trimester.

❑ Using benzodiazepines during labor may cause neonatal flaccidity.

❑ A neonate whose mother took a benzodiazepine during pregnancy may have withdrawal symptoms.

❑ When administered to breast-feeding women, benzodiazepines may cause sedation, feeding difficulties, and weight loss in the infant.

❑ Therapeutic doses of a beta blocker may cause bradycardia, dizziness, and fatigue; some may cause other central nervous system disturbances, such as depression, hallucinations, memory loss, and nightmares.

❑ Toxic doses of a beta blocker can produce severe hypotension, bradycardia, heart failure, or bronchospasm.

❑ Verapamil may cause bradycardia, hypotension, various degrees of heart block, and worsening of heart failure after rapid I.V. delivery.

❑ Prolonged oral verapamil therapy may cause constipation.

❑ Nifedipine may cause flushing, headache, heartburn, hypotension, light-headedness, and peripheral edema.

❑ The most common adverse reactions to diltiazem are anorexia and nausea; it may also induce bradycardia, heart failure, peripheral edema, and various degrees of heart block.

❑ Agranulocytosis, intermittent tachycardia, and seizures are adverse effects of clozapine.

❑ Adverse reactions associated with phentermine are related to its stimulatory effect and include hypertension, palpitations, tachyarrhythmias, urticaria, constipation, diarrhea, dizziness, excitement, insomnia, tremor, and restlessness.

❑ Sibutramine can cause headache, insomnia, constipation, and rash.

❑ Excessive use of systemic corticosteroids may cause cushingoid symptoms and various systemic disorders, such as diabetes and osteoporosis.

❑ The therapeutic dose of a loop diuretic commonly causes metabolic and electrolyte disturbances, particularly potassium depletion.

❏ The therapeutic dose of a loop diuretic also may cause hyperglycemia, hyperuricemia, hypochloremic alkalosis, and hypomagnesemia.

❏ Rapid parenteral administration of a loop diuretic may cause hearing loss (including deafness) and tinnitus.

❏ High doses of a loop diuretic can produce profound diuresis, leading to hypovolemia and cardiovascular collapse.

❏ Photosensitivity may occur with high doses of a loop diuretic.

❏ Hyperkalemia is the most serious adverse reaction associated with spirono-lactone, a potassium-sparing-diuretic, and could lead to arrhythmias.

❏ Adverse reactions to spironolactone include nausea, vomiting, headache, weakness, fatigue, bowel disturbances, cough, and dyspnea.

❏ Long-term effects of estrogen use include benign hepatomas, cholestatic jaundice, elevated blood pressure (sometimes into the hypertensive range), endometrial carcinoma (rare), and thromboembolic disease.

❏ $H_2$-receptor antagonists rarely cause adverse reactions.

❏ Inotropic agents may cause arrhythmias, nausea, vomiting, diarrhea, headache, fever, mental disturbances, visual changes, and chest pain.

❏ Inamrinone and milrinone may cause thrombocytopenia, hypotension, hypokalemia, and elevated liver enzymes.

❏ The most frequently reported adverse effects of the nucleoside reverse transcriptase inhibitors are anemia, leukopenia, and neutropenia; thrombocytopenia is less common.

❏ Respiratory and circulatory depression (including orthostatic hypotension) is the major hazard of opioids.

❏ A neuroleptic malignant syndrome resembling severe parkinsonism may occur, most often in young men taking fluphenazine.

❏ Progestins may cause amenorrhea, breakthrough menstrual flow, breast enlargement and tenderness, alterations in weight, and mood changes.

❏ The most common adverse effects of protease inhibitors, which require immediate medical attention, include kidney stones, pancreatitis, diabetes or hyperglycemia, ketoacidosis, and paresthesia.

❏ Permanent discoloration of teeth occurs if tetracycline is given during tooth formation in children younger than age 8.

## Contraindications

❏ Carbamazepine is contraindicated within 14 days of monoamine oxidase inhibitor use.

❏ Tricyclic antidepressants are contraindicated within 2 weeks of monoamine oxidase inhibitor therapy.

❑ Risk of thromboembolic disease in a client taking estrogen increases greatly with cigarette smoking, especially in women older than age 35.

❑ Thiazide diuretics shouldn't be used for clients with hyperparathyroidism because they decrease renal excretion of calcium, thereby raising serum calcium levels even higher.

❑ Magnesium sulfate shouldn't be administered in normal saline solution.

❑ Aspirin is contraindicated in clients with conditions in which bleeding may be present, such as trauma.

❑ Aspirin is contraindicated in children or young adults with viral illnesses due to the danger of Reye syndrome.

❑ Propranolol and other beta-adrenergic blockers are contraindicated in a client with bronchial asthma.

❑ Opioids may mask changes in the level of consciousness that indicate increased intracranial pressure and shouldn't be given as a first-line drug.

❑ Use alpha-adrenergic blockers cautiously with heart failure, renal failure, and in pregnancy.

❑ Isosorbide can cause hypotension, which reduces brain perfusion; isosorbide should be avoided in a client with a stroke.

❑ Use angiotensin II receptor blockers cautiously in clients with renal impairment and hypovolemia.

❑ Do not administer barbiturates intra-arterially because they may produce arteriospasm, thrombosis, and gangrene.

❑ Clients with allergies to shellfish may be allergic to iodine-containing drugs.

❑ The Food and Drug Administration has assigned a pregnancy risk category to each drug based on available clinical and preclinical information.

❑ The five Food and Drug Administration pregnancy risk categories (A, B, C, D, and X) reflect a drug's potential to cause birth defects.

❑ Although drugs should ideally be avoided during pregnancy, sometimes they're needed; the pregnancy risk category rating system permits rapid assessment of the risk-benefit ratio.

❑ Drugs in Food and Drug Administration pregnancy risk category A are generally considered safe to use in pregnancy; drugs in category X are generally contraindicated.

❑ Drugs in Food and Drug Administration pregnancy risk category A are those in which adequate studies in pregnant women have failed to show a risk to the fetus.

❑ Drugs in Food and Drug Administration pregnancy risk category B are those in which animal studies haven't shown a risk to the fetus, but controlled studies haven't been conducted in pregnant women;

this category also includes those drugs in which animal studies have shown an adverse effect on the fetus, but no adequate studies have been performed in pregnant women to show a risk to the fetus.

❑ Drugs in Food and Drug Administration pregnancy risk category C are those in which animal studies have shown an adverse effect on the fetus, but adequate studies haven't been conducted in humans; the benefits from use in pregnant women may be acceptable despite potential risks.

❑ Drugs in Food and Drug Administration pregnancy risk category D are those in which there is positive evidence of human fetal risk, but the potential benefits of use in pregnant women may be acceptable despite the risks (such as in a life-threatening situation or a serious disease for which safer drugs can't be used or are ineffective).

❑ Drugs in Food and Drug Administration pregnancy risk category X are those in which studies in animals or humans show fetal abnormalities or adverse reaction reports indicate evidence of fetal risk, and the risks involved clearly outweigh potential benefits.

❑ Drugs in Food and Drug Administration pregnancy risk category NR are not rated.

❑ Drug toxicities occur when a drug level rises as a result of impaired metabolism or excretion.

❑ Hepatic dysfunction impairs the metabolism of theophylline, raising theophylline levels.

❑ Renal dysfunction may cause digoxin toxicity because this drug is eliminated from the body by the kidneys.

❑ Tinnitus is usually a sign that the safe dose of aspirin has been exceeded.

❑ Most drug toxicities are predictable, dosage-related, and reversible upon dosage adjustment.

❑ Drugs in controlled substance schedule I have high abuse potential and have no accepted medical use; examples include heroin, marijuana, and LSD.

❑ Drugs in controlled substance schedule II have high abuse potential with severe dependence liability; examples include opioids, amphetamines, and some barbiturates.

❑ Drugs in controlled substance schedule III have less abuse potential than schedule II drugs and moderate dependence liability; examples include nonbarbiturate sedatives, nonamphetamine stimulants, anabolic steroids, and limited amounts of certain opioids.

❑ Drugs in controlled substance schedule IV have less abuse potential than schedule III drugs and limited dependence liability; examples include some sedatives, anxiolytics, and nonopioid analgesics.

❑ Drugs in controlled substance schedule V have limited abuse potential; examples include mainly small amounts of opioids, such as codeine, used as antitussives or antidiarrheals.

❑ Pregnant women should avoid oral antidiabetic agents and use insulin therapy to maintain glucose levels as close to normal as possible.

❑ Because aging is associated with a decline in kidney function and because the kidneys subsequently secrete metformin, metformin should be used with caution in elderly clients.

❑ Because metformin given with iodinated contrast dye can cause acute renal failure, metformin should not be given to clients undergoing procedures that require contrast dye.

❑ Alpha blockers are contraindicated in clients with myocardial infarction, coronary insufficiency, or angina, and in those with hypersensitivity to these drugs or any of their components.

❑ Use alpha blockers cautiously in pregnant or breast-feeding women.

❑ The safety and effectiveness of many alpha blockers in children haven't been established; use cautiously.

❑ In elderly clients taking alpha blockers, hypotensive effects may be more pronounced.

❑ Drugs used to treat Alzheimer disease are contraindicated in clients hypersensitive to any of the drug components.

❑ Use Alzheimer disease drugs cautiously with concomitant drugs that slow heart rate; there is an increased risk for heart block.

❑ Use Alzheimer disease drugs cautiously in clients with moderate hepatic or renal impairment.

❑ Drugs used to treat Alzheimer disease are not recommended for clients with severe hepatic impairment or severe renal impairment (creatinine clearance less than 9 mL/minute).

❑ Use Alzheimer disease drugs cautiously in clients with a history of asthma or chronic obstructive pulmonary disease.

❑ Aminoglycosides are contraindicated in clients hypersensitive to these drugs.

❑ Use aminoglycosides cautiously in clients with a neuromuscular disorder and in those taking neuromuscular blockades.

❑ Use aminoglycosides at lower dosages in clients with renal impairment.

❑ Use aminoglycosides cautiously in pregnant women.

❑ Aminoglycoside safety hasn't been established in breast-feeding women.

❑ In neonates and premature infants, the half-life of aminoglycosides is prolonged because of immature renal systems.

❑ Dosage adjustment of aminoglycosides may be needed in infants and children.

❑ Elderly clients have an increased risk of nephrotoxicity if receiving amino-glycosides; they commonly need a lower dose and longer dosage intervals.

❑ Elderly clients receiving aminoglycosides are also susceptible to ototoxicity and superinfection. Angiotensin-converting enzyme inhibitors are contraindicated in clients hypersensitive to these drugs.

❑ Use angiotensin-converting enzyme inhibitors cautiously in clients with impaired renal function or serious autoimmune disease and in those taking other drugs known to decrease white blood cell count or immune response.

❑ Women of childbearing potential taking angiotensin-converting enzyme inhibitors should report suspected pregnancy immediately to the prescriber.

❑ High risks of fetal morbidity and mortality are linked to angiotensin-converting enzyme inhibitors, especially in the second and third trimesters.

❑ Some angiotensin-converting enzyme inhibitors appear in breast milk.

❑ To avoid adverse effects in infants, instruct the client to stop breast-feeding during angiotensin-converting enzyme inhibitor therapy.

❑ In children, safety and effectiveness of angiotensin-converting enzyme inhibitor use hasn't been established; give drug only if potential benefits outweigh risks.

❑ Elderly clients may need lower doses of angiotensin-converting enzyme inhibitors because of impaired drug clearance.

❑ Ranolazine is contraindicated in clients with clinically significant hepatic impairment.

❑ Beta blockers are contraindicated in clients hypersensitive to them and in clients with cardiogenic shock, sinus bradycardia, heart block greater than first degree, or bronchial asthma.

❑ Calcium channel blockers are contraindicated in clients with severe hypotension or heart block greater than first degree (except with functioning pacemaker).

❑ Nitrates are contraindicated in clients with severe anemia, cerebral hemorrhage, head trauma, glaucoma, or hyperthyroidism.

❑ Nitrates are contraindicated in clients using phosphodiesterase type 5 inhibitors (sildenafil, tadalafil, vardenafil).

❑ Use beta blockers cautiously in clients with nonallergic bronchospastic disorders, diabetes mellitus, or impaired hepatic or renal function.

❑ Use calcium channel blockers cautiously in clients with hepatic or renal impairment, bradycardia, heart failure, or cardiogenic shock.

❑ Use nitrates cautiously in clients with hypotension or recent myocardial infarction.

- ❑ Use beta blockers cautiously in pregnant women.
- ❑ Recommendations for breast-feeding vary by drug; use beta blockers and calcium channel blockers cautiously.
- ❑ Many antiarrhythmics are contraindicated or require cautious use in clients with cardiogenic shock, digoxin toxicity, and second- or third-degree heart block (unless the client has a pacemaker or implantable cardioverter defibrillator).
- ❑ Caspofungin is contraindicated with concomitant use of cyclosporine because of the possibility of elevated liver enzymes.
- ❑ Bile-sequestering drugs are contraindicated in clients with complete biliary obstruction.
- ❑ Fibric acid derivatives are contraindicated in clients with primary biliary cirrhosis or significant hepatic or renal dysfunction.
- ❑ HMG-CoA reductase inhibitors and cholesterol absorption inhibitors are contraindicated in clients with active liver disease or persistently elevated transaminase levels.
- ❑ Use bile-sequestering drugs cautiously in constipated clients.
- ❑ Use fibric acid derivatives cautiously in clients with peptic ulcer.
- ❑ Use HMG-CoA inhibitors cautiously in clients who consume large amounts of alcohol or in those who have a history of liver or renal disease.
- ❑ Sibutramine is contraindicated with concomitant monoamine oxidase inhibitor use.
- ❑ Inamrinone is contraindicated in clients with a sulfite allergy and severe aortic or pulmonic valve disease.
- ❑ Use inamrinone cautiously in clients with hypertrophic subaortic stenosis and acute myocardial infarction.
- ❑ Digoxin is contraindicated in ventricular fibrillation.
- ❑ Use digoxin cautiously in clients with renal insufficiency because of the potential for digoxin toxicity.
- ❑ Use digoxin cautiously in clients with sinus node disease or atrioventricular block because of the potential for advanced heart block.
- ❑ Because of the complexity of human immunodeficiency virus infection, it's often difficult to distinguish between disease-related symptoms and adverse drug reactions.
- ❑ Opioids are contraindicated in clients hypersensitive to these drugs and in those who have recently taken a monoamine oxidase inhibitor.
- ❑ Opioids are contraindicated in those with acute or severe bronchial asthma or respiratory depression.

## Dosage calculations

❑ When converting pounds to kilograms, remember that 2.2 pounds equals 1 kilogram.

❑ To convert a client's weight in pounds to kilograms, divide his weight in pounds by 2.2.

❑ To convert a client's weight in kilograms to pounds, multiply his weight in kilograms by 2.2.

❑ 2 tablespoons equals 1 fluid ounce or 30 milliliters.

❑ 1 teaspoon equals 1 fluidram or 5 milliliters.

❑ 1 pint equals 16 fluid ounces or 480 milliliters.

❑ 1 quart equals 32 fluid ounces.

❑ 1 drop (gtt) equals 1 minim.

❑ To calculate the dose to be administered when a medication is available in units, use this equation:

$$\frac{\text{Amount of drug in mL}}{\text{Dose required in units}} = \frac{1\,\text{mL or other measure}}{\text{Drug available in units}}$$

❑ A meter is the basic unit of length.

❑ A liter is the basic unit of volume.

❑ A gram is the basic unit of weight.

❑ The unit measurement system is used for certain drugs, such as insulin, heparin, penicillin G and V, and some hormones and vitamins.

❑ To calculate the dose to be given when a medication is available in milliequivalents (mEq), use this equation:

$$\frac{\text{Amount of drug in mL or other measure}}{\text{Dose required in mEq}} = \frac{1\,\text{mL or other measure}}{\text{Drug available in mEq}}$$

❑ One inch equals 2.5 centimeters.

❑ You can calculate a pediatric dose by dividing the child's body surface area (BSA) by the average adult BSA (1.73 m²) and multiplying that number by the average adult dose of the drug.

❑ To calculate a pediatric dose using the child's body surface area (BSA) use this formula:

$$\frac{\text{Child's BSA in m}^2}{\text{Average adult's BSA (1.73 m}^2)} \times \text{Average adult dose} = \text{Child's dose in mg}$$

ccurate and common way to calculate pediatric drug doses is dosage per kilogram of body weight method.

❑ You can determine the pediatric dose by using the following formula:

Child's body weight in kg × Required number of mg of the drug per kg

❑ To solve a two-step dosage calculation, use the following formula:

$$\frac{\text{Amount desired}}{\text{Amount you have}} = \frac{\text{Equivalent amount desired}}{\text{Equivalent amount you have}}$$

## Expected actions and outcomes

❑ The half-life of a drug is the time it takes for one-half of the drug dose to be eliminated by the body.

❑ Factors that affect a drug's half-life include its rate of absorption, metabolism, and excretion.

❑ A drug that is given only once is eliminated from the body almost completely after four or five half-lives.

❑ A drug that is administered at regular intervals reaches a steady concentration after about four or five half-lives.

❑ A drug's onset of action refers to the time interval from when the drug is administered to when its therapeutic effect actually begins.

❑ Supplemental or replacement therapy is used to replenish or substitute missing substances in the body.

❑ Enalapril is an angiotensin-converting enzyme inhibitor that directly lowers blood pressure.

❑ Metoprolol is a beta-adrenergic blocker that is used to slow the heart rate and lower blood pressure.

❑ Vasodilators cause dilation of peripheral blood vessels, directly relaxing vascular smooth muscle and decreasing blood pressure.

❑ Most drugs are excreted by the kidneys and leave the body through urine.

❑ Drugs can be excreted through the lungs, exocrine (sweat, salivary, or mammary) glands, skin, and intestinal tract.

❑ Class IA antiarrhythmic drugs include disopyramide procainamide hydrochloride, quinidine gluconate, and quinidine sulfate.

❑ Class IB antiarrhythmic drugs include lidocaine hydrochloride and mexiletine hydrochloride.

❑ Class IC antiarrhythmic drugs include flecainide acetate and propafenone hydrochloride.

❑ Class II antiarrhythmic drugs (beta blockers) include amiodarone hydrochloride, dofetilide, esmolol hydrochloride, ibutilide fumarate, and sotalol hydrochloride.

❑ Class IV antiarrhythmic drugs (calcium channel blockers) include verapamil hydrochloride.

❑ Adrenergic blockers decrease sympathetic cardioacceleration and decrease blood pressure.

❑ Pentoxifylline decreases blood viscosity, increases red blood cell flexibility, and improves flow through small vessels.

❑ Warfarin is an oral anticoagulant that prevents vitamin K from synthesizing certain clotting factors.

❑ Tricyclic antidepressants are used to decrease the frequency of reenactment of the trauma for the client with posttraumatic stress disorder.

❑ Tricyclic antidepressants are used to help the client with memory problems and sleeping difficulties.

❑ Tricyclic antidepressants will decrease numbing in the client with posttraumatic stress disorder.

❑ Heparin is a parenteral anticoagulant that interferes with coagulation by readily binding with antithrombin to prevent clot formation.

❑ Angiotensin-converting enzyme inhibitors are given to reduce blood pressure by inhibiting aldosterone production, which in turn decreases sodium and water reabsorption.

❑ Angiotensin-converting enzyme inhibitors reduce production of angiotensin II, a potent vasoconstrictor.

❑ Inotropic agents increase contractility of the heart.

❑ Negative inotropic agents decrease contractility of the heart.

❑ A client with acute pulmonary edema may be given an angiotensin-converting enzyme inhibitor to reduce blood pressure.

❑ The client's apical pulse should always be checked before giving propranolol.

❑ If the client's pulse rate is extremely low, propranolol should be withheld and the physician notified.

❑ Taking propranolol with food enhances its absorption.

❑ Propranolol is given to control hypertension.

❑ Amiodarone is indicated for ventricular tachycardia, ventricular fibrillation, and atrial flutter.

❑ A calcium channel blocker, such as diltiazem, is indicated in managing Prinzmetal angina.

❑ Diltiazem reduces the incidence of coronary artery spasm.

- ❑ A beta-adrenergic blocker, such as metoprolol, is used to treat angina.

- ❑ Zidovudine is an antiviral drug that suppresses the replication of human immunodeficiency virus (HIV) and is most commonly used for HIV-positive clients in conjunction with other antiretroviral drugs.

- ❑ Zidovudine helps prevent maternal-fetal transmission of human immunodeficiency virus.

- ❑ Corticosteroids suppress eosinophils, lymphocytes, natural killer cells, and the immune response.

- ❑ Inhaled beta-adrenergic agents help promote bronchodilation, which improves oxygenation.

- ❑ Aspirin interferes with platelet aggregation and the action of other anti-platelets, and is used in the treatment of thromboembolic stroke.

- ❑ Supportive therapy does not treat the cause of the disease but maintains other threatened body systems until the client's condition resolves.

- ❑ Palliative therapy is used in end-stage disease or terminal diseases to make the client as comfortable as possible.

- ❑ Maintenance therapy is used in clients with chronic conditions that do not resolve.

- ❑ Empirical therapy is based on practical experience rather than pure scientific data.

- ❑ Insulin is an anabolic or building hormone that helps promote storage of glucose as glycogen; increases protein and fat metabolism; slows the break-down of glycogen, protein, and fat; and balances fluids and electrolytes.

- ❑ Insulin facilitates the movement of potassium from the extracellular fluid into the cell.

- ❑ Selective alpha blockers decrease vascular resistance and increase venous capacity, thereby lowering blood pressure and causing nasal and sclero-conjunctival congestion, ptosis, orthostatic and exercise hypotension, mild to moderate miosis, interference with ejaculation, and pink, warm skin.

- ❑ Selective alpha blockers relax nonvascular smooth muscle, especially in the prostate capsule, which reduces urinary problems in men with benign prostatic hypertrophy.

- ❑ Alkylating drugs are cytotoxic; they alkylate cellular DNA, interfering with the replication of susceptible cells and causing cell death.

- ❑ Alpha$_1$-adrenergic blockers selectively block postsynaptic alpha$_1$-adrenergic receptors, decreasing sympathetic tone on the vasculature, dilating arterioles and veins, and lowering both supine and standing blood pressure.

- ❑ Alpha-adrenergic blockers relax the smooth muscle of the bladder and prostate.

❏ Aminoglycosides are bactericidal antibiotics.

❏ Aminoglycosides inhibit protein synthesis in susceptible strains of gram-negative bacteria and appear to disrupt the functional integrity of the bacterial cell membrane, causing cell death.

❏ Oral aminoglycosides are very poorly absorbed and are used to suppress GI bacterial flora.

❏ By inhibiting angiotensin II, adrenocortical secretion of aldosterone is decreased, thus reducing sodium and water retention and extracellular fluid volume.

❏ Angiotensin II receptor blockers selectively block the binding of angiotensin II to specific tissue receptors found in the vascular smooth muscle and adrenal gland.

❏ Angiotensin II receptor blockers block the vasoconstriction effect of the renin-angiotensin system as well as the release of aldosterone, leading to decreased blood pressure.

❏ Angiotensin II receptor blockers are used to treat heart failure in clients resistant to angiotensin-converting enzyme inhibitors.

❏ Angiotensin II receptor blockers are used to reduce the risk of stroke in clients with hypertension and left ventricular hypertrophy.

❏ Antiarrhythmics act at specific sites to alter the action potential of cardiac cells and interfere with the electrical excitability of the heart.

❏ Most antiarrhythmics may cause new or worsened arrhythmias (pro-arrhythmic effect) and must be used with caution and with continual cardiac monitoring and client evaluation.

❏ Antiarrhythmics are used to treat tachycardia when rapid but short-term control of ventricular rate is desirable, such as in clients with atrial fibrillation, atrial flutter, and in perioperative or postoperative situations.

❏ Antiarrhythmics are used to treat noncompensatory tachycardia when the heart rate requires specific intervention.

❏ Antiarrhythmics are used to treat atrial arrhythmias.

❏ Oral anticoagulants interfere with the hepatic synthesis of vitamin K-dependent clotting factors (factors II, VII, IX, and X and prothrombin), resulting in their eventual depletion and the prolongation of clotting times.

❏ Parenteral anticoagulants interfere with the conversion of prothrombin to thrombin, blocking the final step in clot formation but leaving the circulating levels of clotting factors unaffected.

❏ Sulfonylureas are oral antidiabetic agents that stimulate the release of insulin from functioning beta cells in the pancreas; they may either improve binding between insulin and insulin receptors or increase the number of insulin receptors.

- ❑ Second-generation sulfonylureas (glipizide and glyburide) are thought to be more potent than first-generation sulfonylureas.

- ❑ Thiazolidinedione antidiabetic agents increase insulin receptor sensitivity.

- ❑ The antidiabetic agents acarbose and miglitol delay or alter glucose absorption.

- ❑ Antifungals bind to or impair sterols of fungal cell membranes, allowing increased permeability and leakage of cellular components and causing the death of the fungal cell.

- ❑ Antihistamines competitively block the effects of histamine at peripheral $H_1$ receptor sites and have anticholinergic (atropine-like) and antipruritic effects.

- ❑ Antimetabolites are antineoplastic drugs that inhibit DNA polymerase.

- ❑ Triptans (antimigraine drugs) bind to serotonin receptors to cause vascular constrictive effects on cranial blood vessels, causing the relief of migraine in selective clients.

- ❑ Antiviral drugs inhibit DNA or RNA replication in the virus, preventing replication and leading to death of the virus.

- ❑ Barbiturates act as sedatives, hypnotics, and antiepileptics.

- ❑ Barbiturates are general central nervous system depressants.

- ❑ Barbiturates inhibit impulse conduction in the ascending reticular activating system, depress the cerebral cortex, alter cerebellar function, depress motor output, and can produce excitation, sedation, hypnosis, anesthesia, and deep coma.

- ❑ Benzodiazepines are anxiolytics, antiepileptics, muscle relaxants, and sedative-hypnotics.

- ❑ NPH insulin (Novolin N) is an intermediate-acting insulin with a peak effect of 4 to 15 hours.

- ❑ Humalog and NovoLog are rapid-acting types of insulin with a peak effect of 2 to 3 hours.

- ❑ Humulin R insulin is a short-acting insulin with a peak of 2 to 3 hours.

- ❑ Metformin and sulfonylureas are commonly ordered medications for hyperglycemia.

- ❑ Oxybutynin is a spasmolytic.

- ❑ A client with an overactive neurogenic bladder may be treated with oxybutynin.

- ❑ Dopamine is a selective cardiac stimulant that will increase cardiac output, heart rate, and cardiac contractility in a child with a ventricular septal defect repair.

- ❑ The normal therapeutic range of aminophylline is considered to be 10 to 20 mcg/mL.

❑ Albuterol is a rapid-acting bronchodilator for the treatment of asthma.

❑ Bicalutamide, a nonsteroidal antiandrogen, and leuprolide, a gonadotropin-releasing hormone agonist, decrease the production of testosterone.

❑ Bicalutamide and leuprolide therapy helps to decrease the production of cancer cells involved in prostate cancer.

❑ Atropine blocks vagal impulses to the myocardium and stimulates the cardio-inhibitory center in the medulla, thereby increasing heart rate and cardiac output.

❑ Atropine, an anticholinergic agent, is administered to a child with sinus bradycardia.

❑ Erythromycin should be given with a full glass of water and after meals or with food to lessen GI symptoms.

❑ Angiotensin-converting enzyme inhibitors block the conversion of angio-tensin I to angiotensin II in the kidney, causing decreased aldosterone, vasodilation, and increased sodium excretion.

❑ As vasodilators, angiotensin-converting enzyme inhibitors also act to reduce vascular resistance by the manipulation of afterload.

❑ The capacity of the liver to metabolize phenytoin is affected by slight changes in the dosage of the drug, not necessarily the length of time the client has been taking the drug.

❑ The medication of choice for gonorrhea is a single dose of I.M. ceftriaxone sodium in males and a single oral dose of cefixime in females.

❑ When giving injectable vasopressin, it must be thoroughly re-suspended in the oil by being held under warm running water for 10 to 15 minutes and shaken vigorously before being drawn into the syringe.

❑ With vasopressin, small brown particles indicate drug dispersion and must be seen in the suspension.

❑ Lispro insulin has an onset within 5 minutes.

❑ NPH insulin has an onset within 2 to 4 hours, and Ultralente insulin is the longest acting, with an onset of 6 to 10 hours.

❑ Regular insulin is always drawn up first so it won't become contaminated with NPH insulin

❑ 7 to 21 days may pass before the client notes a change in his mood when taking lithium.

❑ Donepezil is used to improve cognition and functional autonomy in mild to moderate dementia of the Alzheimer type.

❑ Bupropion is used for depression.

- ❏ Haloperidol is used for agitation, aggression, hallucinations, thought disturbances, and wandering.

- ❏ Regular insulin's onset is ½ to 1 hour, peak is 2 to 4 hours, and duration is 3 to 6 hours.

- ❏ Triazolam is used for sleep disturbances.

- ❏ Edrophonium is used for the diagnosis of myasthenia gravis.

- ❏ Pyrostigmine bromide is used for the treatment of myasthenia gravis.

- ❏ Mannitol promotes osmotic diuresis by increasing the pressure gradient, drawing fluid from intracellular to intravascular spaces.

- ❏ Mannitol can reduce intraocular pressure, prevent acute tubular necrosis, and draw water into the vascular system to increase blood pressure.

- ❏ A therapeutic phenytoin level is 10 to 20 mg/dL.

- ❏ Isoniazid is the medication most commonly used for the treatment of tuberculosis, but other antibiotics are added to the regimen to obtain the best results.

- ❏ Preferably, ferrous gluconate should be taken on an empty stomach in the client with iron deficiency anemia.

- ❏ Tenecteplase is a medication used with evolving myocardial infarction to dissolve existing clots.

- ❏ Gargling and rinsing the mouth after cromolyn administration can reduce mouth dryness.

- ❏ Warfarin inhibits clot formation by interfering with clotting factors that are dependent on vitamin K.

- ❏ When a therapeutic level of heparin is established, warfarin is started.

- ❏ It can take up to 3 days before a therapeutic level of warfarin is achieved.

- ❏ Beta-adrenergic blockers aren't indicated in the management of asthma because they may cause bronchospasm.

- ❏ Mannitol promotes osmotic diuresis by increasing the pressure gradient in the renal tubules, thus increasing urine output.

- ❏ Taking phenytoin with food minimizes GI distress.

- ❏ Phenytoin should be administered slowly (50 mg/minute).

- ❏ There's no need to withhold additional anticonvulsants when administering phenytoin.

- ❏ Acetazolamide, a carbonic anhydrase inhibitor, decreases intraocular pressure by decreasing the secretion of aqueous humor.

- ❏ Atropine dilates the pupil and decreases outflow of aqueous humor, causing a further increase in intraocular pressure.

❏ Furosemide is a loop diuretic.

❏ Urokinase is a thrombolytic agent.

❏ Atropine, an anticholinergic drug, has mydriatic effects, causing pupil dilation.

❏ Baclofen is a skeletal muscle relaxant used to decrease spasms in a client recovering from a spinal cord injury.

❏ Lidocaine is an antiarrhythmic and a local anesthetic agent.

❏ Heparin will prevent clot formation and prevent clot enlargement.

❏ Digoxin, diltiazem, and quinidine gluconate are used in the treatment and control of atrial fibrillation.

❏ Nitroglycerin is given to relieve chest pain and reduce preload dysreflexia.

❏ Phenytoin levels are checked before giving the drug; the drug is withheld if levels are elevated to avoid compounding toxicity.

❏ Cephalosporins are chemically and pharmacologically similar to penicillin; they act by inhibiting bacterial cell wall synthesis, causing rapid cell destruction.

❏ Some beta blockers are nonselective: they block both $beta_1$ receptors in cardiac muscle and $beta_2$ receptors in bronchial and vascular smooth muscle.

❏ Nonselective $beta_1$ and $beta_2$ blockers include carvedilol, labetalol, nadolol, sotalol, and propranolol.

❏ Some beta blockers are cardioselective and, in lower doses, inhibit mainly $beta_1$ receptors.

❏ Selective $beta_1$ blockers include atenolol, metoprolol, betaxolol, and esmolol.

❏ Some beta blockers have intrinsic sympathomimetic activity and stimulate and block $beta_2$ receptors and thereby have less effect on slowing heart rate.

❏ Some beta blockers stabilize cardiac membranes, affecting cardiac action potential.

❏ The main physiologic action of calcium channel blockers is to inhibit calcium influx across the slow channels of myocardial and vascular smooth muscle cells, which reduces intracellular calcium levels, which in turn dilates coronary arteries, peripheral arteries, and arterioles and slows cardiac conduction.

❏ When used to treat Prinzmetal variant angina, calcium channel blockers inhibit coronary spasm, which then increases oxygen delivery to the heart, and peripheral artery dilation reduces afterload, which decreases myocardial oxygen use.

❏ By inhibiting calcium flow into specialized cardiac conduction cells in the sinoatrial and atrioventricular nodes, calcium channel blockers slow conduction through the heart.

❑ Verapamil and diltiazem have the greatest effect on the atrioventricular node, slowing the ventricular rate in atrial fibrillation or flutter and converting supraventricular tachycardia to a normal sinus rhythm.

❑ Antiparkinsonian drugs include synthetic anticholinergics, dopaminergics, and the antiviral amantadine.

❑ Anticholinergic antiparkinsonian drugs probably prolong the action of dopamine by blocking its reuptake into presynaptic neurons and by suppressing central cholinergic activity.

❑ Dopaminergic antiparkinsonian drugs act in the brain by increasing dopamine availability, thus improving motor function.

❑ The antiparkinsonian drug entacapone is a reversible inhibitor of peripheral catechol-O-methyltransferase (commonly known as COMT), which is responsible for elimination of various catecholamines, including dopamine.

❑ Amantadine is thought to increase dopamine release in the substantia nigra.

❑ The I.V. antiplatelet drugs abciximab, eptifibatide, and tirofiban antagonize the glycoprotein IIb/IIIA (GPIIb/IIIa) receptors located on platelets, which are involved in platelet aggregation.

❑ The antiplatelet drug clopidogrel inhibits platelet aggregation by inhibiting the binding of adenosine diphosphate (ADP) to its platelet receptor and the subsequent ADP-mediated activation of the glycoprotein IIb/IIIa (GPIIb/IIIa) complex.

❑ The antiplatelet drug ticlopidine inhibits the binding of fibrinogen to platelets.

❑ Sulfonylureas are sulfonamide derivatives that aren't antibacterial.

❑ Sulfonylureas lower glucose levels by stimulating insulin release from the pancreas.

❑ Sulfonylureas work only in the presence of functioning beta cells in the islet tissue of the pancreas.

❑ Centrally acting sympatholytics stimulate central alpha-adrenergic receptors, reducing cerebral sympathetic outflow, thereby decreasing peripheral vascular resistance and blood pressure.

❑ Vasodilators act directly on smooth muscle to reduce blood pressure.

❑ Antilipemics lower elevated lipid levels.

❑ Bile-sequestering drugs (cholestyramine and colesevelam) lower the low-density lipoprotein level by forming insoluble complexes with bile salts, thus triggering cholesterol to leave the bloodstream and other storage areas to make new bile acids.

❑ Gemfibrozil, a fibric acid derivative, reduces cholesterol formation, increases sterol excretion, and decreases lipoprotein and triglyceride synthesis.

❑ HMG-CoA reductase inhibitors (atorvastatin, fluvastatin, lovastatin, pravastatin, rosuvastatin, simvastatin) interfere with the activity of enzymes that generate cholesterol in the liver.

❑ Ezetimibe, a selective cholesterol absorption inhibitor, inhibits cholesterol absorption by the small intestine, reducing hepatic cholesterol stores and increasing cholesterol clearance from the blood.

❑ After prolonged administration, sulfonylureas produce hypoglycemia by acting outside the pancreas, including reduced glucose production by the liver and enhanced peripheral sensitivity to insulin.

❑ Meglitinides, such as nateglinide and repaglinide, are nonsulfonylurea antidiabetic agents that stimulate the release of insulin from the pancreas.

❑ Metformin decreases hepatic glucose production, reduces intestinal glucose absorption, and improves insulin sensitivity by increasing peripheral glucose uptake and utilization.

❑ With metformin therapy, insulin secretion remains unchanged, and fasting insulin levels and all-day insulin response may decrease.

❑ Alpha-glucosidase inhibitors, such as acarbose and miglitol, delay digestion of carbohydrates, resulting in a smaller rise in glucose levels.

❑ Pramlintide, a human amylin analogue, slows the rate at which food leaves the stomach, decreasing postprandial increase in glucose level, and reduces appetite.

❑ Rosiglitazone and pioglitazone are thiazolidinediones, which lower glucose levels by improving insulin sensitivity.

❑ Thiazolidinediones are potent and highly selective agonists for receptors found in insulin-sensitive tissues, such as adipose tissue, skeletal muscle, and liver.

❑ Sitagliptin increases insulin release by inhibiting the enzyme dipeptidyl peptidase-4.

❑ Beta blockers decrease catecholamine-induced increases in heart rate, blood pressure, and myocardial contraction.

❑ Tricyclic antidepressants may inhibit reuptake of norepinephrine and serotonin in central nervous system nerve terminals (presynaptic neurons), thus enhancing the concentration and activity of neurotransmitters in the synaptic cleft.

❑ Tricyclic antidepressants exert antihistaminic, sedative, anticholinergic, vasodilatory, and quinidine-like effects.

❑ Anticonvulsants include six classes of drugs: selected hydantoin derivatives, barbiturates, benzodiazepines, succinimides, iminostilbene derivatives (carbamazepine), and carboxylic acid derivatives.

❑ Magnesium sulfate is a miscellaneous anticonvulsant.

- ❑ Some hydantoin derivatives and carbamazepine inhibit the spread of seizure activity in the motor cortex.

- ❑ Some barbiturates and succinimides limit seizure activity by increasing the threshold for motor cortex stimuli.

- ❑ Selected benzodiazepines and carboxylic acid derivatives may increase inhibition of gamma-aminobutyric acid in brain neurons.

- ❑ Magnesium sulfate interferes with the release of acetylcholine at the myoneural junction.

- ❑ Calcium channel blockers inhibit the flow of calcium through muscle cells, which dilates coronary arteries and decreases systemic vascular resistance, known as afterload.

- ❑ Nitrates decrease afterload and left ventricular end-diastolic pressure, or preload, and increase blood flow through collateral coronary vessels.

- ❑ Activated charcoal is used to treat poisoning or overdose with most orally administered drugs, except caustic agents and hydrocarbons.

- ❑ Aminocaproic acid is the antidote for alteplase, anistreplase, streptokinase, or urokinase toxicity.

- ❑ Amyl nitrite is the antidote for cyanide poisoning.

- ❑ Atropine sulfate is the antidote for anticholinesterase toxicity and organophosphate poisoning.

- ❑ Deferoxamine mesylate is used as adjunctive treatment of acute iron intoxication.

- ❑ Digoxin immune Fab (ovine) is used to treat potentially life-threatening digoxin or digitoxin intoxication.

- ❑ Edetate calcium is used to treat lead poisoning in clients with blood levels greater than 50 mcg/dL.

- ❑ Nalmefene is used to treat known or suspected opioid overdose, but it is not recommended for children or neonates.

- ❑ Pralidoxime chloride is an antidote for organophosphate poisoning and cholinergic overdose.

- ❑ Protamine sulfate is used to treat heparin overdose.

- ❑ All histamine-2 ($H_2$)-receptor antagonists inhibit the action of $H_2$-receptors in gastric parietal cells, reducing gastric acid output and concentration, regardless of stimulants, such as histamine, food, insulin, and caffeine, or basal conditions.

- ❑ Epoetin and darbepoetin stimulate red blood cell production in the bone marrow.

- ❑ Inotropics help move calcium into the cells, which increases cardiac output by strengthening contractility.

❏ Digoxin is an inotropic that moves calcium into the cells, which increases cardiac output by strengthening contractility, but it also acts on the central nervous system to slow heart rate.

❏ Inamrinone and milrinone relax vascular smooth muscle, decreasing peripheral vascular resistance (afterload) and the amount of blood returning to the heart (preload).

❏ Fluoroquinolones are broad-spectrum, systemic antibacterial drugs active against a wide range of aerobic gram-positive and gram-negative organisms.

❏ Estrogens inhibit the release of pituitary gonadotropins and have various metabolic effects, including retention of fluid and electrolytes, retention and deposition in bone of calcium and phosphorus, and mild anabolic activity.

❏ Thiazide and thiazide-like diuretics interfere with sodium transport across the tubules of the cortical diluting segment in the nephron, thereby increasing renal excretion of sodium, chloride, water, potassium, and calcium.

❏ Thiazide diuretics also exert an antihypertensive effect; although the exact mechanism is unknown, direct arteriolar dilation may be partially responsible.

❏ In diabetes insipidus, thiazides cause a paradoxic decrease in urine volume and an increase in renal concentration of urine, possibly because of sodium depletion and decreased plasma volume, which increases water and sodium reabsorption in the kidneys.

❏ Loop diuretics inhibit sodium and chloride reabsorption in the ascending loop of Henle, thus increasing excretion of sodium, chloride, and water.

❏ Like thiazide diuretics, loop diuretics increase excretion of potassium.

❏ Loop diuretics produce more diuresis and electrolyte loss than thiazide diuretics.

❏ Spironolactone, a potassium-sparing diuretic, competitively inhibits aldosterone at the distal renal tubules, also promoting sodium excretion and potassium retention.

❏ Corticosteroids suppress cell-mediated and humoral immunity by reducing levels of leukocytes, monocytes, and eosinophils; by decreasing immunoglobulin binding to cell-surface receptors; and by inhibiting interleukin synthesis.

❏ First-generation cephalosporins act against many gram-positive cocci, including penicillinase-producing *Staphylococcus aureus* and *S. epidermidis*, *Streptococcus pneumoniae*, group B streptococci, and group A beta-hemolytic streptococci.

❏ Second-generation cephalosporins are effective against all organisms attacked by first-generation drugs and have additional activity against *Moraxella catarrhalis*, *Haemophilus influenzae*, *Enterobacter*, *Citrobacter*, *Providencia*, *Acinetobacter*, *Serratia*, and *Neisseria*.

❑ *Bacteroides fragilis* is susceptible to cefoxitin.

❑ Third-generation cephalosporins are less active than first- and second-generation drugs against gram-positive bacteria, but are more active against gram-negative organisms, including those resistant to first- and second-generation drugs.

❑ Third-generation cephalosporins have the greatest stability against beta-lactamases produced by gram-negative bacteria.

❑ Thrombolytics convert plasminogen to plasma, which lyses thrombi, fibrinogen, and other plasma proteins.

❑ Dobutamine increases cardiac output by decreasing peripheral vascular resistance, reducing ventricular filling pressure, and increasing atrioventricular node conduction.

❑ The skeletal muscle relaxant baclofen may reduce impulse transmission from the spinal cord to skeletal muscle.

❑ Dantrolene acts directly on skeletal muscle to decrease excitation and reduce muscle strength by interfering with intracellular calcium movement.

❑ Selective serotonin reuptake inhibitors selectively inhibit the reuptake of serotonin with little or no effects on other neurotransmitters in the central nervous system such as norepinephrine or dopamine.

❑ Proton pump inhibitors reduce stomach acid production by combining with hydrogen, potassium, and adenosine triphosphate in parietal cells of the stomach to block the last step in gastric acid secretion.

❑ Protease inhibitors bind to the protease active site and inhibit human immunodeficiency virus protease activity.

❑ Progestins transform proliferative endometrium into secretory endometrium.

❑ Nucleoside reverse transcriptase inhibitors suppress human immunodeficiency virus (HIV) replication by inhibiting HIV DNA polymerase.

❑ Phenothiazines are believed to function as dopamine antagonists by blocking postsynaptic dopamine receptors in various parts of the central nervous system.

❑ The antiemetic effects of phenothiazines result from blockage of the chemoreceptor trigger zone.

❑ Phenothiazines also produce varying degrees of anticholinergic effects and block alpha-adrenergic receptors.

## Medication administration

❑ Children absorb topical medications at a higher rate than adults due to their thinner stratum corneum, increased skin hydration, and a greater ratio of body surface area to weight.

❑ A subcutaneous injection for a child should contain no more than 1 mL of solution.

❑ An intramuscular injection for a child should contain no more than 1 mL of solution.

❑ When administering intramuscular injections to a child, use the vastus lateralis muscle.

❑ Enteric-coated, buccal, and sublingual tablets should never be crushed or chewed.

❑ When combining insulins in a syringe, always draw the clear regular insulin first to avoid contamination by the cloudy, longer-acting insulin.

❑ Drugs that become unstable in solution are packaged as powders.

❑ Powders come in single-strength or multiple-strength formulas.

❑ A multiple-strength powder can be reconstituted to various dose strengths by adjusting the amount of the diluent.

❑ Single-strength powders can only be reconstituted to one dose strength per administration route.

❑ Check the label on the medication three times before administering it to a client to ensure that you're administering the prescribed medication in the prescribed dose.

❑ If you're administering a unit-dose medication, check the label immediately after pouring the medication and again before discarding the wrapper.

❑ Don't open a unit-dose medication until you're at the client's bedside.

❑ To assess the client's response to medication, be aware of his condition and what the drug's desired or expected effect should be.

❑ Documenting all medications given to a client provides a legal record of drugs the client received during his stay in the facility.

❑ Medication administration involves documenting on a medication administration record as well as in the nurse's notes.

❑ After administering a drug, document on the client's medication administration record or computer files the drug name, dosage, route and time of administration, and your signature and title.

❑ In the nurse's notes, include any assessment data that refer to the client's response to the medication and any adverse effects of the medication.

❑ Apply daily transdermal medications at the same time every day to ensure a continuous effect, but alternate the application sites to avoid skin irritation.

❑ Before applying nitroglycerin ointment, obtain the client's baseline blood pressure and then obtain another blood pressure reading 5 minutes after applying the ointment.

❏ If the client's blood pressure has dropped significantly after applying nitroglycerin ointment and he has a headache, notify the physician immediately.

❏ If the client's blood pressure has dropped after applying nitroglycerin ointment but he has no symptoms, instruct him to lie still until the blood pressure returns to normal.

❏ Before reapplying nitroglycerin ointment, remove any ointment remaining on the skin at the previous site.

❏ When teaching an elderly client how to instill eyedrops, keep in mind that he may have difficulty sensing drops in the eye; suggest chilling the medication slightly to enhance the sensation.

❏ To apply eye ointment, squeeze a small ribbon of medication on the edge of the conjunctival sac, from the inner to the outer canthus.

❏ To maintain the sterility of the drug container, never touch the tip of the dropper or bottle to the eye area.

❏ To administer ear drops to an infant or a child younger than age 3, gently pull the auricle down and back; the ear canal is straighter at this age.

❏ To instill nose drops into the ethmoidal and sphenoidal sinuses, have the client lie on his back, with his neck hyperextended and his head tilted back over the edge of the bed, while supporting his head with one hand to prevent neck strain.

❏ To instill nose drops into the maxillary and frontal sinuses, have the client lie on his back, with his head toward the affected side and hanging slightly over the edge of the bed, and then ask him to rotate his head laterally after hyperextension.

❏ Calcitonin, a hormone used for osteoporosis, should be given in only one nostril daily, with the nostrils alternated each day.

❏ Oral drugs are sometimes prescribed in higher dosages than their parenteral equivalents because, after absorption through the GI system, the liver breaks them down before they reach the systemic circulation.

❏ Some oral respiratory drugs can cause restlessness, palpitations, nervousness, other systemic effects, and hypersensitivity reactions, such as a rash, urticaria, and bronchospasm.

❏ If the client has heart disease, use caution when administering an oral respiratory drug because it can potentiate coronary insufficiency, cardiac arrhythmias, or hypertension; if paradoxical bronchospasm occurs, discontinue the drug and call the physician.

❏ If the client is using a bronchodilator and a steroid, have him use the bronchodilator first, wait 5 minutes, and then use the steroid.

❑ To confirm the placement of a nasogastric tube, place a small amount of gastric contents from the tube on a pH test strip; the appearance of gastric contents and pH ≤ 5 implies that the tube is patent and in the stomach.

❑ When giving medication through a nasogastric tube, as the last of the medication flows out of the syringe, start to irrigate the tube by adding 30 to 50 mL of water (15 to 30 mL for a child).

❑ If you must give a tube feeding as well as instill medication, give the medication first to ensure that the client receives it all.

❑ Tube feedings must be withheld 2 hours before and 2 hours after phenytoin or warfarin administration.

❑ If residual stomach contents exceed 100 mL, withhold the medication and feeding and notify the physician; excessive stomach contents may indicate intestinal obstruction or paralytic ileus.

❑ Drugs that are given buccally include nitroglycerin and methyltestosterone.

❑ Drugs that are given sublingually include ergotamine tartrate, isosorbide, and nitroglycerin.

❑ Translingual drugs, which are sprayed onto the tongue, include nitrate preparations for clients with chronic angina.

❑ Because the intake of food and fluid stimulates peristalsis, a suppository for relieving constipation should be inserted about 30 minutes before mealtime to help soften the stool and facilitate defecation.

❑ A medicated retention suppository should be inserted between meals.

❑ When giving an injection, avoid any site that's inflamed, edematous, or irritated or that contains moles, birthmarks, scar tissue, or other lesions.

❑ The Z-track I.M. injection method prevents leakage, or tracking, into the subcutaneous tissue and is typically used to administer drugs that irritate and discolor subcutaneous tissue, primarily iron preparations such as iron dextran.

❑ The Z-track method for I.M. injection may be used in elderly clients who have decreased muscle mass.

❑ The I.V. bolus injection method allows rapid I.V. drug administration to quickly achieve peak levels in the bloodstream.

❑ The I.V. bolus injection method may be used for drugs that can't be given I.M. because they're toxic or for a client with a reduced ability to absorb these drugs.

❑ The I.V. bolus injection method may also be used to deliver drugs that can't be diluted.

❑ Bolus doses may be injected through an existing I.V. line or through an implanted port.

❑ When giving an epidural analgesic, the physician injects or infuses the drug into the epidural space, and thus into the cerebrospinal fluid, so that the medication can bypass the blood-brain barrier.

❑ After an epidural has been started, assess the client's respiratory rate and blood pressure every 2 hours for 8 hours, every 4 hours for 8 hours, and then once per shift, unless ordered otherwise.

## Parenteral and intravenous therapies

❑ When documenting parenteral medications, be sure to include the injection site and the route used.

❑ A child should receive 120 mL of fluid for every 100 kilocalories (kcal) of metabolism.

❑ Intermittent infusions are used when drugs or fluids need to be administered periodically.

❑ Intravenous fluids may be used to maintain volume or to correct an existing fluid or electrolyte imbalance.

❑ Continuous infusions are used when a client requires around-the-clock continuous fluids, drug therapy, or both.

❑ Extracellular fluid has a higher percentage of water, so fluid exchange rates are two to three times higher for children than adults, making them more susceptible to dehydration than adults.

❑ Transdermal patches administer drugs by passive diffusion at a constant rate.

❑ Parenteral drugs are administered through the skin, subcutaneous tissue, muscle, or veins.

❑ Parenteral means outside the intestines.

❑ Intradermal medications are injected into the dermis, or outer layer of the skin.

❑ Common uses for intradermal injections include anesthetizing skin for invasive procedures and testing for allergies, tuberculosis, and other diseases.

❑ The volume of a drug given intradermally is less than 0.5 mL.

❑ To administer an intradermal injection, use a 1-mL syringe that's calibrated in 0.01-mL increments with a 25- to 27-gauge needle that is $^3/_8$" to $^5/_8$" long.

❑ Drugs commonly injected into the subcutaneous tissue include heparin, insulin, and tetanus toxoid.

❑ A volume of 0.5 to 1 mL can be injected subcutaneously.

❑ Needles used for a subcutaneous injection are 25- to 28-gauge and ½" to $^5/_8$" long.

❑ Injection sites for subcutaneous injection include the lateral upper arm, thigh, abdomen, and upper back.

❑ When giving an intradermal injection, stretch the skin taut with one hand and insert the needle with your other hand at a 10- to 15-degree angle to a depth of about 0.5 cm.

❑ Administer a subcutaneous injection by pinching the skin if the client is thin and inserting the needle at a 45-degree angle; if the client is obese, do not pinch the skin but insert the needle into the fatty tissue at a 90-degree angle.

❑ Do not massage the skin after giving an injection of heparin or insulin.

❑ The intramuscular injection route is used to administer drugs that need to be absorbed quickly, as well as large volumes of drugs, and to prevent tissue irritation that can occur with shallow administration routes.

❑ A volume ranging from 0.5 to 3 mL may be given intramuscularly except to a child, who should only receive a total of 1 mL.

❑ The ventrogluteal site is the safest site for intramuscular injections.

❑ Intramuscular injections should be inserted with the needle at a 75- to 90-degree angle.

❑ After administering an intramuscular injection, pressure should be applied to the site; it should not be rubbed.

❑ Intramuscular injections are given with a 18- to 23-gauge needle that is 1″ to 3″ long.

❑ Tuberculin syringes are commonly used for intradermal injections and to administer small amounts of drugs because they are calibrated to hundredths of a milliliter on the right and minims on the left.

❑ Signs and symptoms of a hematoma with peripheral I.V. therapy include tenderness and the appearance of bruising at the insertion site.

❑ Circulatory overload is a complication of peripheral I.V infusion and may be evidenced by discomfort, engorgement of the jugular veins, respiratory distress, increased blood pressure, and crackles.

❑ Extravasation is leakage of infused solution from a vein into the surrounding tissue.

❑ Extravasation is the result of a needle puncturing the vessel wall or leakage around a venipuncture site and causes local pain and itching, edema, blanching, and decreased skin temperature in the affected extremity.

❑ Extravasation of I.V. solution may be referred to as infiltration because the fluid infiltrates the tissues.

❑ Extravasation of a small amount of isotonic fluid or nonirritating drug usually causes only minor discomfort.

❑ Treatment of extravasation involves routine comfort measures, such as the application of warm compresses.

❑ Extravasation of some drugs can severely damage tissue through irritative, sclerotic, vesicant, corrosive, or vasoconstrictive action, in which case emergency measures must be taken to minimize tissue damage and necrosis, prevent the need for skin grafts or, rarely, avoid amputation.

❑ Check the prescribed I.V. flow rate before each solution change to prevent errors.

## Pharmacologic pain management

❑ Selective nonsteroidal anti-inflammatory drugs (NSAIDs; also called cyclo-oxygenase-2 [COX-2] inhibitors) are NSAIDs that selectively block COX-2, relieving pain and inflammation.

❑ Opioid refers to any derivative of the opium plant or any synthetic drug that imitates natural narcotics.

❑ Opioid agonists, also called narcotic agonists, include opium derivatives and synthetic drugs with similar properties.

❑ Opioid agonists are used to relieve or decrease pain without causing the client to lose consciousness.

❑ Opioid agonists can cause constipation and respiratory depression because of their binding to receptor sites in the peripheral and central nervous system.

❑ Opioid agonists are classified as pregnancy category C, and most appear in breast milk; recommend that the client wait 4 to 6 hours after ingesting before breast-feeding.

❑ A common adverse reaction to opioid agonists is a decreased rate and depth of respirations that worsens as the dose is increased.

❑ The adverse effects of opioid agonists may trigger an asthma attack in a susceptible client.

❑ Some commonly administered opioid agonists are codeine, morphine, fentanyl, hydrocodone, and oxycodone.

❑ Mixed opioid agonist-antagonists are administered to relieve pain while reducing the toxic effects and dependency associated with opioid agonists.

❑ Some commonly used mixed opioid agonist-antagonists are butorphanol, nalbuphine, and pentazocine.

❑ The client with a history of opioid abuse should not receive any mixed opioid agonist-antagonists because they can cause withdrawal symptoms.

❑ Opioid antagonists block the effects of opioids.

❑ Common opioid antagonists are naltrexone and naloxone.

❑ Naloxone is the drug of choice for managing an opioid overdose by reversing respiratory depression and sedation and helps stabilize the client's vital signs within seconds after administration.

❑ An unconscious client abruptly returned to consciousness after naloxone administration may hyperventilate and experience tremors.

❑ Children metabolize drugs differently from adults and may experience the effects of analgesics differently.

❑ When assessing pain in a child, use verbal, numeric, or picture scales to help determine the child's pain level in addition to direct questions.

❑ An older adult may not report pain and may metabolize and experience the effects of analgesic drugs differently than a younger client.

❑ To assess pain in an older client with cognitive dysfunction, use such cues as behavior (motor responses, facial expressions, crying) and physiologic changes (increased blood pressure and heart rate) in addition to self-reporting.

❑ Watch for behavioral cues (facial expressions, crying) and physiologic changes (increased blood pressure and heart rate) to help determine the child's pain level of pain.

❑ During the course of an illness, a client may experience acute pain, chronic pain, or both.

❑ Acute pain is caused by tissue damage from injury or disease; it can vary in intensity from mild to severe and lasts briefly.

❑ Acute pain is considered a protective mechanism because it warns of current or potential damage or organ disease and may result from a traumatic injury, from surgical or diagnostic procedures, or from a medical disorder.

❑ Chronic pain is pain that has lasted 6 months or longer and is ongoing.

❑ Although it may be as intense as acute pain, chronic pain isn't a warning of tissue damage.

❑ The three most common pain assessment tools used by clinicians are the visual analog scale, the numeric rating scale, and the FACES scale.

❑ To use the numeric rating scale, the client rates his pain by choosing a number from 0 (indicating no pain) to 10 (indicating the worst pain imaginable) to reflect his current level of pain.

❑ Two classes of medications are commonly used for pain management: nonopioids and opioids.

❑ Nonopioids are the first choice for managing mild pain because they decrease pain by inhibiting inflammation at the injury site.

❑ Examples of nonopioids are acetaminophen, nonsteroidal anti-inflammatory drugs, and salicylates such as aspirin.

❑ Opioids work by blocking the release of neurotransmitters that are involved in transmitting pain signals to the brain.

❑ Salicylates are contraindicated in clients with glucose-6-phosphate dehydrogenase deficiency or bleeding disorders, such as hemophilia, von Willebrand disease, or telangiectasia.

❑ Salicylates are contraindicated in clients with sensitivity reactions to nonsteroidal anti-inflammatory drugs.

❑ Use salicylates cautiously in clients with GI lesions, impaired renal function, hypoprothrombinemia, vitamin K deficiency, thrombotic thrombocytopenic purpura, or hepatic impairment.

❑ Use salicylates cautiously in clients with a history of GI disease (especially peptic ulcer disease), increased risk of GI bleeding, or decreased renal function.

❑ Use acetaminophen cautiously in clients with a history of chronic alcohol abuse because hepatotoxicity has occurred after therapeutic doses.

❑ Use acetaminophen cautiously in clients with hepatic or cardiovascular disease, impaired renal function, or viral infection.

❑ Know the client's total daily acetaminophen intake, especially if he's taking other prescribed drugs containing the compound such as Percocet (acetaminophen/oxycodone) because toxicity can occur.

❑ Monitor the prothrombin time and International Normalized Ratio values in clients who are receiving oral anticoagulants and long-term acetaminophen therapy.

❑ In a client taking salicylates, periodically monitor the complete blood count, platelet count, prothrombin time, blood urea nitrogen level, serum creatinine level, and the results of liver function studies during salicylate therapy to detect abnormalities.

❑ Assess the client taking salicylates for signs and symptoms of hemorrhage, such as petechiae, bruising, coffee-ground vomitus, and black, tarry stools.

❑ Codeine may delay gastric emptying, increase biliary tract pressure resulting from contraction of the sphincter of Oddi, and interfere with hepatobiliary imaging studies.

❑ Use fentanyl cautiously in elderly or debilitated clients and in those with head injuries, increased cerebrospinal fluid pressure, chronic obstructive pulmonary disease, decreased respiratory reserve, compromised respirations, arrhythmias, or hepatic, renal, or cardiac disease.

❑ Give an anticholinergic, such as atropine or glycopyrrolate, to minimize the possible bradycardic effect of fentanyl.

❑ Ibuprofen is contraindicated right before and right after coronary artery bypass surgery because of the risk of heart attack or stroke.

❑ Monitor auditory and ophthalmic functions periodically during ibuprofen therapy.

# Coordinated care

## Advance directives and client rights

❑ The right to die involves whether to initiate or withhold life-sustaining treatment for a client who is irreversibly comatose, vegetative, or suffering with end-stage terminal illness.

❑ An advance directive is a document used as a guideline for starting or continuing life-sustaining medical care.

❑ The federal Omnibus Reconciliation Act of 1986 mandates that all hospitals establish written protocols for the identification of potential organ and tissue donors.

❑ An organ procurement coordinator is knowledgeable about the organ donation process and should have exceptional interpersonal skills for dealing with grieving family members.

❑ A psychiatric inpatient usually receives a copy of the bill of rights for psychiatric clients, which includes the right to refuse treatment, the right to a written treatment plan, the right to confidentiality, and the right to personal mail.

❑ Any mentally competent adult may legally refuse treatment if he's fully informed about his medical condition and about the likely consequences of his refusal.

❑ Some clients may refuse treatment on the grounds of freedom of religion or cultural beliefs.

❑ The client's right to refuse treatment may be challenged if compelling reasons exist to overrule the client's wishes, such as when the refusal endangers the life of another, when a parent's decision to withhold treatment threatens a child's life, when a client makes statements indicating that he wants to live, and when public interest outweighs the client's right.

❑ The types of advance directives are the living will and the durable power of attorney for health care.

❑ The Patient Self-Determination Act of 1990 requires facilities to provide clients with information about their rights regarding advance directives, living wills, and durable power of attorney for health care as well as about the facility's policy for implementing them.

❑ Jehovah's Witnesses oppose blood transfusions based on their interpretation of a biblical passage that forbids "drinking" blood.

❑ Some Jehovah's Witnesses believe that even a lifesaving transfusion given against their will deprives them of everlasting life.

❏ The courts usually uphold the client's right to refuse treatment because of the constitutionally protected right to religious freedom such as in the case of a Jehovah's Witness or a Christian Scientist.

❏ If the client is a critically ill minor, the court may deny the parents' request to refuse treatment.

❏ Most religious freedom court cases involve Christian Scientists, who oppose many medical interventions, including medicines.

❏ The right-to-die laws recognize the client's right to choose death by refusing extraordinary treatment when he has no hope of recovery.

❏ The courts also recognize several compelling circumstances that justify overruling a client's refusal of treatment. These include when refusal endangers the life of another, when a parent's decision to withhold treatment threatens a child's life, when despite refusing treatment the client makes statements indicating that he wants to live, and when the public interest outweighs the client's right.

❏ If your client tells you he's going to refuse treatment or he simply refuses to give consent, you should stop preparations for treatment at once, notify the physician immediately, and report your client's decision to your supervisor promptly.

❏ If your client has an advance directive, review your nursing or facility manual for specific directions on what to do.

❏ If your client has an advance directive, you may need to inform the client's physician, or you may need to ask your nursing supervisor to inform the facility administration and the legal affairs department.

❏ If the client drafts an advance directive while under your care, document this in your nurses' notes, describing the circumstances under which the advance directive was drawn up and signed.

❏ When a legally competent person draws up a living will, he declares the steps he wants or doesn't want taken when he's incompetent and can no longer express his wishes.

❏ Commonly, a living will authorizes the attending physician to withhold or discontinue certain lifesaving procedures under specific circumstances.

❏ A living will may also address treatment options, such as enteral feedings, blood transfusion, antibiotic administration, and dialysis.

❏ Although living will laws vary from state to state, they generally include such provisions as who may execute a living will, witness and testator requirements, immunity from liability for following a living will's directives, documentation requirements, instructions on when and how the living will should be executed, and under what circumstances the living will takes effect.

❑ A durable power of attorney for health care is a document in which the client designates a person (a proxy) to make medical decisions for him if he becomes incompetent.

❑ A durable power of attorney for health care document differs from the usual power of attorney, which requires the client's ongoing consent and deals only with financial issues.

❑ Most states have laws authorizing durable power of attorney for the purpose of initiating or terminating life-sustaining medical treatment.

❑ The most appropriate action when the client refuses injections for pain is to call the physician to request an oral pain medication; by doing so, the nurse is adhering to the client's wishes.

❑ Administering an injection without client consent is considered battery and may lead to a lawsuit.

❑ When the client refuses injections for pain, withholding the medication without providing an alternative would violate the standards of care.

❑ Any attempt to manipulate the client into taking the medication also would violate the standards of care.

❑ A teenage client should be kept informed about medical decisions, but until he's an adult or emancipated, a parent must give consent for the child's care.

❑ The client has a legal right to see his chart; however, if he asks to see it, the nurse should first ask him if he has any questions about his care and try to clear up any confusion.

❑ The nurse should check the facility's policy to see whether the chart must be read in the nurse's presence when the client wishes to view it.

❑ The nurse should inform the physician and nurse-manager of the client's request if he wishes to see his chart.

❑ If a client requests a discharge against medical advice, the nurse should notify the physician immediately.

❑ If the physician can't convince the client to stay, the physician will ask the client to sign an against medical advice form, which releases the facility from legal responsibility for any medical problems the client may experience after discharge.

❑ If the physician isn't available, the nurse should discuss signing an against medical advice form with the client and obtain the client's signature.

❑ A client who refuses to sign an against medical advice form shouldn't be detained because this would violate the client's rights.

❑ After the client leaves, the nurse should document the incident thoroughly and notify the physician that the client has left.

❑ Ordinary means of medical treatment are medications, procedures and surgeries that offer the client some hope of benefit without incurring excessive pain or expense.

❑ Extraordinary means, sometimes called heroic measures, merely maintain or prolong a client's life, usually at great expense and suffering for the client and his family.

❑ Because of continuing advances in medicine and technology, the distinction between ordinary and extraordinary treatments is becoming less defined.

❑ When deciding whether to terminate life-sustaining treatment, health care providers face incredible emotional pressure; a client can't be brought back after he stops treatment.

❑ The right to refuse treatment is based on the ethical principle of respect for the autonomy of the individual.

❑ The principle of autonomy has led to the concept of informed consent—the obligation of health care providers to inform the client of the risks and benefits of a procedure and to obtain permission before the procedure is carried out.

❑ Because the nursing profession is oriented to saving and prolonging lives, the nurse may find it difficult to go along with a client's decision to withhold life-sustaining treatment.

❑ A client who has chosen to forgo life-sustaining treatment still has the right to receive care that preserves his comfort, hygiene, and dignity; in particular, he has the right to adequate pain control.

❑ If the nurse believes that she will violate her own values by implementing a certain treatment, she has an obligation to arrange for the transfer of the client's care to another provider.

❑ The conscience clause, or conscientious objection, applies to the nurse who does not wish to assist in abortions as well as to the nurse who does not wish to cooperate in noninitiation or withdrawal of life-sustaining treatment or euthanasia.

❑ Many hospitals have used the American Hospital Association's client bill of rights as a model for formulating their own bills of rights.

## Client advocacy

❑ The stages of grief include denial, anger, bargaining, depression, and acceptance.

❑ Denial is the avoidance of death's inevitability and is the first step of the grieving process.

❑ Anger, the most intense grief reaction, arises when people realize that death and loss will actually occur or has occurred for a family member.

❑ Bargaining happens when family members attempt to stall or manipulate the outcome or death.

❑ Depression is a response to loss that's expressed as profound sadness or deep suffering.

❑ Acceptance is the final stage of the grieving process, and it's the ability to overcome the grief and accept what has happened.

❑ The nurse who understands the advocacy role promotes, protects, and advocates for a client's interests and rights in an effort to make the client well.

❑ The nurse doesn't make decisions for clients but provides care for the acutely ill client with the consent of his significant other, or with the direction of a power of attorney, or his living will.

❑ Standards of care are the basis for providing safe, competent nursing care and set minimum criteria for proficiency on the job, enabling the nurse and others to judge the quality of care provided.

❑ Paternalism violates self-determination and advocacy by acting for another.

❑ The nurse has a responsibility to assess, monitor, and communicate the status of a client under her care.

❑ Failure to act as a client advocate has been recognized by the courts when the nurse fails to develop and implement nursing diagnoses and fails to exercise good judgment on the client's behalf.

❑ Failure to communicate with the client refers to not adequately educating him about care, procedures, or discharge instructions.

❑ Failure to protect from harm occurs when health care providers must protect a client because of the client's vulnerable state and inability to distinguish potentially harmful situations.

❑ The neonate's safety and protection is the first priority when the nurse observes an abusive action by the mother. Assessment of the client's strengths and weaknesses in coping mechanisms and the presence of support systems is needed to formulate an appropriate plan of care.

❑ To be an effective advocate, a nurse must understand the ethical and legal principles of informed consent, and that the client's consent isn't valid unless he understands his condition, the proposed treatment, treatment alternatives, potential risks and benefits, and relative chances of success or failure.

❑ When a client must make an ethical decision, the nurse should help him resolve his moral dilemma in ways that enhance personal values, priorities, freedom, dignity, and the quality of life.

❑ By listening carefully to the client and asking thoughtful questions, the nurse may be able to help the client and his family make ethical decisions with which they are most comfortable. The nurse needs to understand what the physician told the client about the situation.

❏ The most difficult ethical decisions in health care involve whether to initiate or withhold life-sustaining treatment for clients who are irreversibly comatose, vegetative, or suffering with end-stage terminal illness.

❏ The nurse cannot make the ultimate medical decisions to initiate or limit treatment, but the nurse can help the client express his wishes about his health care and guide him in translating these desires into advance directives.

❏ The nurse needs to pay attention to the client's questions and misunderstandings, and be especially alert for unexpressed fears.

❏ Effective communication is essential when helping families decide whether to limit or withhold treatment.

❏ Create a quiet, private, and unhurried environment and keep all communication to the family simple, factual, and direct.

❏ Encourage decision makers in the family to ask questions.

❏ Clarify missing or misunderstood information for the client and family.

## Collaboration with interdisciplinary team

❏ The plan of care should be individualized to the client's condition or needs.

❏ The plan of care is developed with the client, partners in care, and health care providers.

❏ The plan of care includes strategies that address each of the nursing diagnoses.

❏ The plan of care should provide for continuity of care, and should also include a pathway or timeline.

❏ The plan of care provides directions to other health care providers.

❏ The plan of care reflects current statutes, rules and regulations, and standards, as well as current trends and research.

❏ The economic impact of the plan needs to be considered.

❏ The plan should be documented using standardized language and terminology.

❏ The nurse coordinates implementation of the plan, and coordination of care should be documented.

❏ Evaluation of the plan of care is systematic, ongoing, and criteria-based.

❏ The client, partners, and health care providers are involved in the evaluation process of the plan of care.

❏ Results of the evaluation of care should be disseminated to the client and other health care providers involved with the client's care in accordance with all laws and regulations.

❏ The nurse interacts with colleagues to enhance her own professional practice.

❏ The nurse maintains compassionate and caring relationships with peers and colleagues.

❏ The nurse contributes to an environment that is conducive to education of health care professionals.

❏ The nurse contributes to a supportive and healthy work environment.

## Client confidentiality

❏ The nurse may lawfully disclose confidential information about a client when the welfare of a person is at stake.

❏ The physician is required to inform the state's department of motor vehicles that a taxi driver has an uncontrolled seizure disorder because it's in the best interest of the public's and client's safety.

❏ The Health Insurance Portability and Accountability Act protects the privacy and security of medical information.

❏ Under the Health Insurance Portability and Accountability Act, only those who have a "need to know" are authorized to access client information.

❏ The privacy rule, which is part of the Health Insurance Portability and Accountability Act, consists of national standards that protect all oral, written, and electronic (computer and fax) health information.

❏ The privacy rule allows health care providers to share any information they need to give high-quality health care at the same time that it protects the public by granting clients rights over their health information.

❏ All types of health information are considered confidential, including the client's chart or medical record, conversations about a client's care or treatment, information in the facility's computer system, and billing information.

❏ Breeches in confidentiality are subject to fines. Specific protected health information that falls under the privacy rule includes individually identifiable information (such as the client's name, date of birth, and Social Security number); past, present, and future health information; demographic information (address, phone number, fax number, or e-mail address); billing and payment information; and information about the client's relatives, household members, and employers.

❏ Photographs of clients are considered protected health information, so the same protections that apply to written information apply to photos.

❏ Permission is needed when the client's name, face, or a unique feature (such as a tattoo) are shown.

❏ However, permission isn't required when pictures are taken as part of the client's medical record or when the photo doesn't show enough information to identify the client.

❏ All members of the health care team are responsible for keeping the client's health care records private, including facilities, nursing homes, pharmacies, and clinics; physicians and dentists; laboratories and radiology centers; insurance companies, health maintenance organizations, and most employer group health plans; and certain government programs that pay for health care, such as Medicare and Medicaid.

❏ To ensure that privacy standards are maintained, health care providers must implement specific strategies to protect their clients' medical information.

❏ Any health or health care information that doesn't reveal a client's commonly identifiable information (including information that could identify him through his relatives, household members, and employers) is considered de-identified health information.

❏ One example of de-identified health information is a case study presented at a conference that uses a fictitious name in place of the client's real name.

❏ There are no limits on the use of de-identified health information; it isn't protected by the privacy rule.

❏ Strategies to protect clients' medical information include such safeguards as not posting lists of clients' names where the public can see them, not allowing staff to discuss client information in public areas where others can overhear, and disposing of protected health information in a proper and confidential manner, usually by shredding it.

❏ Electronic information requires special safeguards to ensure that it's protected, such as assigning computer passwords that allow each employee access only to information necessary to do the employee's job, forbidding employees from sharing or posting passwords, and instructing them to log out of the computer immediately after each use.

❏ Prior written permission is required when a provider must give information to a client's employer such as in a drug test for employment.

❏ Protected health information can be shared without the client's written permission during the course of treatment to coordinate care with other health care providers and services, in the case of a medical emergency, or to aid in accurate diagnosis and treatment.

❏ Protected health information can be shared without the client's written permission for payment (to bill and collect payment for treatment and services provided) and for health care operations—for quality assessment and improvement, legal issues, auditing, training, and evaluating the performance of health care providers.

❑ The facility may also decide to release information to the client's relatives or significant others if the client can't agree to release information because of illness or injury.

❑ Minors have the right to privacy, but in most situations, a parent or legal guardian is authorized to receive and release the minor's protected health information.

❑ In some circumstances, the parent isn't considered the minor's personal representative and therefore doesn't control the minor's protected health information.

❑ Parents cannot control the minor's public health information when there's a reasonable suspicion of parental abuse, neglect, or endangerment; when state (or other applicable) law stipulates that the minor doesn't require the consent of a parent or other person before he can obtain a particular health care service; when a court determines someone other than the parent must make treatment decisions for the minor; and when a parent agrees to a confidential relationship between the minor and the physician.

❑ The Center for Adolescent Health & the Law has stated that it's appropriate for a minor to exercise privacy rights under the Health Insurance Portability and Accountability Act.

❑ It isn't appropriate for the nurse (or the physician) to discuss the client's information with the client's mother without the client's permission.

❑ The Family Educational Rights and Privacy Act, or FERPA, protects the confidentiality of minors by defining the term "education records" to include all material containing information related directly to a student and by giving the parents permission to have some control over disclosure of this information; it doesn't apply to health care situations.

❑ The client's health information is protected regardless of whether she's emancipated.

## Consultation and referrals

❑ Many support services have become available for both abusers and their victims.

❑ If a female victim of abuse is afraid to return to the scene of her abuse, she may find temporary housing in a women's shelter.

❑ If no shelter is available for the abuse victim, she may be able to stay with a friend or family member.

❑ Social workers or community liaison workers may also be able to offer the abuse victim suggestions for shelter.

❑ Another possible place for the abuse victim to take refuge is a church, synagogue, or mosque, which may have members willing to take the client in.

❑ The police department should be called to collect evidence if the client wants to press charges against the abuser.

❑ If the client is a child, the law usually requires filing a report with a government family-service agency.

❑ The nurse needs to evaluate the abuser's ability to handle stress.

❑ In some cases of abuse, you may be able to refer the abuser to an appropriate local or state agency that can offer help.

❑ In most cases, an abuser poses a continued threat to others until he gets help in understanding his behavior and how to change it.

❑ For abusive fathers or mothers, a local chapter of Parents Anonymous may be helpful.

❑ Parents Anonymous, a self-help group made up of former abusers, attempts to help abusing parents by teaching them how to deal with their anger.

❑ Besides helping short-circuit abusive behavior, a self-help group takes abusing parents out of their isolation and introduces them to individuals who can understand their feelings.

❑ A self-help group provides help in a crisis, when members may be able to prevent an abusive incident.

❑ Telephone hot lines to crisis intervention services give abusers someone to talk with in times of stress and crisis and may help prevent abuse.

❑ Commonly staffed by volunteers, telephone hot lines provide a link between those who seek help and trained counselors.

❑ By becoming familiar with national and local resources, you'll be able to respond quickly and authoritatively when an abuser or victim needs your help.

❑ Consider calling on social workers, psychologists, the clergy, and ethics committee members to help resolve difficult ethical problems.

❑ Except in emergencies, information for informed consent should include but is not necessarily limited to the specific procedure or treatment, the medically significant risks involved, and the probable duration of incapacitation.

❑ The client has the right to refuse treatment to the extent permitted by law and to be informed of the medical consequences of his action.

❑ The client has the right to considerate and respectful care, as well as the right to obtain from his doctor complete current information about his diagnosis, treatment, and prognosis in terms he can reasonably understand.

❑ The client has the right to know, by name, the doctor responsible for coordinating his care.

❑ The client has the right to every consideration of his privacy concerning his own medical care program.

❑ Case discussion, consultation, examination, and treatment are confidential and should be conducted discreetly; those not directly involved in the case must have permission of the client to be present.

❑ The client has the right to expect that all communications and records pertaining to his care should be treated as confidential.

❑ The client has the right to expect that within its capacity a hospital will make reasonable response to the client's request for services.

❑ The client has the right to obtain information about the existence of any professional relationships among individuals, by names, who are treating him.

❑ The client has the right to be advised if the hospital proposes to engage in or perform human experimentation affecting his care or treatment; the client has the right to refuse to participate in such research projects.

## Continuity of care

❑ Discharge planning and client teaching go hand in hand; one can't be accomplished without the other.

❑ If the client is admitted to the hospital as an emergency, client teaching should begin as soon as the client's condition stabilizes.

❑ Discharge planning should begin before hospitalization for clients with planned admissions. For example, a client planning to undergo a nonemergency surgical procedure should be taught about the procedure and his postoperative care in the physician's office before admission to the hospital.

❑ Complete, accurate, and timely documentation is crucial to the continuity of each client's care.

❑ A well-documented record allows interdisciplinary exchange of information about the client and reflects professional and ethical conduct and responsibility.

❑ A well-documented record provides evidence of the nurse's legal responsibilities toward the client and also demonstrates standards, rules, regulations, and laws of nursing practice.

❑ A well-documented record supplies information for analysis of cost-to-benefit reduction analysis.

❑ A well-documented record furnishes information for continuing education, risk management, diagnosis-related group assignment and reimbursement, continuous quality improvement, case management monitoring, and research.

❑ Common documentation errors include omissions, personal opinions, vague entries, late entries, improper corrections, unauthorized entries, erroneous or vague abbreviations, illegibility, and lack of clarity.

❑ If the medication administration record doesn't provide space to document the drug omission, the nurse should document the reason in the progress notes.

❑ Any time a drug is omitted, the reason for withholding the medication must be documented.

❑ Discharge planning should begin as soon as the client is admitted.

❑ Beginning the planning for discharge as soon as possible gives the staff time to allocate necessary resources the client will require at discharge.

❑ Waiting until the client stabilizes, the day before discharge, or after the order is written doesn't allow adequate time for planning for the client's discharge.

❑ Health teaching should include healthy lifestyles, risk-reducing behaviors, developmental needs, activities of daily living, and preventive self-care.

❑ Health promotion and teaching are appropriate to the client's needs and feedback should be received on the effectiveness of health promotion and teachings.

## Delegation, supervision, and prioritization

❑ If a serious problem occurs on the unit, the nurse-manager should be notified as soon as possible.

❑ If the nurse-manager of a unit isn't on duty when a staff nurse makes a serious medication error, the nursing supervisor on duty will call the nurse-manager at home and apprise her of the problem.

❑ Delegation involves entrusting a task to another staff member.

❑ Delegation helps free the nurse-manager from tasks that can be completed successfully by someone else and also enables the manager to prepare a staff member for career advancement.

❑ Notify your immediate supervisor if you believe an assignment is unsafe.

❑ Inspect all equipment and machinery regularly, and make sure that subordinates use them competently and safely.

❑ If someone under your supervision isn't familiar with a piece of equipment, teach how to properly operate it before the subordinate uses it for the first time.

❑ Report incompetent health care personnel to superiors through the institutional chain of command.

❑ A nurse may delegate to the nursing assistant such tasks as taking vital signs, documenting intake and output, and performing blood glucose checks.

❑ The nursing process is a continuous, interdependent, systematic organization of cognitive behaviors designed to resolve problems and promote well-being.

❑ Priority of data collection activities is determined by the client's immediate condition or needs.

❑ Pertinent data are collected using appropriate evidence-based assessment techniques and instruments; analytical models and problem-solving tools are used.

❑ The care, treatment, and rehabilitation planning process should ensure that care is appropriate to the client.

## Ethical practice

❑ In the data collection process, the nurse gathers facts, perceptions, and opinions about the ethical problem and talks with the client and his family, other health care providers, and anyone who may be familiar with the client's values.

❑ Identify the people involved in any problem, and assess their roles, responsibilities, authority, and decision-making abilities.

❑ When making an ethical decision, identify available resources; these may include the ethics committee, chaplain, nurse ethicist, counselors, and facilitators; resources may also include institution policies, as well as literature on similar cases.

❑ Help decision makers participate in values clarification.

❑ Investigate the nature of the conflict by examining the rights, duties, and values that are in dispute; identify possible courses of action, along with their probable and possible risks and benefits.

❑ The nurse practice act is a series of statutes, enacted by each state legislature, that outline the legal scope of nursing practice within a particular state.

❑ The nurse practice act sets educational requirements for the nurse, distinguishes between nursing practice and medical practice, and defines the scope of nursing practice.

❏ Facility policies and procedures govern the practice in that particular facility.

❏ Standards of care, which are criteria that serve as a basis for comparison when evaluating the quality of nursing practice, are established by federal, accreditation, state, and professional organizations.

❏ Each state has a nurse practice act designed to protect both the nurse and the public by defining the legal scope of nursing practice and excluding untrained or unlicensed people from practicing nursing.

❏ Your state's nurse practice act is the most important law affecting your nursing practice.

❏ You're expected to care for clients within defined practice limits; if you give care beyond those limits, you become vulnerable to charges of violating your state's nurse practice act.

❏ Make sure that you're familiar with the legally permissible scope of your nursing practice as defined in your state's nurse practice act and that you never exceed its limits; otherwise, you're inviting legal problems.

❏ There are no automatic guidelines for solving all ethical conflicts.

❏ Legally, nurses are responsible for using their knowledge and skills to protect the comfort and safety of their clients.

❏ Laws are binding rules of conduct enforced by authority.

❏ In many situations, laws and ethics overlap; when they diverge, you have to identify and examine the fine lines that separate them.

❏ When a law is challenged as unjust or unfair, the challenge usually reflects some underlying ethical principle.

❏ When clients believe they haven't been treated with respect and dignity or that their needs and rights have been ignored or violated, they're more likely to initiate legal action.

❏ At times, the nurse may not know what the right or ethical course of action should be.

❏ A moral dilemma may be further complicated by psychological pressures and personal emotions, especially when a choice is a forced one at best and, in many cases, results in an uncomfortable compromise.

❏ Many moral dilemmas in nursing involve choices about justice or fairness, when scant resources (such as bed space or limited staffing) must be divided among clients with equal needs.

❏ Dilemmas of beneficence are those that involve deciding what is good as opposed to what is harmful; they often occur when health care providers, clients, or family members disagree about what course of action is in the client's best interest.

❑ Dilemmas of nonmaleficence are those that involve the avoidance of harm; these issues often involve a nurse's responsibility to "blow the whistle" if she sees others compromising the client's safety.

❑ Dilemmas of autonomy are those that involve deciding what course of action maximizes the client's right of self-determination.

❑ Autonomy issues are often closely related to beneficence issues, especially when individuals other than the client must determine (or attempt to determine) what is best for the client.

❑ Dilemmas of justice are ethical issues of fairness and equality, such as dilemmas that involve dividing limited health care resources fairly.

❑ Dilemmas of fidelity are those that involve honoring promises; these include the extent and limits of a nurse's role and duties to a client that might conflict with other duties, such as the nurse's duties to the physician.

❑ Fidelity involves confidentiality, respecting privileged information; a client's right to privacy must be balanced against society's right to be informed of potential threats to public health.

❑ Fidelity involves a commitment to veracity: telling the truth and fully informing a client of his medical condition.

❑ Active decisions by the nurse are ethical decisions that lead directly to actions and bring about change.

❑ Passive decisions are ethical decisions that deny, delay, or avoid action and maintain the status quo by denying or shifting responsibility to avoid change.

❑ Programmed decisions are those decisions that use precedents, established guidelines, procedures, and rules to resolve anticipated, routine, and expected types of moral dilemmas.

❑ Nonprogrammed decisions are those that require a unique response to complex and unexpected moral dilemmas.

❑ Most commonly, a nurse's programmed decisions are also active ones.

❑ The nurse is likely to encounter many conflicting sets of values in the course of her professional career. The nurse must choose among competing values to establish her own ethical beliefs.

❑ The nurse needs to incorporate chosen values into everyday thoughts and actions, to be better prepared to act on chosen values when confronted with difficult ethical choices.

❑ The nurse acts as a client advocate and assists clients in developing skills so that they can advocate for themselves.

❑ The nurse maintains a therapeutic and professional client-nurse relationship within professional role boundaries.

❏ The nurse is committed to practicing self-care, managing stress, and connecting with self and others.

❏ The nurse helps resolve ethical issues, including participating in ethics committees.

❏ The nurse reports illegal, incompetent, or impaired practices.

## Informed consent

❏ The client must be fully informed regarding treatment, tests, surgery, and the risks and benefits prior to giving informed consent.

❏ The professional nurse only witnesses the informed consent process and doesn't actually obtain the consent.

❏ Only a minor who is married or emancipated can give informed consent.

❏ Legally, the client must be mentally competent to give consent for procedures.

❏ Responsibility for obtaining informed consent rests with the person who will perform the treatment or procedure (usually the physician).

❏ The client should be told that he has a right to refuse the treatment or procedure without having other care or support withdrawn and that he can withdraw consent after giving it.

❏ Carrying out a procedure without informed consent can be grounds for charges of assault and battery.

❏ Informed consent involves providing the client (or someone acting on his behalf) with enough information to know what the client is getting into if he decides to undergo the treatment or procedure, as well as the anticipated consequences if consent is refused or withdrawn.

❏ Nurses may provide clients and their families with information that's within a nurse's scope of practice and knowledge base.

❏ A nurse can't substitute her knowledge for the physician's input.

❏ The basics of informed consent should include a description of the treatment or procedure; a description of inherent risks and benefits that occur with frequency or regularity (or specific consequences significant to the given client or his designated decision maker); explanation of the potential for death or serious harm (such as brain damage, stroke, paralysis, or disfiguring scars) or for discomforting adverse effects during or after the treatment or procedure; explanation and description of alternative treatments or procedures; name and qualifications of the person who is to perform the treatment or procedure; and discussion of the possible effects of not undergoing the treatment or procedure.

❑ If you witness a client's signature on a consent form, you attest to three things: the client voluntarily consented, the client's signature is authentic, and the client appears to be competent to give consent.

❑ If you believe a client is incompetent to participate in giving consent because of medication or sedation given to him, or you learn that the practitioner has discussed consent issues with the client when the client was heavily sedated or medicated, you have an obligation to bring it to the practitioner's attention immediately.

❑ Every state allows an emancipated minor to consent to his own medical care and treatment.

❑ Most states allow teenagers to consent to treatment, even though they aren't emancipated, in cases involving pregnancy or sexually transmitted infection.

❑ Informed consent should include an explanation of alternative treatments or procedures.

❑ The client's next of kin can only sign the consent form if the client is deemed incompetent.

❑ In medical malpractice cases that involve consent issues, expert testimony is usually required to establish whether or not the information given to the client was reasonable, understandable, presented at a time when the client was functionally able to process the information (as opposed to being sedated or medicated), and complete enough to allow the client to knowledgeably agree to proceed.

❑ If the health care practitioner knows that specific consequences are particularly significant to the client, those must be discussed before true informed consent may be obtained.

## Information technology

❑ As with the manual record system, the computerized medical record provides a detailed account of the client's clinical status, diagnostic tests, treatments, and medical history.

❑ Unlike the manual system, the computerized record stores all of the client's medical data in a single, easily accessible source.

❑ A hospital's computer system typically consists of a large, centralized computer to store information, linked to smaller video display terminals in each work area.

❑ The nurse may access care plans, vital signs, medication records, general progress notes, laboratory and diagnostic test results, assessment findings, discharge plans, and other information.

❑ The nurse can order a printed copy of the client's record.

❏ Health care reform legislation may further transform the documentation process, with the creation of a universal medical record that follows a client throughout his life.

❏ By improving legibility, computers reduce the risk of misinterpretation.

❏ Computers reduce misinterpretation by offering standardized, structured input formats and mandatory charting fields for assessment reports, flow charts, and care plans.

❏ Use of an incorrect descriptive prompt or phrase can give a misleading assessment.

❏ If the prompts aren't exactly descriptive, it's important to type or write out the assessment.

❏ Your liability when working with computer documentation is exactly the same as when working with a manual system.

❏ You may be liable for any client injuries associated with charting errors.

❏ To minimize legal risks, always double-check all client information.

❏ Don't divulge signature codes.

❏ Inform your supervisor if you suspect that someone is using your signature code.

❏ Know your state's rules and regulations and your facility's policies and procedures regarding privileged data, confidentiality, and disclosure.

❏ To learn about state rules and regulations, consult your facility's policy and procedure manual, check with your facility's attorney, or consult your state board of nursing or the state statutory and administrative codes.

❏ The primary safeguard, the signature code, limits access to the records; for example, a nurse's code would call up a client's entire record, but a technician's code would produce only part of the record.

❏ Care must be taken to safeguard client information sent by fax machine.

❏ Policies and procedures should be established to prevent confidential client information, such as a positive result on an HIV test, from being transmitted by fax machine, especially one that's centrally located and easily seen by staff members or the general public.

❏ Hospitals must show that their computer systems are trustworthy enough to be used in court.

❏ The hospital should use software that automatically records the date and time of each entry and each correction, as well as the name of the author or anyone who modifies a record.

## Legal rights and responsibilities

❑ A nurse may not knowingly administer or perform tasks that will harm a client.

❑ It's within a nurse's scope of practice to refuse to carry out orders that would harm a client.

❑ Administering medications and initiating I.V. therapy aren't within the scope of practice for nursing assistants.

❑ A staff nurse isn't licensed to fill prescriptions.

❑ Assault occurs when a person puts another person in fear of harmful or threatening contact.

❑ Battery is the actual contact with one's body.

❑ A detailed description of physical findings of abuse in the medical record is essential if legal action is pursued.

❑ Discovery rule is the actual term for the client's discovery of the injury.

❑ Alternative dispute resolution refers to any means of settling disputes outside the courtroom setting.

❑ Any professional negligence action must meet four demands—commonly known as the four D's—to be considered negligence and result in legal action: a duty for the health care professional to provide care to the person making the claim, a dereliction (breach) of that duty, a breach of duty that resulted in damages, and evidence that the damages were a direct result of the negligence (causation).

❑ Incident reports are internal to the facility and are used to evaluate care, determine potential risks, or examine system problems that could have contributed to the error.

❑ The responsibility of a nurse in a domestic abuse situation is to document the situation and provide support for the victim.

❑ In a case of suspected abuse, the nurse's responsibility is to document the client's statement and complete a body map indicating size, color, shape, location, and type of injuries.

❑ Safe, effective nursing practice requires becoming fully aware of the many legal and ethical issues surrounding professional practice.

❑ Negligence is failure to exercise the degree of care that a person of ordinary prudence would exercise under the same circumstances.

❑ Malpractice is a specific type of negligence; it is a violation of professional duty or a failure to meet a standard of care, or failure to use the skills and knowledge of other professionals in similar circumstances.

❑ It is your responsibility to ask the physician if you're confused about an order.

❑ If the physician fails to correct the error or answer your questions, inform your immediate supervisor or nurse-manager of your doubts.

❑ Follow the chain of command established in your facility.

❑ Conflicts of duty can arise if your state's nurse practice act disagrees with your facility's policies.

❑ Policies and procedures usually specify the allowable scope of nursing practice within the facility.

❑ You have a legal obligation to practice within your nurse practice act's limits.

❑ To protect yourself, compare your facility's policies with your nurse practice act.

❑ To align nurse practice acts with current nursing practice, professional nursing organizations and state boards of nursing generally propose revisions to regulations.

❑ Nurse practice acts are statutory laws subject to the inevitably slow legislative process, so the law sometimes has trouble keeping pace with medicine.

❑ Administering drugs to clients continues to be one of the most important and, legally, one of the riskiest tasks you perform.

❑ When administering drugs, one easy way to guard against malpractice liability is to remember the long-standing "five rights" formula: the right drug to the right client at the right time in the right dosage by the right route.

❑ The law expects you to know a drug's safe dosage limits, toxicity, potential adverse effects, and indications and contraindications for use.

❑ The law expects you to refuse to accept an illegible, confusing, or otherwise unclear drug order and also to seek clarification of a confusing order from the physician rather than trying to interpret it yourself.

❑ It is your responsibility to follow your facility's policies if you question a drug order.

❑ If unsure about a medication, you can ask the prescribing physician's supervisor (service chief) or get in touch with the facility administration and explain your problem.

❑ It is your responsibility to document your findings objectively; try to keep your emotions out of your charting.

❑ Breach of duty means that the nurse provided care that didn't meet the accepted standard.

❑ When investigating breach of duty, the court asks: How would a reasonable, prudent nurse with comparable training and experience have acted in comparable circumstances?

❑ During a malpractice trial, the court will measure the defendant-nurse's action against the answer it obtains to the following question: What would a reasonable prudent nurse, with like training and experience, do under these circumstances?

❑ The plaintiff-client and his attorney have the burden to prove that certain standards of care exist and that the defendant-nurse failed to meet those standards in her treatment of him, as well as having to prove the appropriateness of those standards, how the nurse failed to meet them, and how that failure caused the client injury.

❑ When the standard of care is at issue, the plaintiff-client must present expert witness testimony to support the claims.

❑ The defendant-nurse and her attorney need to produce expert witness testimony to support her claim that her actions didn't fall below accepted standards of care and that she acted in a reasonable and prudent manner.

❑ The court seeks information about all the national and state standards applicable to the defendant-nurse's actions.

❑ The court may seek applicable information about the policies of the defendant-nurse's employer.

❑ Nurses who perform the same medical services are subject to the same standard of care and liability as physicians.

❑ During a malpractice trial, non-nursing professionals who are trained and educated in medicine, are familiar with standards of nursing care, and delegate nursing orders may provide expert witness testimony with regard to standards of nursing care.

## Performance and quality improvement

❑ If a nurse-manager has received complaints from discharged clients about inadequate instructions for performing home care, knowing the importance of good, timely client education, the nurse-manager should work with the staff to evaluate current client education practices and revise as needed.

❑ Client education is the responsibility of all nurses providing care to the client, and the nurses must work together to establish the best methods.

❑ Evaluating client education in only one setting doesn't consider the entire process and the staff providing it. No complaint should be ignored.

❑ Client education is an important nursing responsibility.

❑ Benchmarking is a good approach for the nurse-manager to take; it's the process of comparing the delivery of client care practices in one organization to those in the best health care organizations.

❑ If the nurse-manager has contacts at the best facilities, she's the most appropriate person to obtain the necessary information from those institutions.

❑ The nurse-manager should evaluate the policies to determine which ones might be implemented at her facility, and then make recommendations for change in conjunction with her staff.

❑ Asking the staff to form a task force is a good idea, but benchmarking is a practice that saves time and effort and allows information to be obtained from excellent resources.

❑ Performance improvement is an important component of continuous quality improvement.

❑ In quality management, there is continuous quality improvement; it is used to continually assess and evaluate the effectiveness of client care.

❑ Quality management also involves performance improvement, which establishes a system of formal evaluation of job performance and recommends ways to improve performance and promote professional growth.

❑ Resource management involves the use of equipment, finances and budgets, and staff.

❑ Areas that need improvement can be identified by reviewing such incidents as medication errors, client fall reports, treatment errors, and treatment omissions.

❑ Incidents are investigated and a plan is devised to minimize or eliminate the risk of recurrence.

❑ The performance improvement committee identifies problems that don't meet an established standard and then recommends changes in the facility's policies, procedures, or documentation forms in an effort to improve client care.

❑ The Joint Commission is a private agency that establishes guidelines for the operation of hospitals and other health care facilities.

❑ Unit council is a group of individuals who represent the nursing unit and voice concerns of other staff members.

❑ Quality is demonstrated by documenting the application of nursing process in a responsible, accountable, and ethical manner.

❑ The nurse uses the results of quality-of-care activities to initiate changes in nursing practice and throughout the health care delivery system.

❑ The nurse collects data to monitor quality and effectiveness of nursing care and analyzes quality data to identify opportunities for improving care.

❑ The nurse can assist in developing policies, procedures, and practice guidelines to improve quality of care.

❑ The nurse participates on interdisciplinary teams that evaluate clinical practice or health services.

❑ The nurse incorporates new knowledge to initiate change in nursing practice if outcomes aren't achieved.

# Patient safety

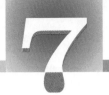

## Accident and injury prevention and home safety

❑ A low center of gravity helps you keep your balance and distributes your weight evenly between the upper and lower parts of your body when lifting objects.

❑ Teach the client proper body mechanics by telling him to keep the center of gravity low, flex the hips and knees, and not to bend at the waist.

❑ Try to keep your work (such as the client you will transfer or the object you will lift) close to your body, which aligns your back properly and lets your leg muscles—the body's strongest muscle group—do most of the work to avoid undue strain on your back.

❑ A wide base of support lowers your center of gravity and provides lateral (side-to-side) stability.

❑ To widen your base of support, stand with your feet spread about 8" to 12" (20.3 to 30.5 cm) apart, or roughly the width of your shoulders.

❑ Proper body alignment helps prevent muscle fatigue and overstretched ligaments; keep your head above your shoulders so your ears line up vertically with the top of your shoulders, and keep the top of your shoulders over your hips.

❑ To prevent back injuries, instruct the client to use an assistive or mechanical device as a first option to move a large or heavy object.

❑ If an assistive device is not available, instruct the client to slide or push the object, when possible, rather than pulling or lifting it and to use his arms or legs to provide leverage as he begins sliding or pushing the object.

❑ Sliding and pushing make use of your entire body weight—not just a few muscle groups—requiring less energy than lifting and resulting in less likelihood of an injury.

❑ Pulling is *not* the preferred method to move large or heavy objects.

❑ If you must pull a large object, stand close to it, tighten your leg, stomach, and buttock muscles, and keep a low center of gravity over a stable base.

❑ Back belts may cause problems by giving workers a false sense of security or making them think they can lift heavier loads; therefore, back belts should not be relied on as personal protective equipment and should not be recommended for use in the workplace.

❑ Gait belts (also called transfer belts) are used to assist a client with walking; they have handles at the waist that the health care worker can grasp to support and stabilize the client.

❑ Gait belts are used for partially dependent clients who can bear weight and need minimal assistance; they should never be used to help lift a client.

❑ Poor body mechanics, improper lifting or transfer technique, and workplace injuries can lead to musculoskeletal disorders.

❑ Musculoskeletal disorders are conditions that involve the nerves, tendons, muscles, and supporting structures (such as the disks in your spine).

❑ The nurse can help avoid musculoskeletal disorders by maintaining good posture, practicing good body mechanics, using appropriate assistive and mechanical devices, asking for help from coworkers, exercising regularly, and wearing supportive footwear.

❑ Your client should avoid postures that can lead to injury, which include swayback (exaggerated inward curve of the lower back), slouching, holding the head too high, looking down too much, carrying a heavy object on one side of the body, and cradling a phone between the neck and shoulder.

❑ Never lift more than you're able to; seek help from coworkers, or use appropriate assistive or mechanical devices.

❑ Always bend at the knees and hips—never at the waist.

❑ Use your leg muscles, not back muscles, to lift.

❑ When lifting and carrying a heavy object, keep it close to your body.

❑ Move heavy objects in one smooth, continuous motion.

❑ Avoid awkward postures, especially when lifting.

❑ Avoid repetitive motions. If you can't avoid them, take frequent rests.

❑ If the client uses a walker, make sure that he moves it about 6″ to 8″ (15 to 20 cm) at a time and then steps forward on his weaker leg while using his arms for support.

❑ Encourage the client using a walker to take steps of equal length with each leg.

❑ Instruct the client using a walker that to sit down he should back up so his stronger leg is against the chair and the weaker is right in front of him; then he can lower himself into the chair using his stronger leg and the opposite arm.

❑ Many factors contribute to the high incidence of falls in older adults, including changes related to aging, risks from mobility aids, adverse effects from medications, environmental hazards, unsafe caregiving, clothing that trips the client, and the effects of disease.

❑ Medications, particularly those that can cause dizziness, vertigo, drowsiness, orthostatic hypotension, and incontinence (such as antihypertensives, antipsychotics, sedatives, and hypnotics), can increase the risk for falls.

❑ The National Highway Traffic Safety Administration recommends that infants should be kept in the back seat, in rear-facing child safety seats, as long as possible up to the height or weight limit of the particular seat; at a minimum, keep infants rear-facing until a at least age 1 and at least 20 pounds (9 kg).

❑ The National Highway Traffic Safety Administration recommends that when children outgrow their rear-facing seats (at a minimum of age 1 and at least 20 pounds [9 kg]), they should ride in forward-facing child safety seats, in the back seat, until they reach the upper weight or height limit of the particular seat (usually around age 4 and 40 pounds [18 kg]).

❑ The National Highway Traffic Safety Administration recommends that once children outgrow their forward-facing seats (usually around age 4 and 40 pounds [18 kg]), they should ride in booster seats, in the back seat, until the vehicle seat belts fit properly.

❑ For a child age 8 or 4'9" (145 cm) tall, seat belts fit properly when the lap belt lays across the upper thighs and the shoulder belt fits across the chest.

❑ The National Highway Traffic Safety Administration recommends that when children outgrow their booster seats, (usually at age 8 or when they are 4'9" [145 cm] tall), they can use the adult seat belt in the back seat, if it fits properly (lap belt lays across the upper thighs and the shoulder belt fits across the chest).

❑ Instruct the client using a walker to get up from a chair by putting the walker in front of the chair and using both hands on the arms of the chair to push himself up; once standing he can support himself with the stronger leg and opposite arm and grab onto the walker with his free hand and then with the other hand.

❑ If the client needs a cane to walk, make sure he holds it close to his body, about 4" (10 cm) to the side of his stronger foot.

❑ Help the client keep a slow and even pace when he walks with a cane.

❑ When the client with a cane needs to sit, make sure he does not lean on the cane for support but stands with the backs of his legs against the chair, holds the arm rests with both hands, and lowers himself into the seat.

❑ Make sure that the client getting out of bed puts on shoes or nonskid slippers to prevent falling.

❑ When transferring a client from his bed to a wheelchair, bring the wheelchair as close to the bed as possible and make sure you lock the wheelchair wheels before the client transfers.

❑ When assisting a client who is walking, walk beside him with one arm around his waist for support in the event he starts to fall.

❑ If a client begins to fall as you are walking beside him, try to break his fall with your body and guide him to the floor as gently as possible while supporting his upper body and head as best you can.

❑ To help prevent falls from happening in the client's home environment, instruct the client to remove clutter from hallways and stairs, secure electrical cords, remove throw rugs, replace burnt-out light bulbs, remove loose stair treads, and trim frayed carpet.

❑ To prevent falls in the client's home bathroom, instruct the client to make sure he uses a bath stool or shower chair with nonskid feet; ask if he needs a raised toilet seat or grab bars.

❑ Warn the client against climbing on a chair or an unsteady stool to reach high cabinets; instead use a reacher pole or grips.

❑ To prevent fires in a client's home, instruct the client to install smoke and carbon dioxide alarms on each level of the home and to make sure to check the alarms once a month and to change the batteries every 6 months whether they work or not.

## Emergency response plan

❑ An emergency is a natural or man-made event that impacts your hospital's ability to provide care, treatment, and services and causes a sudden, major increase in the number of people who need the hospital's services.

❑ During an emergency, your hospital must maintain the safety of clients, staff, and visitors and each worker must respond quickly and efficiently.

❑ If an emergency occurs, listen for the announcement of the disaster code, stay calm, avoid tying up lines of communication, and provide clients, families, and visitors with emotional support.

❑ During an emergency, maintain client confidentiality.

❑ Always follow your hospital's emergency operation plan and the instructions of your emergency coordinator.

❑ Instructions to follow during an emergency will originate from the Incident Commander, located in the Command Center, who will spread information using the chain of command.

❑ Being prepared for emergencies is the responsibility of all health care workers.

❑ The nurse must be able to assess for possible hazards in the work area.

❑ Each health care worker should understand and carry out their role in an emergency.

❑ Health care workers should know how to obtain and use equipment required for their emergency response role.

❑ Health care workers should be able to show correct use of emergency communication equipment, such as emergency phones, fax machines, and radios.

❑ Health care workers should communicate well with other employees, clients, families, and the public in an emergency.

❑ Health care workers should know how to seek help through the chain of command in an emergency.

❑ The hospital develops an emergency operation plan that is put into effect by hospital administrators and identifies leadership's role and the chain of command during an emergency.

❑ The hospital develops procedures for establishing a Command Center, where the Incident Commander will lead the emergency operation.

❑ The hospital develops procedures for responding to and recovering from the emergency, including the type of evacuation and exit route and ways to notify external authorities of emergencies.

❑ The hospital develops ways to identify and assign staff to cover all vital duties, including accounting for all employees after evacuation.

❑ An emergency operation plan identifies procedures for evacuating the entire hospital and ways to establish an alternative care site.

❑ An emergency operation plan identifies roles and responsibilities of staff during emergencies and ways to recognize care providers and other staff during emergencies.

❑ An emergency operation plan identifies plans for combining efforts with other local health care facilities and backup communication systems in case primary communication fails.

❑ An emergency operation plan identifies an alternative plan for meeting utility needs and ways to isolate and decontaminate those exposed to biological, chemical, and radioactive agents.

❑ Make sure you're familiar with your hospital's emergency operation plan, and be prepared to participate in regular drills.

❑ Personal protective equipment helps protect the nurse from illness or injury caused by contact with hazardous materials.

❑ Personal protective equipment, depending on the situation, may include a face shield, goggles or safety glasses, safety shoes or boots, splash apron or coveralls, hood, gloves, respirator or breathing apparatus, nonencapsulating or fully encapsulating suit, and a radiation-protective suit.

❑ External emergencies include biological incidents, chemical incidents, radiation incidents, gas leaks, explosions, power or water outages, water main breaks, and airplane, train, or motor vehicle crashes.

❑ External emergencies include natural disasters and severe weather (for instance, earthquakes, hurricanes, tornadoes, floods, snowstorms, tsunamis, and severe heat or cold) or other mass casualty incidents (including domestic war).

❑ Internal emergencies include fires, power or water outages, gas leaks, explosions, flooding, internal telephone or communication systems failure, airplane or motor vehicle crashes into the hospital, workplace violence, bomb threats, and hostage situations.

❑ If an internal emergency occurs, you should remove people from immediate danger, call the appropriate number according to your hospital policy, and contact your supervisor.

❑ Follow your internal emergency response plan according to the type of internal emergency.

❑ During some emergencies, staff, clients, and visitors may need to evacuate.

❑ Evacuation may be horizontal, vertical, or external.

❑ In horizontal evacuation, staff, clients, and visitors are moved to a different area on the same floor.

❑ In vertical evacuation, staff, clients, and visitors are moved to a different floor in the facility.

❑ In external evacuation, staff, clients, and visitors are moved to another hospital or site.

❑ Biological emergencies are life-threatening diseases or outbreaks resulting from contact with dangerous biological agents.

❑ Biological emergencies may be accidental (natural) or planned.

❑ Bioterrorism is a planned biological emergency caused by terrorists.

❑ Bioterrorism is also called germ warfare or biological warfare.

❑ Biological agents used by bioterrorists include the germs that cause anthrax, botulism, plague, smallpox, tularemia, Ebola virus infection, Marburg virus infection, and brucellosis.

❑ Biological emergency victims (and, possibly, caregivers and other persons in close contact with victims) may require immediate decontamination (such as removing the person's clothing and showering with soap and water), isolation precautions, immunization, and treatment that cures the disease or eases symptoms.

❑ An industrial chemical spill is an example of an accidental chemical emergency.

❑ Toxic chemical release by terrorists is an example of a planned chemical emergency.

❑ Agents that may be involved in chemical emergencies include cyanide, sulfur mustard, ricin, sarin, organophosphates (such as certain insecticides), and other toxins.

❑ In a chemical emergency, exposure occurs when a person breathes air, drinks water, eats food, or touches soil that contains a hazardous agent.

❑ Most deaths from chemical incidents result from inhalation (breathing in the chemical).

❑ Health care workers who care for clients who have been exposed to toxic chemical liquids are at risk when the chemical evaporates if they don't wear the proper personal protective equipment.

❑ Depending on their injuries, victims of a chemical emergency may require immediate decontamination before entering the emergency department to remove the hazardous chemical agent, preventing it from being further absorbed into the victim's body and from spreading to other people and surfaces.

❑ Victims of a chemical emergency may require measures to keep their airway open and maintain breathing and circulation, as well as medications to reverse the effects of chemical agents.

❑ Never induce vomiting if the victim ingested a toxic chemical.

❑ If the victim of a chemical emergency enters the hospital before decontamination takes place, be sure to cover the victim with a blanket or sheet right away, if one is available, to keep others and the area from becoming exposed; then take the victim to the decontamination area.

❑ Chemical decontamination involves three steps: removing clothing, washing the victim, and disposing of clothing and belongings.

❑ In a chemical decontamination, quickly remove any clothing with the toxic chemical on it and cut away clothing that would have to be pulled overhead.

❑ In a chemical decontamination, if solid material remains on the skin, brush or wipe it off (some materials react with water) and then quickly wash the area with running water for at least 15 minutes.

❑ In a chemical decontamination, if the eyes are burning or vision is blurred, rinse the eyes with water or an approved eyewash solution for 15 minutes and wash the victim's eyeglasses or remove contact lenses, as applicable, but don't put contacts back in the eyes.

❑ In a chemical decontamination, place the victim's clothing and belongings in a plastic bag, being careful not to touch any contaminated areas as you do this; then seal the bag, place it inside another bag, and (if appropriate) dispose of it according to your hospital's policy.

❏ In a chemical decontamination, you must maintain the chain of custody for all clothing and valuables, keeping in mind that these articles may be evidence if the contamination was crime-related.

❏ Radiation emergencies can result from release of or exposure to radioactive material, as in explosion of a nuclear device, nuclear weapons testing, or nuclear power plant accidents.

❏ Radiation emergencies can result from radioactive material in the food or water supply, accidental release of radioactive material from a medical or industrial device, or accidental overexposure to a client undergoing radiation therapy.

❏ Radiation emergencies can result from accidents involving the transport of radioactive materials or terrorist acts, such as blowing up a truck carrying radioactive material, bombing a nuclear facility, or blowing up a "dirty" bomb.

❏ Radiation emergencies may contaminate or expose hundreds of people to radioactive material.

❏ If the radiation emergency involves an explosion, thermal burns and blast injuries also may occur.

❏ External radioactive contamination occurs when a radioactive material lands on a person's hair, skin, or clothing.

❏ Internal radioactive contamination occurs when a person breathes in or swallows radioactive material, or absorbs such material through the skin or an open wound.

❏ People with external radioactive contamination may contaminate other people or surfaces they physically contact, caregivers who touch or move them, equipment used to assess and treat them, and the surrounding area.

❏ If a radiation victim is admitted to your hospital, a radiologic emergency response team or radiation officer should manage the response.

❏ The radiation victim should be checked using a radiation meter to determine if he or she is contaminated.

❏ A person contaminated with radioactive material must be decontaminated to prevent or reduce internal contamination, to reduce the radiation dose from the contaminated site, and to prevent radioactive material from spreading to other people.

❏ Before radioactive decontamination, the victim's clothing and belongings are removed and double-bagged.

❏ The bags containing the radioactive decontaminated victim's clothing are sealed, a radioactive material label is placed on the outside bag, and the bag is then placed in a designated storage area until it can be properly discarded.

❑ To decontaminate a person with radioactive contamination, clean wounds and body openings first, followed by intact skin areas; then wash each area gently under a stream of warm tap water while scrubbing gently with a surgical sponge or soft brush.

❑ If plain-water washing is ineffective when decontaminating a person with radioactive contamination, use a mild soap or surgical scrub soap.

❑ To help keep the facility functioning during an emergency, you must know your responsibilities for reporting to work during a natural disaster.

❑ To help keep your facility functioning during an emergency, you must plan other ways to get to work and be prepared to report to another area in the facility, depending on where your skills are needed most.

❑ Know which types of natural disasters are most likely to strike your area.

❑ Participate in emergency preparedness drills to gain knowledge and experience.

❑ Learn how to use emergency communication equipment in case land and cell phone lines are overloaded during the disaster.

❑ During high-wind weather, such as a tornado or hurricane, keep all exterior doors and windows closed, unplug unnecessary equipment, keep people and vital equipment away from doors and windows, and be prepared to move clients to hallways or the basement, if ordered.

❑ Make sure key equipment is connected to an emergency (red) power outlet at all times.

❑ Know where to locate and how to use an alternative communication method, such as a two-way radio or an emergency phone system.

❑ Although most health care facilities have backup generators, these generators may not meet all energy needs (such as air conditioning).

❑ If a fire occurs in your hospital, you must act quickly. Use the memory aid RACE to help you remember what to do.

❑ In the memory aid RACE, **R** is for *Rescue*; rescue anyone in danger, and move them to a safe area.

❑ In the memory aid RACE, **A** is for *Alarm;* activate the fire alarm system, and call the phone number chosen by your hospital to report the fire.

❑ In the memory aid RACE, **C** is for *Contain;* contain the smoke and fire by closing all doors and windows in both client and nonclient areas.

❑ In the memory aid RACE, **E** is for *Extinguish* or *Evacuate;* extinguish the fire, if possible. If you can't extinguish the fire, evacuate clients, starting with those nearest the fire.

❑ During a fire remember to use the stairs—not the elevator.

❑ If a telephone caller reports a bomb in your hospital, stay calm and try to have someone else notify security while you stay on the line with the caller.

❑ In the event of a bomb threat, prepare to evacuate—usually a distance of at least 300 to 400 feet (92 to 122 m) from the bomb's location.

❑ In the event of a bomb threat, don't touch or move any suspicious packages or objects you encounter while evacuating. Instead, notify authorities of their location.

❑ In the event of a bomb threat, don't reenter the hospital until you get permission from law enforcement personnel.

❑ If someone has been taken hostage in your hospital, notify security personnel immediately (if this hasn't been done already) and try to stay calm and reassure others around you.

❑ If someone has been taken hostage in your hospital, expect the hospital to be either evacuated or "locked down" (meaning no one can enter or leave).

## Error prevention

❑ Always ask the client if he is allergic to any medications, plants, or herbal supplements, even if he is in distress.

❑ A client who has a peanut allergy could have an anaphylactic reaction to ipratropium given by a metered-dose inhaler because it contains soy lecithin.

❑ Client teaching is a crucial aspect of the client's responsibility in minimizing medication errors and their consequences.

❑ Teach the client about his diagnosis and the purpose of his drug therapy and provide this information in writing.

❑ Always ask the client if he takes over-the-counter medications as well as herbal remedies or nutritional supplements at home in addition to his prescribed drugs.

❑ Instruct the client what types of drug-related problems warrant notifying his physician.

❑ Encourage the client to report anything about his drug therapy that concerns or worries him.

❑ Always check the client's identification using two client identifiers according to your facility policy every time you give a medication or perform a procedure on a client.

❑ In addition to the traditional "five rights" of medication administration, best practice researchers have added three additional "rights": the right reason, the right response, and the right documentation to help prevent medication errors.

❑ To help prevent medication errors, always verify that the drug prescribed is appropriate to treat the client's condition.

❏ To help prevent medication errors, monitor the client's response to the drug administered.

❏ To help prevent medication errors, completely and accurately document in the client's medical record the drug administered; the monitoring of the client, including his response; and any other nursing interventions.

❏ The National Coordinating Council for Medication Error Reporting and Prevention defines a medication error as "any preventable event that may cause or lead to inappropriate medication use or patient harm while the medication is in the control of the health care professional, patient, or consumer."

❏ Medication errors can occur from process problems within any one stage or within multiple stages of drug administration.

❏ Medication errors that occur as part of ordering or prescribing can include incomplete or illegibly written orders by the prescriber; prescription of contraindicated drugs (such as drugs to which the client is allergic); prescription of the wrong drug, dose, route, or frequency; or using inappropriate or inadequate verbal orders to prescribe drugs.

❏ Medication errors that occur as part of transcribing and verifying include transcribing the incorrect drug, dose, route, time, or frequency into the medication administration record (MAR) by the pharmacist or nurse or inadequate drug verification and documentation in the MAR by the pharmacist or nurse.

❏ Medication errors that occur as part of dispensing include incorrect filling of the prescribed drug and failure to deliver the right drug to the right place for the right client.

❏ Medication errors that occur as part of administering include giving the wrong drug to the wrong client by the nurse or other licensed professional; the nurse or other licensed professional calculating and giving or infusing the wrong dose, or preparing the right drug incorrectly (such as crushing a drug that shouldn't be crushed) that is then given by the nurse or other licensed professional. Medication errors that occur as part of administering can also include the nurse or other licensed professional administering the correct drug by the wrong route (such as an oral drug that is injected intravenously) and the nurse or other licensed professional giving the correct drug at the wrong time or frequency.

❏ Medication errors that occur as part of monitoring and reporting include inadequate monitoring of the client by the nurse before and after medication administration and inadequate documentation and reporting of the client's condition by the nurse before and after medication administration.

❏ Medication errors that occur as part of monitoring and reporting can also include inadequate hand-off communication between licensed professionals and inadequate reporting of medication errors.

## Handling hazardous materials

❑ The Occupational Safety and Health Administration created the Hazard Communication Standard, which protects workers who use or come in contact with hazardous materials in their workplace.

❑ The Hazard Communication Standard states that workers must be taught about hazardous materials and their proper use.

❑ The Hazard Communication Standard states that workers have the "right to know" about the possible risks to their health and safety and the right to tell their physician this information.

❑ The manufacturer who makes the hazardous materials must label the material with the product name, a warning, and the manufacturer's name and address.

❑ The manufacturer who makes the hazardous materials must provide information about how to safely use the product.

❑ Hospitals often purchase hazardous materials in large volumes and then transfer them to smaller containers.

❑ Your hospital may use a coding system to help you identify hazards that uses color-coded diamonds and a rating scale to identify the hazards: blue (health hazard), red (flammability), yellow (reactivity; risk for causing an explosion or reaction), and white (special hazard; includes oxidizers and substances that are water-reactive, radioactive, corrosive, acidic, or alkaline).

❑ The material safety data sheet contains the name of the substance, the physical and health hazards associated with the substance, and ways in which the substance can enter the body.

❑ Hazardous materials are any substances or chemicals that pose a physical or health hazard and include hazardous chemicals (including some drugs), infectious wastes, and radioactive materials, all of which can be found in your workplace.

❑ The Occupational Safety and Health Administration's Hazard Communication Standard classifies hazards into two major categories: health hazards and physical hazards.

❑ Health hazards may cause serious health problems.

❑ Health hazards include carcinogens, teratogens, toxic or highly toxic agents, irritants, corrosives, and sensitizers.

❑ Carcinogens are substances that can cause cancer.

❑ Teratogens are substances that may cause birth defects.

❑ Toxic or highly toxic agents are substances that cause health problems with even the smallest exposure.

❏ Irritants are substances that cause redness or swelling of the skin or eyes on contact.

❏ Corrosives are substances that cause damage and burns when they contact the skin or eyes.

❏ Sensitizers are substances that cause allergic reaction after repeat contact.

❏ Physical hazards threaten a person's safety; the most common types of physical hazards include materials that are likely to burn, explode, or react with water.

❏ Physical hazards include flammables, combustibles, pyrophobics, explosives, water reactives, unstable reactives, oxidizers, and organic peroxides.

❏ Flammables are substances that easily catch on fire.

❏ Combustibles are substances that burn, but don't easily catch on fire.

❏ Pyrophobics are substances that can burst into flames on their own.

❏ Explosives are substances that can cause a sudden release of pressure and heat that's harmful.

❏ Water reactives are substances that may explode or release a gas that easily burns when in contact with water.

❏ Unstable reactives are substances that may react with pressure or temperature changes.

❏ Oxidizers are substances that cause other substances to change and burn.

❏ Organic peroxides are substances that contain oxygen, which may cause other substances to burn.

❏ Infectious wastes place you at risk for getting an infection.

❏ Radioactive materials may be present in your workplace.

❏ You may be exposed to radioactive materials through contact with X-ray machines and other testing equipment, through contact with clients who need radioactive materials for testing or treatment, and through radioactive materials that have spilled.

❏ Hazardous materials are only dangerous when they come in contact with and enter the body. Hazardous materials can get into your body if you breathe them in, if you eat or drink them, or if your skin absorbs them.

❏ Your hospital's respiratory protection program helps to protect you from hazards that can be breathed in, such as vapors, gases, fumes, dusts, and infections (such as tuberculosis).

❏ The Occupational Safety and Health Administration requires that respirators be "fit-tested" every year.

❏ To protect yourself from contact with hazardous materials, clean work surfaces before and after working with hazardous materials, wash your hands before eating, don't eat or drink near hazardous materials, and dispose of all sharp instruments immediately.

❑ When working with radioactive materials, observe the principles of time (limiting the amount of time exposed to the material), distance (keeping distance between you and the radioactive material), and shielding (using a lead barrier between you and the radioactive material whenever possible).

❑ When working with radioactive materials, wear a personal radiation dosimeter, such as a film badge, to monitor your exposure to radiation and wear lead protection whenever handling radioactive wastes.

❑ Place all radioactive waste in a special radiation container with a radiation label; immediately notify the appropriate person in your hospital to help clean up a radiation spill or other accident with radioactivity.

❑ Eyewash stations should be located in hospital areas where there is a risk of eye contamination, such as the laboratory and emergency department.

❑ If your eye comes in contact with a hazardous material, go immediately to the nearest eyewash station and flush the eye with clear water or an approved eyewash solution for 15 minutes while holding the eyelid open and moving your eyes so the water or solution flows onto the entire surface of the affected eye and into the surrounding folds.

## Infection control

❑ One of the most important things that you must do as a health care worker is to keep infection from spreading.

❑ Infections can increase the amount of time that clients spend in the hospital, increase health care costs, and cause workers to miss time at work.

❑ An infection occurs when an organism enters the body and the body's immune system is unable to fight it off, causing illness.

❑ Infections can be caused by different types of organisms, including bacteria, viruses, fungi, and parasites.

❑ For an infection to occur, a six-part chain, known as the chain of infection, must be present.

❑ The chain of infection includes the infectious agent, reservoir, exit route, mode of transmission, portal of entry, and susceptible host.

❑ The infectious agent is the organism responsible for the infection.

❑ The reservoir is the place where the infectious agent lives and grows, such as food, water, soil, an animal, an insect, or a human.

❑ The exit route is the way in which the infectious agent leaves the living being, such as through secretions, excretions, skin, or droplets.

❏ The mode of transmission is the way in which the infectious agent spreads to another location, such as by direct contact, through droplets in the air, by eating or drinking contaminated food or water, or through insect or animal bites.

❏ The portal of entry is where the infectious agent finds its way onto or into another person, such as through an opening in the skin or through the airway or eyes.

❏ The susceptible host is a person who is at risk for getting the infection.

❏ The best way to control the spread of infection is to break the weakest link in the chain of infection, which is usually the mode of transmission, or the way in which the infectious agent spreads.

❏ You can break the weakest link by performing good hand hygiene, using barriers, such as personal protective equipment, and following isolation precautions.

❏ Performing hand hygiene is one of the most important things you can do to prevent the spread of infection.

❏ Wash your hands with soap and water whenever they are visibly soiled, before eating, and after using the restroom.

❏ Clean your hands before and after direct client contact.

❏ Clean your hands before putting on sterile gloves to perform any procedure.

❏ Clean your hands after removing gloves.

❏ Clean your hands if moving from one body site to another during client care.

❏ Clean your hands after contact with any object that is near a client.

❏ When using an alcohol-based hand rub, first apply the product to the palm of your hand and rub your hands together, covering all surfaces, until they're completely dry.

❏ Be sure to get the alcohol-based hand rub under your fingernails.

❏ When washing your hands with soap and water, first wet your hands with water then apply soap to your hands; rub your hands together briskly for at least 15 seconds, covering all surfaces of the hands and fingers; and then rinse your hands with water while pointing them downward.

❏ After washing your hands with soap and water, dry them with a paper towel and use another paper towel to turn off the faucet.

❏ Don't wear artificial nails if you have direct contact with client equipment or clients who are at risk for infection, or if you prepare food.

❏ Keep natural nail tips less than ¼" (6 mm) long.

❏ Avoid using hot water when washing your hands; repeated use of hot water may increase your risk of developing skin problems.

❑ Use hospital-supplied hand lotions and creams to prevent your skin from drying and cracking.

❑ Personal protective equipment can help you prevent the spread of infection by acting as a barrier between you and the infectious agent.

❑ Personal protective equipment available in your workplace includes gloves, gowns, eye and face shields, surgical mask, an N-95 respirator, hoods, caps, and shoe covers.

❑ Choose the right size and type of gloves (gloves that contain powdered latex can cause allergic reactions in clients or staff with latex allergies).

❑ Check to see that there are no holes or tears in gloves when you first put them on.

❑ Change gloves whenever moving from one body site to another.

❑ If your gloves become torn, remove them, perform hand hygiene, and put on a new pair.

❑ Avoid touching your face and adjusting other personal protective equipment.

❑ Wash your hands (if visibly soiled) or use an alcohol-based hand rub (if not visibly soiled) right after discarding gloves.

❑ When wearing a gown, make sure the gown covers your torso, fits well when it's tied in the back at the waist and neck, and the sleeves fit snugly at the wrist.

❑ Remove the gown right before leaving the client's room by untying the waist strings first, then the neck strings, and then allowing the gown to fall forward (down toward your wrists), turning it inside out as it falls.

❑ When removing a gown, make sure the soiled portion of the gown doesn't touch your clothing.

❑ Place a used gown in a laundry bag or discard a disposable gown in an appropriate container inside the client's room.

❑ Wash your hands or use an alcohol-based hand rub right after removing a gown.

❑ Goggles protect your eyes and the areas just above, below, and next to them.

❑ Goggles should fit snugly over and around your eyes (or eyeglasses).

❑ A face shield protects your skin as well as your eyes, nose, and mouth; the shield should cover your forehead, extend below your chin, and wrap around the side of your face.

❑ When removing eyewear, make sure you don't touch the outer surface; if eyewear is reusable, clean it after use according to your hospital's policy.

❑ Wash your hands or use an alcohol-based hand rub right after removing the eyewear.

❑ Always wear an N-95 respirator to protect yourself against airborne diseases, and make sure it fits properly before each use.

❑ Avoid touching the N-95 respirator once it's in place and change it when it becomes damaged.

❑ Remove the N-95 respirator outside the client's room when the door is closed, touching only the straps of the N-95 respirator during removal.

❑ Wash your hands or use an alcohol-based hand rub right after removing the N-95 respirator.

❑ When wearing a regular surgical mask to protect against diseases that require droplet precautions, always make sure the mask fits properly before use.

❑ When wearing a surgical mask, avoid touching the face mask once it's in place and change it when it becomes damp.

❑ Touch only the straps or strings of the mask during removal; remove the face mask when you exit the client's room and discard it in the appropriate waste container.

❑ Wash your hands or use an alcohol-based hand rub right after removing a face mask.

❑ During mouth-to-mouth resuscitation, use a mouthpiece or a pocket mask.

❑ When there's a risk that blood or body fluids could be splashed or sprayed, you may need to use a hood, surgical cap, shoe covers, face mask, or eye shield in addition to a gown and gloves.

❑ If you're wearing several types of personal protective equipment at once, always remove gloves first because they're the most contaminated items.

❑ Remove a face shield or goggles after you remove your gloves.

❑ Remove your gown (after your gloves and face shield or goggles) by pulling from the back toward your front, turning it inside out as you disrobe.

❑ When removing personal protective equipment, remove the face mask or N-95 respirator last, making sure to remove the N-95 respirator when you are outside of the client's room. If only gloves are worn, you can safely remove and discard them in the client's room.

❑ You can safely remove a gown inside the client's doorway just before exiting the room, or you can remove it in the anteroom (for contact and droplet isolation precautions only).

❑ Once you've removed all personal protective equipment, remember to perform good hand hygiene.

❑ Two major types of infection control procedures can help you break the chain of infection: standard and transmission-based precautions.

❑ Standard precautions are based on the idea that the blood and body fluids of any client may carry infection.

❑ Health care workers must follow standard precautions whenever they may come in contact with blood, body fluids (breast milk, feces, fluid from the lungs, saliva, semen, urine, vaginal secretions, wound drainage, and other fluids, such as excretions and secretions except sweat), broken skin, and mucous membranes.

❑ As part of standard precautions, always perform hand hygiene.

❑ As part of standard precautions, always wear gloves when touching blood, body fluids, broken skin, or soiled items.

❑ As part of standard precautions, always change gloves between clients.

❑ As part of standard precautions, always wear a mask and eye protection or a face shield to protect the eyes, nose, and mouth when splashing is likely.

❑ As part of standard precautions, always wear a gown to protect skin and prevent soiling of clothing when splashing or spraying is likely.

❑ As part of standard precautions, always use hospital safety sharps and dispose of them in a puncture-resistant sharps container.

❑ Always use mouthpieces or resuscitator bags under standard precautions when cardiopulmonary resuscitation is needed.

❑ As part of standard precautions, always clean and disinfect equipment and surfaces.

❑ As part of standard precautions, always handle soiled linen correctly.

❑ Transmission-based precautions are used in addition to standard precautions for clients with certain types of infections.

❑ Transmission-based precautions include airborne isolation precautions, droplet precautions, and contact precautions.

❑ Airborne isolation precautions are used for clients with known or suspected diseases that spread through the airborne route.

❑ Diseases that spread through the airborne route include tuberculosis, chickenpox, measles, and severe acute respiratory syndrome.

❑ Diseases that spread through the airborne route are spread through small droplet nuclei that float in the air or attach to dust; the droplet nuclei exit the body when an infected person coughs, sneezes, or speaks.

❑ During airborne isolation precautions, the client must be placed in an airborne isolation room.

❑ An airborne isolation room is a special isolation room with negative pressure.

❑ During airborne isolation precautions, the door of the room must be kept closed except when entering or exiting the room.

❑ During airborne isolation precautions, everyone who enters the room must wear an N-95 respirator that has been properly fit-tested.

❑ During airborne isolation precautions, the N-95 respirator should be removed outside of the client's room when the door to the isolation room is closed.

❑ During airborne isolation precautions, procedures and treatments should be done in the client's room, if possible.

❑ During airborne isolation precautions, if the client needs to go to another area, he should wear a surgical mask; if the client can't wear a mask, he should be taught to cover his mouth with a tissue if he needs to cough or sneeze.

❑ Droplet precautions are used to prevent the spread of infections through droplets.

❑ When droplet precautions are needed, the client should be placed in a private room; if one isn't available, he or she can be placed in a room with another client who has the same infection.

❑ When droplet precautions are needed, the door to the client's room may be open or closed.

❑ When droplet precautions are needed, everyone who enters the client's room must wear a regular surgical mask and other personal protective equipment according to hospital policy.

❑ When droplet precautions are needed, the client must stay in the room except when special testing or a procedure is needed; then the client should wear a surgical mask, if able.

❑ When droplet precautions are needed and the client cannot wear a surgical mask, procedures should be done in the client's room if feasible.

❑ Contact precautions reduce the spread of infectious agents through direct (skin-to-skin) or indirect contact (by touching surfaces or client care items that contain the germ).

❑ When contact precautions are needed, make sure the client is placed in a private room; if one isn't available, the client can be placed in a room with someone who has the same infection.

❑ When contact precautions are needed, put on gloves and a gown before entering the client's room.

❑ When contact precautions are needed, make sure gloves cover the cuffs of the gown; none of your hand, wrist, or arm should be exposed.

❑ When contact precautions are needed, change gloves after contact with germ-containing material.

❑ When contact precautions are needed, remove gloves before leaving the client's room.

❑ When contact precautions are needed, remove your gown just before leaving the client's room or in the anteroom, making sure your clothing doesn't touch anything that may contain germs after the gown is removed.

❑ You must wash your hands or use an alcohol-based hand rub after removing personal protective equipment.

❑ Always wear gloves when handling used client items because many different client items, including towels, bed linens, and used dressings, tubing, or equipment, could contain infectious agents.

❑ A sharp is anything that could cut or puncture someone who handles it, such as a needle, scalpel, scissors, or broken glass.

❑ Never bend, break, or shear a contaminated sharp.

❑ Never place a sharps container in a biohazard plastic bag for disposal.

❑ Never reach into a sharps container.

❑ Always use tongs to pick up a contaminated sharp.

❑ Change out sharps containers when they are three-quarters full.

❑ Discard contaminated sharps as soon as possible in a rigid, puncture-resistant container. These containers must be marked with a biohazard symbol and clearly labeled as a sharps container.

❑ The Centers for Disease Control and Prevention recommends that all health care workers get immunized against influenza, hepatitis B (only if at risk for blood or body fluid exposure), and varicella (chickenpox).

❑ If you've never had chickenpox and don't know if you're immune to the infection, you should have a blood test; if you aren't immune, you need to receive the varicella vaccine.

❑ If you experience a needle-stick injury or a cut from a sharp, flood the needle stick or cut with water, and clean the wound with soap and water.

❑ If you become exposed to blood or body fluid splashes to the nose, mouth, or skin, flush with water and then wash your skin with soap and water.

❑ If your eyes become exposed to blood or body fluid, flush them with clean water or another approved eyewash fluid using the nearest eyewash station.

❑ If you become exposed to blood or body fluids, seek medical care as soon as possible after you have cleaned the exposed site.

❑ Report any exposure to blood or body fluids right away to the appropriate supervisor and to your employee health coordinator, risk management coordinator, or both.

❑ If you become exposed to blood or body fluids, complete the proper forms according to your hospital's policy and follow your hospital's policy concerning treatment options.

❑ If you think you've been exposed to tuberculosis in the workplace, notify the appropriate supervisor and the infection control or employee health department right away, and fill out reports according to your hospital's policy.

❑ If you think you've been exposed to tuberculosis in the workplace, notify the employee health department in your hospital to schedule a tuberculin skin test right away; they will notify the local or state health department as required by law.

❑ If the tuberculin skin test taken after exposure to tuberculosis is negative, you'll need to schedule repeat testing and symptom screening in 8 to 10 weeks after exposure.

❑ If the tuberculin skin test is positive or you have symptoms, you'll need to have a chest X-ray; make sure you report any symptoms right away.

❑ If you don't know that you've been exposed and the employee health department is informed that a client you had contact with was diagnosed with tuberculosis, your hospital must notify you right away to schedule testing.

❑ Health care workers play an important role in stopping the spread of infection.

❑ Follow standard precautions at all times with all clients and especially whenever you might come in contact with blood, body fluids, broken skin, or mucous membranes.

❑ Contact the infection control or employee health department for treatment options if you are exposed to an infectious agent.

## Restraint use

❑ Restraint is defined as the direct use of force against a person's body; the force may be applied by the use of hands, mechanical devices, seclusion, or a combination of each.

❑ Restraint can include drugs that are used to restrict or manage a client's behavior or restrict his freedom of movement.

❑ Restraint can happen with or without the client's permission.

❑ Restraint in the clinical setting is commonly defined as use of any single or combined force that limits a client's freedom of movement, access to his body, or access to the environment.

❑ Less restrictive measures should be attempted before resorting to the use of restraint.

❑ Always choose the least restrictive method of restraint.

❑ The goal is to use restraints only when absolutely necessary.

❑ Seclusion is described as involuntary confinement of a person to a room or a specific area from which he is told not to leave or is physically prevented from exiting.

❑ Seclusion is used to provide a safe, desensitized environment to support the client's efforts to regain control over unacceptable behavior.

❑ Seclusion eliminates stimulation when less-restrictive approaches have failed and imminent danger to the client or staff is likely.

❑ Restraint use has many associated risks for the client, including death, neurovascular injury, fractures, psychological harm, bruising, skin breakdown, loss of dignity, and violation of the client's rights.

❑ According to Centers for Medicare & Medicaid Services standards, seclusion may only be used for the management of violent or self-destructive behavior that jeopardizes the immediate physical safety of the client, staff members, or others.

❑ Restraints can be used in acute medical-surgical care for the nonviolent, non-self-destructive client during treatment of certain conditions, such as acute brain injury.

❑ Restraints can be used in acute medical-surgical care for the nonviolent, non-self-destructive client during certain clinical procedures, such as endotracheal intubation.

❑ Restraints can be used in acute medical-surgical care for the nonviolent, non-self-destructive client to prevent client injury (for example, to prevent the client from discontinuing treatment or dislodging medical equipment that is necessary for his care).

❑ Restraints and seclusion can be used for behavioral health purposes for the violent or self-destructive client to protect the client from injuring himself or to prevent the client from injuring others.

❑ When restraint is the only alternative, maintain the client's safety, protect the client's rights, preserve the client's dignity, and preserve the client's physical and psychological well-being.

❑ When restraints are initiated, the registered nurse caring for the client must immediately notify the physician or licensed independent practitioner, who will evaluate the situation and who must see the client face to face within 24 hours.

❑ When the initiation of restraints is warranted because of a significant change in the client's condition, the registered nurse caring for the client must immediately notify the physician or licensed independent practitioner, who will then evaluate the client.

❑ If the physician or advanced practitioner is unavailable to give an order, the registered nurse can initiate restraints based on her assessment of the client; the physician or licensed independent practitioner must be notified of the restraint use immediately, and a written or telephone order must be obtained.

❑ If a telephone order is obtained for restraint use, the order must be signed within 24 hours of the initiation of restraint.

❑ If medical-surgical restraint is necessary beyond the 24 hours authorized by the original order, the physician or licensed independent practitioner must provide a new order.

❑ Renewal of the restraint order must occur each calendar day that the restraint is needed after the client is examined by the physician or advanced practitioner.

❑ When behavioral restraint or seclusion is necessary, an order must be obtained from the physician or licensed independent practitioner responsible for the client's care as soon as possible, but no longer than 1 hour after the initiation of restraint use.

❑ The physician or licensed independent practitioner must perform a face-to-face assessment of the client placed in behavioral restraints or seclusion within 1 hour if the hospital is required to follow guidelines established by the Centers for Medicare & Medicaid Services.

❑ At the time of the face-to-face assessment, the physician or licensed independent practitioner must collaborate with the client and staff to identify measures to help the client gain control of his behavior.

❑ At the time of the face-to-face assessment, the physician or licensed independent practitioner must collaborate with the client and staff to revise the client's plan of care and provide a new written order, if indicated.

❑ If the client's condition changes, the restraint can be discontinued before the order expires.

❑ Mechanical extremity restraints may be applied to the wrists and ankles.

❑ Commonly used mechanical extremity restraints include soft restraints and leather restraints.

❑ Soft restraints are commonly made of foam or lamb's wool and are applied over padded bony prominences.

❑ When applying soft or leather restraints, make sure that two fingers can be inserted between the wrist or ankle and the restraint.

❑ Leather restraints are used only when soft restraints aren't sufficient and sedation is dangerous or ineffective.

❑ Upper extremity restraints include elbow restraints and hand mitts.

❑ Elbow restraints are commercially made devices that keep the elbow immobilized.

❑ Hand mitts are netted devices that may be tied down and are used to restrain the client's hands.

❑ Elbow restraints are especially helpful in protecting the surgical incision in small children after cleft lip or palate repair.

❑ Hand mitts prevent the client from scratching or removing invasive equipment or dressings and also prevent combative clients from hurting themselves or others.

❑ Hand mitts are considered restraints regardless of whether they are tied down because they prevent the client from having normal access to the body.

❑ A roll belt restraint may be used to prevent falls from a bed or chair while permitting movement of the arms and legs; they allow the client to turn freely in bed.

❑ Restraint ties must be secured to the movable portion of the bed frame, not the side rails.

❑ Using a restraint solely to keep a client in bed or to keep the client from falling is not an acceptable use.

❑ Always document what the client is doing and why the behavior presents a safety risk to the client and requires the use of restraint or seclusion.

❑ Belt restraints are used to prevent falls from a chair and can also be used as a seatbelt for the client who is out of bed in a wheelchair.

❑ Bed side rails can be considered another form of restraint.

❑ Maintaining all of the client's bed side rails in the "up" position limits the client's movement within his environment, making the side rails a form of restraint.

❑ Keeping one side rail in the "down" position allows the client access to his environment; in this situation, the side rails are no longer considered a form of restraint.

❑ Mummy restraints are commonly used for infants and small children; they help maintain an infant or a small child in a fixed position during examinations or procedures.

❑ When using a mummy restraint on a child or infant, always make sure that the infant's or child's arms are kept in proper alignment with the body.

❑ Always use a quick-release knot when tying any type of restraint.

❑ Client monitoring during restraint use is important because it maintains the client's physical and emotional well-being and protects the client's rights, dignity, and safety.

❑ Client monitoring during restraint use allows for periodic inspection of devices to ensure that restraints are secure and properly applied, released, and reapplied as necessary.

❑ All restraints used for nonviolent, non-self-destructive medical-surgical purposes must be removed at least every 2 hours, or as indicated by your hospital's policy.

❑ A client who is being restrained for medical-surgical purposes must be monitored and assessed at least every 2 hours.

❑ Client monitoring during restraint use enables frequent reassessment and opportunities to use less-restrictive alternatives whenever possible.

❑ Client monitoring during restraint use allows staff-client interaction and opportunities to assist the client to change his behavior so that restraints can be removed.

❑ Clients being restrained for violent or self-destructive behavioral reasons require direct observation by an assigned staff member.

❑ Monitor the restrained client's vital signs and recognize the psychophysiologic effects that restraint or seclusion might have on them.

❑ Monitor the restrained client's nutritional and hydration needs, and ensure that these needs are met.

❑ Check the restrained client's circulation, and perform range-of-motion exercises with each extremity.

❑ Make sure that the restrained client's hygiene and toileting needs are met.

❑ Assess the restrained client's skin for any sign of restraint-related injury, such as bruising or skin breakdown.

❑ The client who is being restrained should be assessed more frequently if policy dictates or the client's condition warrants more frequent assessment; become familiar with your hospital's policy on this issue.

❑ Restraints must be discontinued at the earliest possible time, according to the Centers for Medicare & Medicaid Services.

❑ According to The Joint Commission standards, restraints used for medical-surgical purposes can be discontinued when the client's condition improves and he no longer poses a threat to his medical healing, when the client's condition improves and less restrictive measures prove effective, or when the client's medical condition deteriorates and restraints are no longer necessary.

❑ Restraints used for behavioral purposes can be discontinued when the client is able to develop a safety plan, when the client is reoriented to place and time, or when the client is no longer making threats.

❑ After discontinuing restraints or seclusion, a debriefing should occur that should involve the staff, the client, and (if appropriate) the client's family to reduce the risk of recurrent restraint or seclusion use.

## Safe equipment use

❑ Insulated cords and other coverings prevent the electricity inside electrical equipment from touching you; if there's a problem with any of these parts, you might not be able to see it from the outside as the electrical problem may remain hidden until it becomes very dangerous.

❑ Everyone who works in the hospital is responsible for electrical safety, and all workers need to know about the dangers of electricity and must take steps to maintain safety.

❑ Electricity can cause serious or deadly injuries, including electrocution, electrical shock, burns, falls, and blast injuries.

❑ If you find a person who is suffering an electrical shock, don't touch the victim, or you could get shocked, too; unplug the appliance or turn off the power at the control panel.

❑ If you find a person who is suffering an electrical shock and you can't reach the wall outlet to unplug the appliance, use a dry object that isn't made of metal, such as a dry piece of wood, to move the appliance away from the victim; don't pull the appliance away with your hands or kick it away with your shoe because you could get shocked.

❑ Some client care areas pose a high risk for electrical hazards; these include operating rooms, intensive care units, emergency departments, procedure units, and postanesthesia care units.

❑ The operating room is a very high-risk area because electricity travels the path of least resistance, and an open surgical wound would be a path of least resistance.

❑ Before using any electrical equipment, read the manufacturer's directions.

❑ Look at electrical equipment before use to see if you notice any problems.

❑ Don't use electrical equipment that isn't grounded.

❑ Remove unsafe equipment from use right away, and report it to the engineering department.

❑ If a hazard alarm sounds, unplug the equipment right away and remove it from use; tag it with the date, time, and reason that you are removing it from use and tell the engineering department.

❑ Keep floors and other surfaces dry.

❑ Don't allow clients to use electrical equipment from home.

❑ If a client's personal equipment is brought to the hospital, it must be checked by the engineering department.

❑ Outlets, plugs, and power cords used in the hospital should be of heavy-duty, hospital-grade quality.

❑ Keep in mind that even high-quality electrical equipment isn't always hazard-free.

❑ In the hospital, ivory outlets are for general equipment use.

❑ In the hospital, red emergency outlets are for equipment that needs nonstop power.

❑ Only lifesaving equipment (such as ventilators and life-safety equipment) should be plugged into red outlets; these outlets connect to generators that operate when the hospital's main electricity system fails.

❑ Electrical equipment used in the hospital should be polarized and grounded.

❑ Never try to remove the third prong of a three-prong plug.

❑ Don't use a "cheater" adapter plug because it can overheat or overload a circuit.

❑ Don't use a plug with a bent or broken prong.

❑ Always insert the plug all the way so that no part of a prong is exposed.

❑ Make sure the plug fits into the socket and doesn't become loose or fall out.

❑ A damaged or worn power cord can cause electrocution or shock.

❑ Always check the cord before use, and don't use it if it's cut, frayed, or broken.

❑ Don't roll equipment or furniture over the cord.

❑ Keep the cord out of the path of foot traffic.

❑ Don't attach the cord to a wall, baseboard, or other surface using staples or other fasteners.

❑ Keep the cord away from door and window edges, which may cause kinking.

❑ Keep some slack in the cord to reduce tension.

❑ Clients should be taught proper electrical safety for home use, especially when using equipment usually found in a hospital, such as intravenous pumps or nebulizers.

❑ Don't pull on the cord to disconnect a device from an electrical outlet; always grip the plug and then pull it out.

❑ Keep cords away from heat sources, moisture, and metal pipes.

❑ After use, don't wrap an electrical cord around the equipment until the equipment has cooled.

❑ Avoid using extension cords whenever possible.

❑ Extension cords are dangerous because they retain heat when covered, which can lead to fire; are likely to become looped, kinked, or otherwise mangled, causing the wires inside the cord to touch and spark a fire; and often become overloaded, which can overload the circuit.

❑ Water conducts electricity, making water and electricity a deadly mix.

❑ Never use wet electrical equipment or ungrounded equipment near water.

❑ Never touch anything electrical if your hands are wet—even if the electrical device is turned off.

❑ Never use electrical devices or touch switches, wires, or metal when any part of your body is touching water.

❑ Don't use electrical equipment, cords, or wall outlets in wet weather or a damp environment.

❑ If you can't avoid working in a damp environment, make sure all the equipment is properly grounded.

❑ If liquid spills onto an electrical device, unplug the device immediately—if this can be done safely.

❑ If an electrical device drops into water, don't touch it until you've unplugged it; after it's unplugged, remove the device from use and notify the engineering department.

❑ Stay alert for the warning signs of electrical hazard which can include flickering lights, warm light switches or wall outlets, loose electrical connections, equipment that "trips" a circuit breaker or blows a fuse, equipment that causes a shock or even a slight tingle, and equipment that smokes, sparks, or emits a burning odor.

❑ The Food and Drug Administration states that a medical device is an item used to help diagnose, treat, cure, or prevent disease.

❑ Examples of medical devices include man-made heart valves, ventilators, X-ray machines, defibrillators, bandages, I.V. pumps, and hospital beds.

❑ The Safe Medical Devices Act of 1990 requires hospitals to assess the client right away to find the cause of a serious injury or death and report any death or serious injury that may have been caused by a medical device to the Food and Drug Administration and the company that made the device within 10 work days.

❑ The Safe Medical Devices Act of 1990 requires hospitals to send a yearly review to the Food and Drug Administration about all medical device reports submitted during the previous year.

❑ Client entrapment in a bed is rare, but when it occurs it can be fatal; it involves clients being caught, trapped, entangled, or strangled in hospital beds.

❑ The seven zones of a hospital bed that are potential risks for client entrapment include within the rail, under the rail (between the rail supports or next to a single rail support), between the rail and the mattress, between the rail (at the ends of the rail), between split bed rails, between the end of the rail and the side edge of the head or foot board, and between the head or foot board and the mattress end.

❑ If you find a problem with an electrical device in your hospital, don't use the device, don't let anyone else use the device, and don't try to fix the problem yourself. Remove the equipment from service, and tag it with the date, time, and reason it is being removed from service; keep the settings the same on the piece of equipment; or if you can't, then write down the original settings; and report the problem to the engineering department right away.

❑ A lockout or tagout is a system that's used to lock or tag equipment so that it can't cause injury by starting up or releasing energy by mistake.

❑ With a lockout system, a lock is placed on the device to keep it in a safe or "off" position; in a tagout system, a tag is placed on the device warning workers not to use it.

❑ An I.V. pump that doesn't work properly would be "tagged out," but a computed tomography scanner that doesn't work properly would be "locked out."

❑ The Occupational Safety and Health Administration requires putting a lock or tag on any equipment that needs service or repair to help protect workers from injury.

❑ Make sure you know your hospital's policy about using locks or tags, and who is allowed to place and remove them.

## Security

❑ Violence in a hospital may be committed by a client, worker, visitor or other stranger, or a worker's relative or friend (when domestic violence spills over into the workplace).

❑ The most common type of violence in health care facilities is client-on-worker violence.

❑ Types of workplace violence include threats (which may be verbal, written, or expressed through body language); verbal abuse or harassment; sexual harassment; stalking; mugging; hostage taking; physical assaults, such as punching, hitting, biting, pushing, and kicking; rape; homicide; and terrorist attacks.

❑ Among hospital settings, the highest rates of workplace violence occur in drug and alcohol rehabilitation units, geriatric units, emergency departments, mental health departments, and in admitting or triage areas.

❑ In emergency departments and mental health settings, the greatest threat comes from clients who are agitated or have substance abuse problems.

❑ In geriatric units, clients with dementia pose the main threat of violence.

❑ The hospital uses codes to announce emergency security situations. The operator typically announces these codes over the hospital intercom system.

❑ Make sure you know what number to call to report each type of emergency, what each code means, and how to respond to each code.

❑ If your hospital has other security devices, such as panic buttons or other security alarms, make sure you know where they are located and how to use them.

❑ Security measures include special identification badges for restricted access areas, such as maternity or pediatric units.

❑ Make sure you know your hospital's policies on restricted access areas.

❑ According to the National Institute of Occupational Safety and Health, more than 9,000 health care workers are assaulted on the job, either physically or verbally, every day.

❑ Violence in a hospital may be committed by a client, a worker, a visitor or other stranger, or a worker's relative or friend (when domestic violence spills over into the workplace).

❑ Ask for a security escort when transporting an agitated or hostile client; ask the security officer to stay with you until the client is under control.

❑ Within the hospital and on its grounds, use special care in dimly lit or isolated, out-of-the-way areas, such as stairwells, hallways, elevators, restrooms, and parking lots or garages; avoid being alone in these areas.

❑ Discourage coworkers, clients, and visitors from being alone in dimly lit or isolated, out-of-the-way areas, such as stairwells, hallways, elevators, restrooms, and parking lots or garages.

❑ Don't get into an elevator with someone who behaves in an odd or threatening way or who looks out of place; call security.

❑ If someone on an elevator makes you nervous, get off as soon as possible and call security.

❑ When leaving work, ask a coworker or security officer to escort you to your car if you're working late hours.

❑ If you are working late hours, have your cell phone within easy reach and consider programming security's number for quick access.

❑ Stay alert for possible violence in anyone who shows or claims to have a weapon, makes a threat, verbally expresses anger or frustration, looks angry or defiant, paces back and forth, speaks in a loud voice, clenches his fists, has shifting eyes, states that people are out to get him, or shows signs of drug or alcohol use.

❑ In the hospital, some situations can trigger violence in people who might not otherwise become violent.

❑ Clients or family members may turn violent when they are frustrated with treatment delays, don't know the cause of a health problem, don't know if their loved one will recover, or are worried about the cost of treatment.

❑ Certain behaviors may signal whether a person may become violent, including holding grudges, reacting defensively to criticism, becoming easily frustrated or angered, and abusing drugs or alcohol.

# Understanding the question

NCLEX questions are usually long. As a result, it's easy to feel overwhelmed with information. To focus on the question, apply proven strategies for answering NCLEX questions, including:

❑ determining what the question is asking

❑ determining relevant facts about the client

❑ rephrasing the question in your mind

❑ choosing the best option(s) before entering your answer.

## Determine what the question is asking

Read the question twice. If the answer isn't apparent, rephrase the question in simpler, more personal terms. Breaking down the question into easier, less intimidating terms may help you to focus more accurately on the correct answer.

For example, a question might be, "A 20-year-old female with cystic fibrosis has a small-bowel obstruction. She's admitted to the medical-surgical unit for treatment, which involves placement of an intestinal tube connected to intermittent suction. Which nursing intervention would be most effective for this client?"

The options for this question—numbered from 1 to 4—may be:

1. Record intake and output to accurately keep track of fluid status.

2. Turn the client from side to side every hour to facilitate passage of the tube through the bowel.

3. Give the client sips of water to facilitate passage of the tube through the bowel.

4. Add antacids to the intestinal tube to reduce bowel reaction.

## Read the question again

Read the question again, ignoring all details except what's being asked. Focus on the last line of the question. It asks you to select the most effective nursing intervention for this client.

Determine what facts about the client are relevant. Next, sort out the relevant client information. Start by asking whether any of the information provided about the client isn't relevant. For instance, do you need to know that the client has been admitted to the medical-surgical unit? Probably not; her care plan won't be affected by her location in the hospital.

## Determine what you do know about the client

In the example, you know that:

❑ she is a 20-year-old female

❑ she has a small-bowel obstruction

❑ she has cystic fibrosis (a fact that may be relevant).

## Rephrase the question

After you've determined relevant information about the client and the question being asked, consider rephrasing the question to make it clearer. Eliminate jargon and put the question in simpler, more personal terms. Here's how you might rephrase the question in the example: "My client has a small-bowel obstruction. She requires placement of an intestinal tube, which will be connected to intermittent suction. She's 20 years old and has a history of cystic fibrosis. Which nursing intervention would be most effective for this client?"

## Choose the best option

Armed with all the information you now have, it's time to select an option. You know the client will have an intestinal tube in place that will be connected to intermittent suction. You know that while the tube is being advanced into the intestine, the client will lie quietly on her right side for about 2 hours to promote the tube's passage, eliminating option 2. You also know that nothing but normal saline solution should be instilled into the intestinal tube, a fact that eliminates option 4. In addition, you know it isn't likely that the client will be permitted anything by mouth, eliminating option 3. By process of elimination, option 1 (record intake and output to accurately keep track of fluid status) is the best option because monitoring fluid balance is the most effective nursing intervention for this client.

## Understanding alternate-format questions

The NCLEX examination includes the standard, four-option, multiple-choice items to assess candidate ability. In addition, the examination also includes alternate format questions that include multiple-response, fill-in-the-blank, hot spot, chart/exhibit, drag-and-drop, audio, and graphic options.

The National Council of State Boards of Nursing hasn't yet established a percentage of alternate-format items to be administered to each candidate. In fact, your exam may contain only one alternate-format item.

## Multiple-response question

Unlike a traditional multiple-choice question, each multiple-response, multiple-choice question may contain five or six answer options with a minimum of two correct options. You'll recognize this type of question because it will ask you to select *all* answers that apply—not just the best answer (as may be requested in the more traditional multiple-choice questions).

### Sample multiple-response, multiple-choice question

The nurse is caring for a 45-year-old married client who has undergone hemicolectomy for colon cancer. The client has two children. Which concepts about families should the nurse keep in mind when providing care for this client? Select all that apply:

1. Illness in one family member can affect all members.

2. Family roles don't change because of illness.

3. A family member may have more than one role in the family.

4. Children typically aren't affected by adult illness.

5. The effects of an illness on a family depend on the stage of the family's life cycle.

6. Changes in sleeping and eating patterns may be signs of stress in a family.

---

**Correct answer: 1, 3, 5, 6**

## Fill-in-the-blank question

The second type of alternate-format item is the fill-in-the-blank. These questions require you to provide the answer yourself, rather than select it from a list of options. You will perform a calculation, and then type your answer (a number without any words, units of measurement, commas, or spaces) in the blank space provided after the question. Rules for rounding are included in the question stem if appropriate. A calculator button is provided so you can easily do your calculations electronically.

### Sample fill-in-the-blank calculation question

An infant who weighs 8 kg is to receive ampicillin 25 mg/kg I.V. every 6 hours. How many milligrams should the nurse administer per dose? Record your answer using a whole number.

_____ milligrams

**Correct answer: 200**

## Hot spot question

The third type of alternate-format item is a question that asks you to identify an area on an illustration or graphic. For these questions, the computerized exam will ask you to place your cursor and click over the correct area on an illustration. Try to be as precise as possible when marking the location. As with the fill-in-the-blank items, the identification questions on the computerized exam may require extremely precise answers to be considered correct.

### Sample hot spot question

A client has a history of aortic stenosis. Identify the area where the nurse should place the stethoscope to best hear the murmur.

**Correct answer:**

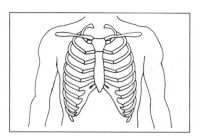 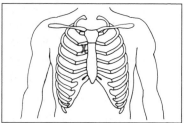

## Chart/exhibit question

The fourth type of alternate-format item is the chart/exhibit format. Here you'll be given a problem, then a series of small screens containing additional information you'll need in order to answer the question. By clicking on the Tab button, you can access each screen in turn. Your answer can then be chosen from four multiple-choice answer options.

### Sample chart/exhibit question

A 3-year-old client is being treated for severe status asthmaticus. After reviewing the progress notes (shown on page 271), the nurse should determine that this client is being treated for which condition?

**Progress notes**

| | |
|---|---|
| 8/1/11 | Pt. was acutely restless, diaphoretic, and with SOB |
| 0600 | at 0530. Dr. T. Smith  notified and ordered ABG |
| | analysis. ABG drawn from right radial artery. Stat |
| | results as follows: pH 7.28, $Paco_2$ 55 mm Hg, |
| | $HCO_3^-$ 26 mEg/L. Dr. Smith with pt. now. |
| | —————————— J. Collins, R.N. |

1. Metabolic acidosis

2. Respiratory alkalosis

3. Respiratory acidosis

4. Metabolic alkalosis

**Correct answer: 3**

*Drag-and-drop question*

You may also see an alternate-format item that involves prioritizing or placing in correct order a series of statements, using a drag-and-drop technique. You'll decide which of the given options is first, click and hold it with the mouse, then drag it into the first box given underneath and drop it into place. You'll repeat this process until you've placed all the available options in the lower boxes.

**Sample drag-and-drop question**

When teaching an antepartal client about the passage of the fetus through the birth canal during labor, the nurse describes the cardinal mechanisms of labor. Place these events in the sequence in which they occur. Use all the options.

**Correct answer:**

| |
|---|
| 1. Flexion |
| 2. External rotation |
| 3. Descent |
| 4. Expulsion |
| 5. Internal rotation |
| 6. Extension |

| |
|---|
| 3. Descent |
| 1. Flexion |
| 5. Internal rotation |
| 6. Extension |
| 2. External rotation |
| 4. Expulsion |

## *Audio question*

The sixth alternate-format item type is the audio item format. You'll be given a set of headphones and will be asked to listen to an audio clip and select the correct answer from four options. You'll need to select the correct answer on the computer screen as you would with the traditional multiple-choice questions.

### Sample audio question

Listen to the audio clip. What sound do you hear in the bases of this client with heart failure?

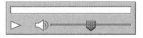

- ○ 1. Crackles
- ○ 2. Rhonchi
- ○ 3. Wheezes
- ○ 4. Pleural friction rub

**Correct answer: 1**

## *Graphic option question*

The final alternate-format item type is the graphic option question. This varies from the exhibit format type because in the graphic option, your answer choices will be graphics, such as ECG strips. You'll have to select the appropriate graphic to answer the question presented.

### Sample graphic option question

Which electrocardiogram strip should the nurse document as sinus tachycardia?

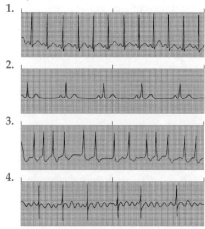

**Correct answer: 1**

# *Key strategies for answering correctly*

Regardless of the type of question, four key strategies will help you determine the correct answer for each question. These strategies are:

❑ considering the nursing process

❑ referring to Maslow's hierarchy of needs

❑ reviewing client safety

❑ reflecting on principles of therapeutic communication.

## Nursing process

One of the ways to answer a question is to apply the nursing process. Steps in the nursing process include:

❑ data collection

❑ diagnosis

❑ planning

❑ implementation

❑ evaluation.

The nursing process may provide insights that help you analyze a question. According to the nursing process, data collection comes before diagnosis, which comes before planning, which comes before implementation, which comes before evaluation. You're halfway to the correct answer when you encounter a four-option, multiple-choice question that asks you to collect data and then provides two data collection options and two implementation options. You can immediately eliminate the implementation options, which then gives you, at worst, a 50-50 chance of selecting the correct answer. Use the following sample question to apply the nursing process:

A client returns from an endoscopic procedure during which he was sedated. Before offering the client food, which action should the nurse take?

1. Monitor the client's respiratory status.

2. Check the client's gag reflex.

3. Place the client in a side-lying position.

4. Have the client drink a few sips of water.

According to the nursing process, the nurse must collect client data before performing an intervention. Does the question indicate that data have been properly collected? No, it doesn't. Therefore, you can eliminate options 3 and 4 because they're both interventions. That leaves options 1 and 2, both of which demonstrate data collection. Your nursing knowledge should tell you the correct answer—in this case, option 2. The sedation required for an endoscopic procedure may impair the client's gag reflex, so you would check the gag reflex before giving food to the client to reduce the risk of aspiration and airway obstruction.

Why not select option 1, monitoring the client's respiratory status? You might select this option, but the question is specifically asking about offering the client food, an action that wouldn't be taken if the client's respiratory status was at all compromised. In this case, you're making a judgment based on the phrase, "before offering the client food." If the question was trying to test your knowledge of respiratory depression following an endoscopic procedure, it probably wouldn't mention a function—such as giving food to a client—that clearly occurs only after the client's respiratory status has been stabilized.

## Maslow's hierarchy

Knowledge of Maslow's hierarchy of needs can be a vital tool for establishing priorities on the NCLEX. Maslow's theory states that physiologic needs are the most basic human needs of all. Only after physiologic needs have been met can safety concerns be addressed. Only after safety concerns are met can concerns involving love and belonging be addressed, and so forth.

Apply the principles of Maslow's hierarchy of needs to the following sample question:

A client complains of severe pain 2 days after surgery. Which action should the nurse perform first?

1. Offer reassurance to the client that he will feel less pain tomorrow.

2. Allow the client time to verbalize his feelings.

3. Check the client's vital signs.

4. Administer an analgesic.

In this example, two of the options—3 and 4—address physiologic needs. Options 1 and 2 address psychosocial concerns. According to Maslow, physiologic needs must be met before psychosocial needs, so you can eliminate options 1 and 2.

Now, use your nursing knowledge to choose the best answer from the two remaining options. In this case, option 3 is correct because the client's vital signs should be checked before administering an analgesic (assessment before intervention). When prioritizing according to Maslow's hierarchy, remember your ABCs—airway, breathing, circulation—to help you further prioritize. Check for a patent airway before addressing breathing. Check breathing before checking the health of the cardiovascular system.

Just because an option appears on the NCLEX doesn't mean it's a viable choice for the client referred to in the question. Always examine your choice in light of your knowledge and experience. Ask yourself, "Does this choice make sense for this client?" Allow yourself to eliminate choices—even ones that might normally take priority—if they don't make sense for a particular client's situation.

## Client safety

As you might expect, client safety takes high priority on the NCLEX. You'll encounter many questions that can be answered by asking yourself, "Which answer will best ensure the safety of this client?" Use client safety criteria for situations involving laboratory values, drug administration, activities of daily living, or nursing care procedures.

You may encounter a question in which some options address the client and others address the equipment. When in doubt, select an option relating to the client; never place equipment before a client. For example, suppose a question asks what the nurse should do first when entering a client's room where an infusion pump alarm is sounding. If two options deal with the infusion pump, one with the infusion tubing, and another with the client's catheter insertion site, select the one relating to the client's catheter insertion site. Always check the client first; the equipment can wait.

## Therapeutic communication

Some NCLEX questions focus on the nurse's ability to communicate effectively with the client. Therapeutic communication incorporates verbal or nonverbal responses and involves:

❑ listening to the client

❑ understanding the client's needs

❑ promoting clarification and insight about the client's condition.

Like other NCLEX questions, those dealing with therapeutic communication commonly require choosing the best response. First, eliminate options that indicate the use of poor therapeutic communication techniques, such as those in which the nurse:

❏ tells the client what to do without regard to the client's feelings or desires (the "do this" response)

❏ asks a question that can be answered "yes" or "no," or with another one-syllable response

❏ seeks reasons for the client's behavior

❏ implies disapproval of the client's behavior

❏ offers false reassurances

❏ attempts to interpret the client's behavior rather than allow the client to verbalize his own feelings

❏ offers a response that focuses on the nurse, not the client.

When answering NCLEX questions, look for responses that:

❏ allow the client time to think and reflect

❏ encourage the client to talk

❏ encourage the client to describe a particular experience

❏ reflect that the nurse has listened to the client, such as through paraphrasing the client's response.

# Selected references

Alfaro-LeFevre, R. (2010). *Applying nursing process* (7th ed.). Philadelphia: Lippincott Williams & Wilkins.

Dudek, S. (2011). *Nutrition essentials for nursing practice* (6th ed.). Philadelphia: Lippincott Williams & Wilkins.

Ford, S., and Roach, S. (2010). *Roach's introductory clinical pharmacology* (9th ed.). Philadelphia: Lippincott Williams & Wilkins.

Hockenberry, M. J., & Wilson, D. (2009). *Wong's essentials of pediatric nursing* (8th ed.). St. Louis: Mosby.

Karch, A. (2011). *2012 Lippincott's nursing drug guide.* Philadelphia: Lippincott Williams & Wilkins.

Kurzen, K. (2011). *Contemporary practical/vocational nursing* (6th ed.). Philadelphia: Lippincott Williams & Wilkins.

*LPN facts made incredibly quick!* (2010). (2nd ed.). Philadelphia: Lippincott Williams & Wilkins.

*NCLEX-PN questions and answers made incredibly easy* (2009). (3rd ed.). Philadelphia: Lippincott Williams & Wilkins.

Nettina, S. M. (2009). *Lippincott's manual of nursing practice* (9th ed.). Philadelphia: Lippincott Williams & Wilkins.

*Nursing 2012 drug handbook* (2011). Philadelphia: Lippincott Williams & Wilkins.

*Pediatric facts made incredibly quick!* (2010). (2nd ed.). Philadelphia: Lippincott Williams & Wilkins.

Pillitteri, A. (2010). *Maternal and child health nursing: Care of the childbearing and childrearing family* (6th ed.). Philadelphia: Lippincott Williams & Wilkins.

Porth, C. M. (2010). *Essentials of pathophysiology* (2nd ed.). Philadelphia: Lippincott Williams & Wilkins.

Timby, B. (2009). *Fundamental nursing skills and concepts* (9th ed.). Philadelphia: Lippincott Williams & Wilkins.

Timby, B., and Smith, N. (2010). *Introductory medical-surgical nursing* (10th ed.). Philadelphia: Lippincott Williams & Wilkins.

Womble, D. (2011). *Introductory mental health nursing* (2nd ed.). Philadelphia: Lippincott Williams & Wilkins.